Handbook of Cardiovascular Magnetic Resonance Imaging

Fundamental and Clinical Cardiology

Editor-in-Chief
Samuel Z. Goldhaber, M.D.
Harvard Medical School
and Brigham and Women's Hospital
Boston, Massachusetts, U.S.A.

1. Drug Treatment of Hyperlipidemia, *edited by Basil M. Rifkind*
2. Cardiotonic Drugs: A Clinical Review, Second Edition, Revised and Expanded, *edited by Carl V. Leier*
3. Complications of Coronary Angioplasty, *edited by Alexander J. R. Black, H. Vernon Anderson, and Stephen G. Ellis*
4. Unstable Angina, *edited by John D. Rutherford*
5. Beta-Blockers and Cardiac Arrhythmias, *edited by Prakash C. Deedwania*
6. Exercise and the Heart in Health and Disease, *edited by Roy J. Shephard and Henry S. Miller, Jr.*
7. Cardiopulmonary Physiology in Critical Care, *edited by Steven M. Scharf*
8. Atherosclerotic Cardiovascular Disease, Hemostasis, and Endothelial Function, *edited by Robert Boyer Francis, Jr.*
9. Coronary Heart Disease Prevention, *edited by Frank G. Yanowitz*
10. Thrombolysis and Adjunctive Therapy for Acute Myocardial Infarction, *edited by Eric R. Bates*
11. Stunned Myocardium: Properties, Mechanisms, and Clinical Manifestations, *edited by Robert A. Kloner and Karin Przyklenk*
12. Prevention of Venous Thromboembolism, *edited by Samuel Z. Goldhaber*
13. Silent Myocardial Ischemia and Infarction: Third Edition, *Peter F. Cohn*
14. Congestive Cardiac Failure: Pathophysiology and Treatment, *edited by David B. Barnett, Hubert Pouleur and Gary S. Francis*
15. Heart Failure: Basic Science and Clinical Aspects, *edited by Judith K. Gwathmey, G. Maurice Briggs, and Paul D. Allen*
16. Coronary Thrombolysis in Perspective: Principles Underlying Conjunctive and Adjunctive Therapy, *edited by Burton E. Sobel and Desire Collen*

Handbook of Cardiovascular Magnetic Resonance Imaging

Edited by

Gerald M. Pohost
University of Southern California
Los Angeles, California, U.S.A.

Krishna S. Nayak
University of Southern California
Los Angeles, California, U.S.A.

With Special Assistance from Steven M. Stevens, M.D.

informa
healthcare

New York   London

Informa Healthcare USA, Inc.
270 Madison Avenue
New York, NY 10016

© 2007 by Informa Healthcare USA, Inc.
Informa Healthcare is an Informa business

No claim to original U.S. Government works
Printed in the United States of America on acid-free paper
10 9 8 7 6 5 4 3 2 1

International Standard Book Number-10: 0-8247-5841-2 (Hardcover)
International Standard Book Number-13: 978-0-8247-5841-7 (Hardcover)

Visit the Informa Web site at
www.informa.com

and the Informa Healthcare Web site at
www.informahealthcare.com

Series Introduction

Informa Healthcare has developed various series of beautifully produced books in different branches of medicine. These series have facilitated the integration of rapidly advancing information for both the clinical specialist and the researcher.

In the current monograph, Drs. Gerald Pohost and Krishna Nayak have written and edited a much-needed practical and timely handbook, which provides a quick start for those practitioners who have ordered cardiovascular magnetic resonance imaging studies on their patients. The Handbook gains much of its strength from its clear outline and organization. It is a coherent work because Dr. Pohost himself has coauthored 5 of the 20 chapters. As a cardiovascular generalist, I find that the detailed images from magnetic resonance imaging are unsurpassed. However, interpreting the findings, sorting through the vast array of data, and understanding the strengths and limitations of MR can be a bit daunting. Therefore, I intend to carry this Handbook with me whenever I see inpatients or outpatients. The Handbook will help me determine which patients are most likely to benefit from this elegant imaging technique and will guide me to a better understanding of the images that I am reviewing.

My goal as Editor-In-Chief of the Fundamental and Clinical Cardiology Series is to assemble the talents of world-renowned authorities to discuss virtually every area of cardiovascular medicine. Future contributions to this series will include books on molecular biology, interventional cardiology, and clinical management of such problems as coronary artery disease, venous thromboembolism, peripheral vascular disease, and cardiac arrhythmias.

Samuel Z. Goldhaber, MD
Professor of Medicine
Harvard Medical School
Staff Cardiologist
Brigham and Women's Hospital
Boston, Massachusetts, U.S.A.

Editor-in-Chief
Fundamental and Clinical Cardiology Series

Foreword

Cardiovascular magnetic resonance (CMR) has recently evolved from a cardiovascular research tool to become a clinical mainstay of noninvasive diagnostic imaging for several cardiovascular disciplines. Furthermore, such an amazing technology continues to provide new innovative approaches for better understanding of cardiovascular disease progression and clinical management algorithms. Thus, the most recent advances in hardware and pulse sequence design now allow for an impressive range of cardiac and vascular imaging opportunities that have extended CMR well beyond anatomic diagnostic studies. In addition, CMR is a safe technology, which benefits from not using harmful radiation or nephrotoxic dyes.

However, despite its noninvasive nature, its continued progress in the diagnostic clinical studies, its rapidly evolving advances guiding management, and its outstanding safeness, CMR has yet to play a primary role in the clinical management of patients with cardiovascular disease. As we recently pointed out, the lack of complete clinical acceptance may in part be related to the "often intimidating technical enigma of CMR and/or the dizzying array of new and evolving applications that appear in the literature on a weekly to a monthly basis." Therefore, concise and simple education and dissemination approaches of this new and rapidly evolving body of information seem to be critical for the acceptance and widespread growth of CMR in the clinical cardiovascular community.

This excellent book, edited by a cardiologist and an electrical engineer who have substantial experience with CMR, provides a very pragmatic approach to the use of such a powerful tool. Specifically, cardiovascular practice requires different abilities, including the ability to select the best test in each clinical setting; this means that the cardiologist or cardiovascular specialist as well as the radiologist interested in cardiovascular medicine should know the possibilities, advantages, and limitations of CMR in the setting to be tested. Within this context, I found rewarding that the various chapters were written by combining cardiovascular clinicians and radiologists, including biomedical engineers and MR technologists, all with practical experience in the field of CMR. Indeed, I agree with the editors, as they point out in their preface, that individual CMR applications such as perfusion, myocardial injury, metabolism, coronary angiography, and peripheral angiography are described in their own chapters in such a practical fashion that will be understandable to those medical personnel who would like to use or support CMR on a clinical or research basis. Overall, and in my judgment, the book fulfills the above mentioned "concise and simple education and dissemination" needs of CMR for the cardiovascular community of today.

In summary, Gerald M. Pohost, MD, Krishna S. Nayak, PhD, and colleagues have put together a very didactic and practical book. It is designed to provide the most recent and practical information on established foundational applications in cardiovascular diagnosis, understanding and management by CMR, as well as to give the reader a look into the future through the presentation of various states of rapid development (Chapter 20). I believe the information will serve to stimulate the interest not only of the cardiovascular specialist ready to become familiarized with this important technological tool, but also of a broad range of professionals and students of cardiovascular medicine. I warmly congratulate the editors and authors.

Valentin Fuster, MD, PhD
Director, Mount Sinai Heart
Mount Sinai School of Medicine,
New York, New York, U.S.A.
Past President, American Heart Association
President, World Heart Federation

Preface

Cardiovascular magnetic resonance, also known as CMR, is an amazing technology that continues to provide new innovative approaches for evaluating the heart and blood vessels. However, it uses a complex technology that includes magnetic and radiofrequency fields, making it considerably different from other imaging approaches. Accordingly, it is among the most complex of all cardiovascular diagnostic approaches. It can assess cardiac morphology, function, perfusion, viability, coronary and peripheral arteries, and metabolism. CMR is uniquely capable of assessing virtually every important diagnostic facet currently available with any diagnostic modality. Furthermore, CMR is a safe, noninvasive technology, which benefits from not using potentially harmful ionizing radiation or nephrotoxic dyes.

The present book provides a practical approach to the use of CMR. It presents a straightforward means to provide physicians and technologists with an understanding of CMR applications and imaging methods. The book discusses the basic physics of magnetic resonance imaging, the instruments involved, how to do a basic CMR exam, and safety considerations. Individual CMR applications such as perfusion, myocardial injury, metabolism, coronary angiography, and peripheral angiography are described in their own chapters. Each chapter describes the indications and presents the methods in a practical fashion that will be understandable to those medical personnel who would like to use or support CMR on a clinical or research basis, including physicians (such as adult and pediatric cardiologists, radiologists, nuclear medicine specialists, internists, and pediatricians), technologists in magnetic resonance and other imaging disciplines (ultrasound, nuclear medicine, and radiology), nurses, and physician assistants. Throughout the book, the reader will find descriptions of key research and historical information that has incrementally made CMR the valuable asset to clinical cardiology that it is today. Recent applications are described, including the imaging of microvascular disease and the use of 3T instruments. Finally, the book contains a chapter on the future applications of CMR, which at this point seem limitless.

The book has been edited by a cardiologist and an electrical engineer who have substantial experience with CMR, both developing new methods and performing clinical studies. Organization and substantial contributions to the book were also made by a medical student, Steven Stevens, number one in his graduating class at the University of Southern California, (now a postgraduate physician in internal medicine at the University of California at San Francisco), who ensured that the technical and applications descriptions were readily understandable. Further, important organizational contributions were made by Dr. Radha Sarma. The chapters were written by cardiovascular specialists including engineers, physicists, and physicians, all with substantial experience in the field of CMR.

The editors thank Vanessa Sanchez and Sandra Beberman from Informa Healthcare, without whom this volume would not have become a reality. We also thank our families for their patience and support. We finally thank the persistent efforts of many of the chapter authors for their patience and updating of their contributions, to make this book representative of the current state of the art. We truly hope that you enjoy this book. We look forward to hearing your comments on this volume and/or your suggestions for the next volume.

Gerald M. Pohost
Krishna S. Nayak

Contents

Contents xi

19. **Risks and Safety** *413*
  Mark Doyle and Robert W. W. Biederman

20. **CMR: The Future** *425*
  Gerald M. Pohost and Krishna S. Nayak

Abbreviations *435*
Index *439*

Contributors

Robert W. W. Biederman Division of Cardiology, Cardiovascular MRI Laboratory, Allegheny General Hospital, Pittsburgh, Pennsylvania, U.S.A.

Hakki Bolukoglu Division of Cardiology, Cardiovascular MRI Laboratory, Allegheny General Hospital, Pittsburgh, Pennsylvania, U.S.A.

Mark Doyle Division of Cardiology, Cardiovascular MRI Laboratory, Allegheny General Hospital, Pittsburgh, Pennsylvania, U.S.A.

Anthony R. Fuisz Cardiac MRI Laboratory, Washington Hospital Center, Washington, D.C., U.S.A.

Jaime O. Henriquez Division of Cardiovascular Medicine, University of Southern California, Los Angeles, California, U.S.A.

Lynne Hung Department of Medicine, Division of Cardiovascular Medicine, LACUSC Medical Center, Keck School of Medicine, University of Southern California, Los Angeles, California, U.S.A.

Uzma Iqbal Cardiology and Internal Medicine, Syracuse, New York, U.S.A.

Hee-Won Kim Department of Medicine, Division of Cardiovascular Medicine, Keck School of Medicine, University of Southern California, Los Angeles, California, U.S.A.

Mark A. Lawson   Division of Cardiovascular Medicine, Vanderbilt University Medical Center, Nashville, Tennessee, U.S.A.

Agostino Meduri   Department of Radiology, Catholic University of Rome, Rome, Italy

Mazda Motallebi   Division of Cardiovascular Medicine, University of Southern California, Los Angeles, California, U.S.A.

Luigi Natale   Department of Radiology, Cardiovascular Magnetic Resonance Unit, Catholic University of Rome, Rome, Italy

Krishna S. Nayak   Departments of Electrical Engineering and Medicine, Division of Cardiovascular Medicine, Viterbi School of Engineering, Keck School of Medicine, University of Southern California, Los Angeles, California, U.S.A.

Gerald M. Pohost   Department of Medicine, Division of Cardiovascular Medicine, Keck School of Medicine, University of Southern California, Los Angeles, California, U.S.A.

Vikas K. Rathi   Division of Cardiology, Cardiovascular MRI Lab, Allegheny General Hospital, Drexel University College of Medicine, Philadelphia, Pennsylvania, U.S.A.

Ronald M. Razmi   Cardiovascular MR/CT Center and Heart Center of Indiana, The Care Group, LLC, Indianapolis, Indiana, U.S.A.

Radha J. Sarma   Department of Medicine, Division of Cardiovascular Medicine, Keck School of Medicine, University of Southern California, Los Angeles, California, U.S.A.

Benigno Soto   Department of Radiology and Medicine, Cardiovascular MRI Laboratory, University of Alabama, Birmingham, Alabama, U.S.A.

Steven M. Stevens   Department of Medicine, Division of Cardiovascular Medicine, Keck School of Medicine, University of Southern California, Los Angeles, California, U.S.A.

Szilard Voros   Cardiovascular MRI and CT, Fuqua Heart Center of Atlanta, Piedmont Hospital, Atlanta, Georgia, U.S.A.

Edward Walsh   Department of Neuroscience, Brown University, Providence, Rhode Island, U.S.A.

1

Physical Principles of Magnetic Resonance Imaging

Mark Doyle

Division of Cardiology, Cardiovascular MRI Laboratory, Allegheny General Hospital, Pittsburgh, Pennsylvania, U.S.A.

ORIGIN OF THE MRI SIGNAL

Of all major imaging modalities, the physical origin of the magnetic resonance (MR) signal is quite possibly the least intuitive to comprehend. In brief, magnetic resonance imaging (MRI) forms a "map" or "image" of the body's water content. Fortunately for the modality, the body is composed of approximately 70% water, thus the "raw material" of MRI is naturally abundant. However, the body does not spontaneously generate an MRI signal, and an elaborate and complex configuration of equipment is required to access this rich signal source. In this chapter, the physical principles of MRI will be addressed in three distinct sections:

- the signal source,
- image formation,
- cardiovascular imaging.

SIGNAL SOURCE

The signal source for MRI has its origin in the discipline of nuclear magnetic resonance (NMR). The phenomenon of NMR was discovered more than 60 years ago, at which time it received widespread attention from chemists due to its ability to probe the structure of molecules (1,2). Bloch and Purcell received the Nobel Prize for Physics in 1952 for their discovery of the NMR phenomenon. Physically, the NMR procedure involves placing a sample (usually in the form of a liquid contained in a test tube) in a strong uniform magnetic field and irradiating it with radiofrequency (RF) electromagnetic energy. The atomic nuclei of the sample absorb the RF irradiation and re-emit it, forming the NMR signal. This re-emitted signal has encoded in it unique sample-specific information that reveals information concerning the molecular composition and structure of the sample. The information is encoded in the frequency and amplitude of the re-emitted RF electromagnetic signal. In 1991, Ernst received the Nobel Prize for Chemistry for his contribution to processing the NMR signal, allowing high-resolution spectroscopy to be performed.

In MRI, the NMR signal is modified to additionally encode information describing the spatial distribution of nuclei within the sample. Configuring the NMR signal to encode spatial information required several innovative steps, and in 2003, the Nobel Prize for Medicine was awarded to Lauterbur and Mansfield for their formulation of the MRI procedure. It can be appreciated that the progression of major innovative steps that have contributed to MRI in its present form rank among the highest achievements in science and medicine.

MAGNETISM, SPINS, AND VECTORS

At one level, the phenomenon of NMR can be understood using quantum-mechanical concepts, although to appreciate many aspects of MRI, a classical physics approach is commonly used. Consider the constituents of a water molecule: two hydrogen atoms and one oxygen atom. The nucleus of an individual hydrogen atom is composed of a single proton. The proton has several commonly acknowledged properties including mass and charge and the less intuitive property of "spin." Physically, this spin property can be regarded as originating from the proton spinning on its axis, just as does the earth. However, the "spin" property is quantized, and has the same value for all protons, each characterized as a "spin ½" system. Just as an electric current circulating in a wire loop produces a small magnetic field, so does the spinning electrically charged nucleus generate a magnetic field, referred to as a magnetic moment (Fig. 1). As the spin quantity is quantized, the magnetic moment is also quantized and has a uniform value for all protons. The important concepts concerning the atomic nucleus are that they have a magnetic moment and a spin and that each of these properties is quantized and is the same for all protons in water molecules.

Within the human body, nuclei are randomly oriented, causing cancellation of any net magnetization vector and thus no magnetization properties

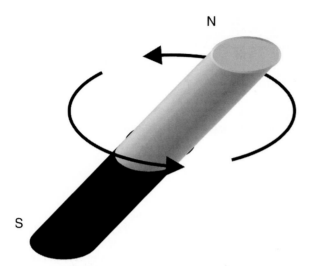

Figure 1 Nuclear spin is a quality of protons that is quantized, the hydrogen nucleus is a "spin half" system. Associated with the spinning, electrically charged nucleus, is a magnetic field, referred to as a dipole, which effectively makes the nucleus appear as a spinning bar magnet with a North (N) and South (S) pole.

are apparent in the body. However, when the body is positioned within a strong magnetic field ($\mathbf{B_0}$), a detectable magnetic moment is generated. Intuitively, one might expect all nuclei to align with the magnetic field. Instead, two quantum mechanical energy states are produced, namely parallel and antiparallel to $\mathbf{B_0}$. Occupancy of these energy states is almost equal, and thus magnetization formed from the aligned spins is canceled by the counter-aligned spins. However, as parallel alignment has a slightly lower energy level, for every million nuclei there will be a few more aligned parallel to $\mathbf{B_0}$ than there are anti-aligned, there is a resultant weak magnetization vector formed within the body (Fig. 2). The strength of the magnetization vector is proportional to the strength of $\mathbf{B_0}$, thus higher fields (e.g., 3 T compared to 1.5 T) generate higher magnetization levels and hence higher signal strengths.

When equilibrium is established within the magnetic field, the body's net magnetization ($\mathbf{M_0}$) is established but does not spontaneously result in the generation of an electromagnetic signal. To generate a signal, $\mathbf{M_0}$ must be perturbed from equilibrium, e.g., by "tipping" $\mathbf{M_0}$ from alignment with $\mathbf{B_0}$, a detectable signal is emitted from the body. When $\mathbf{M_0}$ is tilted from alignment with $\mathbf{B_0}$, the magnetization vector experiences a torque due to its interaction with the magnetic field. This torque propels $\mathbf{M_0}$ to process. The phenomenon of nuclear precession is analogous to the precession exhibited by a spinning top tilted from alignment with the earth's gravitational

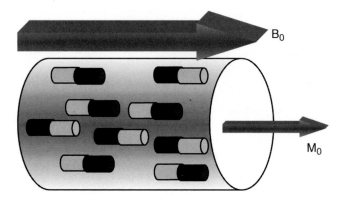

Figure 2 When the body (represented by the large cylinder) is placed in a large external magnetic field, $\mathbf{B}_0$, the spins (represented by the small cylindrical "bar magnets") either aligned or anti-aligned with the magnetic field. There are a few more per million spins aligned with $\mathbf{B}_0$ than are anti-aligned. This small net alignment of spins results in the body exhibiting a net magnetization vector $\mathbf{M}_0$.

field (Fig. 3). Importantly, the precession frequency (ω) is proportional to the field strength $\mathbf{B}_0$. This relationship is referred to as the Larmor equation:

$$\omega = \gamma \mathbf{B}_0$$

where the constant of proportionality (γ), termed the gyromagnetic ratio, is unique for each nuclear species.

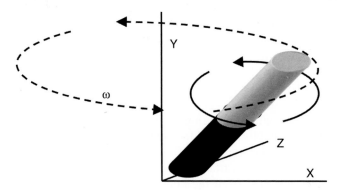

Figure 3 Spin precession is exhibited when spins are tipped from alignment with $\mathbf{B}_0$ (i.e., from the Z-axis towards the X–Y-plane). Note that the precession phenomena (dashed line) is expressed in a lower frequency (ω) than the inherent spin frequency (solid line) of the nucleus.

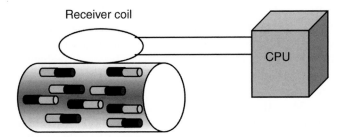

Figure 4 The NMR signal is detected by placing a "receiver" coil in close proximity to the sample, amplifying the received signal voltage and digitizing it for computation and storage purposes. *Abbreviations*: NMR, nuclear magnetic resonance; CPU, central processing unit.

THE RESONANCE PHENOMENON

To tilt the net magnetization (M_0) from alignment with the main magnetic field (B_0), a small magnetic field (B_1) is applied such that B_1 rotates in a plane perpendicular to B_0 at the Larmor frequency. By applying B_1 at the Larmor frequency, it exploits the resonance phenomenon to "tip" M_0 with application of very little energy. The resonance frequency of the B_1 field is in the RF range and contributes the term "resonance" to NMR and MRI. Further, it is only necessary to apply the B_1 RF field for a time sufficient to tilt the spins by several degrees. Typically, M_0 can be tilted into the transverse plane (i.e., through 90°) by application of B_1 for about 1 msec. Once M_0 is tilted, the B_1 field is turned off and the spins are free to precess in the presence of the B_0 field. The act of precession of M_0 generates a time-varying electromagnetic field. This electromagnetic field can be detected by placing a conductive "receiver coil" in close proximity to the body sensitive to the RF frequency of the spins (not unlike a household antenna to receive a radio signal). When amplified and digitized, the signal forms the basis of the MR signal. Importantly, the MRI signal originates with the body itself, and is detected by the receiver coils (Fig. 4).

RELAXATION

The spin signal decays over a matter of a few tens of milliseconds due to the phenomenon of "relaxation" which returns the spin system to equilibrium, i.e., the spins return to their natural state of alignment and anti-alignment with B_0. There are two relaxation processes that act on the spin system, termed T1 and T2.

T1 Relaxation

The body forms a "network" that effectively embeds the nuclei, providing a structure with which the spins can interact. This "structure" is referred to as the "lattice." The lattice and spin system are in a constant state of energy exchange, providing a mechanism for nuclei to give up their energy, that was imparted by the B_1 RF pulse, to the lattice. As the spins exchange energy with the lattice, the net magnetization gradually becomes realigned along the B_0-axis. The mechanism whereby nuclei exchange energy with the lattice is governed by randomly occurring energy exchanges and consequently, realignment of M_0 with B_0 occurs in an exponential manner (similar to random processes that characterize radioactive decay). The Tl relaxation time is the half-life of this decay process and is the time for 63% of the nuclei to return to their equilibrium status. Tl is frequently referred to as the spin-lattice relaxation time. After a perturbation of the spin system, a time interval of approximately five times T1 is regarded as necessary for the spins to return to equilibrium. As spin-lattice relaxation requires an exchange of energy, the process is dependent on field strength with higher fields generally resulting in increasing the T1 value (Fig. 5).

T2 Relaxation

The instant that the spins are tipped into the "transverse plane" (i.e., the plane orthogonal to B_0), they begin to interact with each other. Owing to the energy exchange between spins, they effectively lose phase coherence, i.e., the spins gradually get out of phase relative to each other. Thus, the

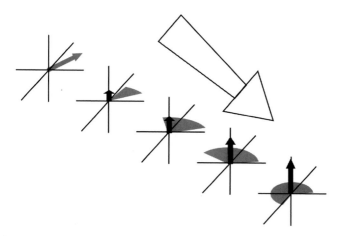

Figure 5 The T1 and T2 relaxation processes are illustrated here. The large arrow represents the passage of time, with time equal to zero represented in the first frame, where the net magnetization vector M_0 is tipped into the transverse plane (*gray arrow*). As time progresses, the spins comprising M_0 gradually dephase (represented by the increasingly dispersing gray shading). This represents the T2 decay process and is responsible for decay of the detected signal. The black arrow in each panel represents spins that have returned to alignment with the B_0 axis, representing T1 relaxation.

net magnetization vector decays due to the increasing loss of phase coherence. The result of these interactions is referred to as spin–spin or T2 relaxation. The spin–spin interaction does not require any net energy loss from the spin system, because spins exchange energy with each other and not with the external lattice. Hence, the T2 process is essentially independent of field strength. As with the T1 process, the spin–spin energy exchange is governed by random events and hence the T2 decay curve is also exponential in character (Fig. 5).

T2* Relaxation

It should be re-stated that the net magnetization vector comprises spins that are physically distributed throughout the body. Owing to this distribution, and to the fact that the B_0 field is not perfectly homogeneous, there is an additional phenomenon that contributes to effectively reducing the perceived T2. Owing to field inhomogeneities, nuclei in different parts of the body are exposed to slightly different magnetic fields and consequently will precess at slightly different frequencies. Thus, the process of loss of phase coherence is accelerated and the perceived T2 decay is faster than expected due to pure T2 considerations. The decreased T2 value (i.e., faster signal loss) is termed as $T2^*$ ("T2 star") and is a combination of the sample characteristics and instrumentation imperfections. It is possible to design imaging sequences to be sensitive to either $T2^*$ or T2.

Tissues are characterized by their T1 and T2 relaxation properties, which are influenced by a variety of physical conditions including: the proximity and mobility of molecules in the surrounding environment, the hydrogen concentration of the tissue, and the degree of "shielding" of the local magnetic field at the molecular level. MR image contrast can be made sensitive to these conditions using specialized imaging sequences. Image contrast is generally described in terms of the level of T1 or T2 "weighting" (described later in this chapter). Additionally, image contrast can be made sensitive to motion, either of the blood or myocardium. These different contrast mechanisms can be understood in terms of the image formation process of MRI techniques used to image cardiovascular structures.

MAGNETIC RESONANCE IMAGING

The concept of using the NMR signal to generate images was introduced by Lauterbur (3) and independently by Mansfield and Grannell (4) in the early 1970s. Mansfield's approach was to exploit the inherent regular structure of matter to generate "interference patterns" using the NMR signal. The intention was that these patterns would differentiate physical regions, forming the basis of an imaging approach. The approach developed by Lauterbur was to impose order on the sample by applying an external magnetic gradient. The latter approach proved more practical and was rapidly developed into the imaging systems that we have today. Advances in computer technology and superconducting magnets now permit routine clinical NMR imaging of the cardiovascular system (5). As NMR imaging becomes a mainstream clinical modality, the term "nuclear" was dropped, in part to distinguish MR imaging from nuclear tomography and the terminology "MRI" is now employed universally. MRI has gained such a widespread acceptance that several sub-specialties in nomenclature have evolved including MRA (angiography), FMR (functional), and CMR (cardiovascular). In general, when MRI has been applied to a clinical situation, it has quickly become regarded as the "gold standard." The reason for this rapid acceptance of MRI by the medical community is multifactorial and reflects the high level of patient acceptance, the exquisite resolution that can be obtained in a 3D manner, and the intrinsic contrast that permits differentiation of normal from pathologic tissue states. Establishment of clinical MRI has been particularly rapid for non-cardiac applications. However, the requirement to accommodate cardiac and respiratory motions, combined with the complexity of cardiac anatomy and function, has resulted in CMR developing at a slower rate compared to non-cardiac applications. Currently, both MRI instrumentation and imaging techniques are sufficiently advanced to allow MRI to become a major modality in evaluation of the cardiovascular system.

Gradients

As indicated above, the key to performing imaging was the introduction of externally applied magnetic gradients to distinguish between spatial regions. This is a direct consequence of the Larmor equation, i.e., that the resonant frequency is proportional to the local magnetic field strength. Thus, if the magnetic field varies linearly across the body (i.e., via application of a gradient), then so will the resonant frequency of the NMR signal (Fig. 6). This mechanism effectively encodes spatial information in the MR signal. The magnetic gradients of an MRI system are of the electromagnetic design, requiring activation by driving electrical currents through the coil systems which are integral to the scanner. For imaging applications, it is necessary to rapidly switch the gradients on and off, and the electromagnetic design allows this to be accomplished in time-scales of considerably less than a millisecond. Three orthogonal gradients are incorporated into the scanner system: one in the cranio-caudal direction (Z), one in the right–left direction (X), and one in the anterior–posterior direction (Y). The currents to drive these gradients are controlled by the scanners' computer system. By combining these three gradients, it is possible to generate a gradient in any desired orientation. This aspect permits slice selection and image formation to be accomplished in any required orientation with great precision.

Field strength

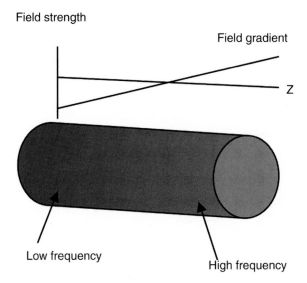

Figure 6 Application of a magnetic field gradient along the length of the sample (patient) results in modification of the local resonance frequencies, i.e., the gradient imposes a linear range of resonant frequencies along the body relative to the central Larmor frequency.

Slice Selection

The most basic step towards image generation is accomplished by restricting the MR signal to a slice. Slice selection is realized by application of a linear magnetic gradient across the body, in such a manner that its direction is orthogonal to the required slice direction. Again, as a consequence of the Larmor equation, the gradient effectively imposes a range of resonant frequencies along its length. Within the body, these families of resonant frequencies form parallel planes, each distinguished from the other by their unique resonant frequency. Applying a B_1 RF pulse at a frequency corresponding to the required slice position ensures that only those spins in a narrow frequency range experience the effects of the RF pulse (Fig. 7). Thus, slice selection is achieved by simultaneous application of a magnetic gradient and an RF pulse. Slice orientation is determined by the direction of the gradient, whereas slice thickness is controlled by adjusting either the characteristics of the RF pulse or by adjusting the strength of the gradient (a weaker gradient results in a lower range of resonant frequencies and will select a wider slice). Thus, in MRI, slice selection can be accomplished with great precision with the orientation, thickness, and position being user selectable via the control interface (i.e., the scan console). Importantly, the spatial relationship between slices is known, allowing integration of data from multiple slices to be combined for a unified 3D volumetric analysis.

Field strength

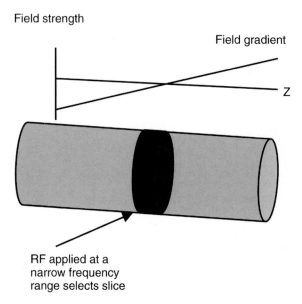

Field gradient

RF applied at a
narrow frequency
range selects slice

Figure 7 Slice selection is accomplished by application of a magnetic gradient oriented perpendicular to the required slice direction. This gradient forms planes of spins with narrow frequency distributions. Application of an RF pulse within a narrow frequency range selects only those spins falling within that narrow frequency range and can be used to define a slice. *Abbreviation*: RF, radiofrequency.

This aspect allows MRI to not only visualize 3D structures, but also allows measurements to be performed, generating accurate volumes in addition to linear dimensions.

Spatial Encoding

To accomplish slice selection, a linear gradient is applied across the body, imposing a linear progression of resonant frequencies. Following slice selection, application of a gradient within the selected plane similarly generates parallel columns of spins, each column characterized by a unique resonant frequency (Fig. 8). In the presence of a magnetic gradient, the signal emitted from the selected slice contains information relating to the multiple frequencies present. It can be appreciated that it is possible to distinguish one column from the another based on their differences in frequency. In this manner, spatial differentiation (column-wise in this case) within the slice is realized. However, it is still not intuitively obvious how the detected MRI signal that contains this "spatial" information is processed to form an image. Spatial information extraction is accomplished by subjecting the NMR signal to the mathematical process of Fourier transformation (this was a key contribution introduced by Ernst). By this procedure, the

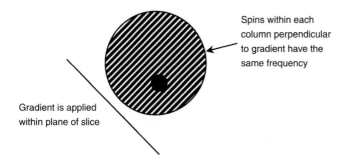

Spins within each
column perpendicular
to gradient have the
same frequency

Gradient is applied
within plane of slice

Figure 8 Following slice selection, a gradient applied along a direction within the plane produces a frequency distribution across the slice such that columns of spins are established in a direction perpendicular to the applied gradient.

intensity associated with each resonant signal is obtained (Fig. 9). From Figure 9, it is apparent that the Fourier-processed signal forms a projection of the spin density across the slice, the direction of the projection being perpendicular to the applied gradient. By systematically rotating the gradient, sampling the data, and Fourier processing it, a series of projections can be formed. It is possible to acquire a sufficient number of projections to form an image by the filtered back-projection reconstruction method similar to that used in computed tomography (CT) and radionuclide applications (Fig. 10). This was the original reconstruction method used by Lauterbur.

k-space

The "projection reconstruction" approach has several disadvantages, namely the spatial resolution towards the periphery is lower compared to the center and bright image features can generate "star" artifacts. Nevertheless, projection reconstruction has found widespread application in clinical modalities such as nuclear medicine, CT, and PET imaging. These modalities rely on the physical placement of a detector (or array of detectors)

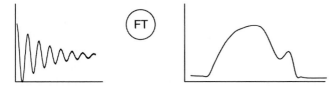

Figure 9 For the sample shown in Figure 8, the signal sampled in the presence of the in-plane gradient has the form shown in the first panel. This is termed the time domain signal or "free induction decay." After digitizing, the Fourier transform (FT) process is applied to generate the "frequency domain" signal shown in the second panel. This may be recognized as a "projection" of the sample in Figure 8, i.e., a circular object with a low signal circle on one side.

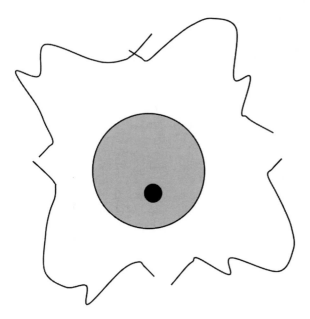

Figure 10   For the sample shown in Figure 8, a series of four projections are represented, positioned in the orientation of each projection. Conceptually, an image can be generated by "back-projecting" each profile across the image plane in the orientation that they were acquired. The back-projection approach essentially smears the signal from each projection across the image plane. The summation of all projections produces an image.

relative to the body to acquire signals directly in the "spatial" domain. This format of signal is almost exclusively processed into images by the projection reconstruction method. However, the NMR signal has to be transformed (via the Fourier transform) into the spatial domain. In this respect, the placement of the MRI signal receiver (which is a coil sensitive to RF signals) does not directly relate to the encoding of spatial information. This dissociation of the position of the receiver coil and the orientation of the image allows MRI the potential to generate images by alternate means, which have the advantage of providing uniform resolution, independent of signal intensity or position within the image field.

The MRI signal is acquired in the "time domain" (i.e., the signal is sampled for a number of milliseconds) and requires transformation (Fourier) into the spatial domain (e.g., projection data). Generation of a projection requires knowledge of the amplitude of the frequency information, which is extracted by performing the Fourier transform. However, there is another property that can be extracted from the time domain MRI signal, namely the relative phase of each frequency component. The amplitude and phase are important when forming MR images.

To form an image, we require data to be resolved along two dimensions. Thus, the phase information has potential to differentiate spins along each column of a projection. Consider applying a gradient across the selected slice, e.g., in the X-direction, resulting in columns of spins with uniform resonant frequency perpendicular to the applied gradient, i.e., along the Y-axis. Immediately prior to application of the X gradient, consider applying the Y gradient for a short time. The Y gradient alters the relative phase of the spins along the Y-axis. This relative change of phase can be detected in the Fourier-transformed data by changes observed in the phase of the frequency data (e.g., a sine and cosine wave may have the same frequencies, but they are 90° out-of-phase relative to each other). However, a single application of the Y gradient is not sufficient to uniquely differentiate all spins along the Y-axis. In practice, the number of pixels that are required along the Y dimension determines the number of separate applications required for the Y gradient. Diagrammatically, a 2D imaging sequence is represented in Figure 11. The signals generated by each application of the

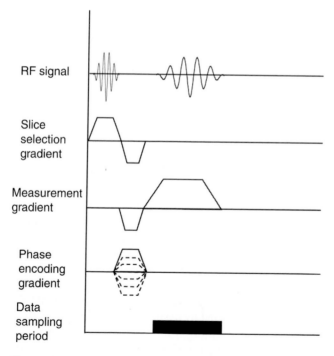

Figure 11   The basic elements of an MR imaging sequence are shown, with gradients applied along the "measurement," "phase encoding," and "slice selection" axis as illustrated. The RF pulse is applied at the same time as the slice selection gradient and the MRI signal is detected in the form of an RF signal. *Abbreviations*: MR, magnetic resonance; RF, radiofrequency; MRI, magnetic resonance imaging.

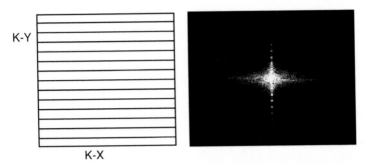

K-Y

K-X

Figure 12 Conceptually, successive signals from the MRI sequence are arranged in a matrix termed k-space comprising the $K{-}Y$-direction and the $K{-}X$-direction. Each $K{-}X$ line of k-space corresponds to the signal read out in the presence of the measurement gradient. The $K{-}Y$ lines correspond to different values of the phase-encoding gradient (Fig. 11). A k-space data set is shown in the left panel. *Abbreviation*: MRI, magnetic resonance imaging.

"imaging sequence" are arranged systematically in a 2D matrix termed "k-space" (Fig. 12) (6). Each time the sequence is applied, the Y gradient is applied at a slightly different level, each level corresponding to one line of k-space. The advantage of arranging the sampled NMR signals in the order required by k-space is that an image can be generated directly by Fourier transformation of the k-space data. The terminology used to describe k-space is that data are read in the presence of one imaging gradient (e.g., X) referred to as the "frequency encoding" or "measurement gradient" and the gradient required to step between lines of k-space (e.g., Y) is referred to as the "phase encoding" gradient.

Echo Formation

In the above discourse, a rudimentary imaging sequence was depicted. From this, it can be appreciated that a preparation period is required (i.e., to apply the phase-encoding gradient) prior to reading out the signal (i.e., in the presence of the measurement gradient). This preparation period requires that signal detection be delayed relative to slice selection. However, when the net magnetization vector is tipped into the transverse plane, it immediately starts to decay due to the relaxation processes. Thus, to accommodate the signal preparation period, it is necessary to recall the signal at a later time. This procedure is referred to as recalling an "echo." In an echo recall, the signal initially decays and is recalled during a period of signal growth. There are three possible modes of echo formation:

- gradient echo,
- spin echo,
- stimulated echo.

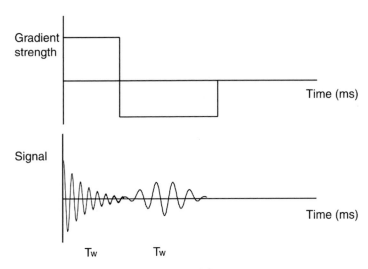

Figure 13 The elements of the gradient echo are shown. A positive gradient is applied for a time T_w during which time the signal decays due the "dephasing" aspect of the gradient. Immediately following this time, the gradient is reversed in polarity, which reverses the dephasing that it initially caused. As the spins rephase, the signal increases in magnitude, until a further time T_w has elapsed, at which time an echo peak is formed.

Gradient Echo

Application of a gradient causes spins to dephase relative to each other causing the signal to rapidly decay in amplitude (Fig. 13). At this stage, if no additional gradients are applied, the spins retain their relative phase differences, but even these relationships are gradually disrupted due to T2 relaxation. However, after termination of the initial gradient a second gradient is applied with opposite polarity, which causes the spins to reverse their relative phase dispersion, coming back into phase with each other (Fig. 13) (7). As the spins regain phase coherence, the MRI signal increases. However, the spins never completely refocus because of the continuous disruption exerted by the T2* processes which serve to decrease the signal amplitude in proportion to the time required to form the echo. The elements of a gradient echo are:

- excitation of spins by application of an RF pulse at time $t = 0$,
- application of a gradient with one polarity,
- application of a second gradient with opposite polarity.

During the slice excitation process, the point in time when the spins are in-phase with each other is at the mid point of the RF excitation and this time is generally taken as the "zero" time point of the system. The interval between the "zero" time point and the time at which spins refocus as an echo is referred to as the "echo time" or TE. For gradient echo sequences, TEs of less than 4 msec are commonly achievable.

Spin Echo

As indicated above, the gradient echo procedure cannot completely refocus spins due to the effects of T2*, i.e., due to the underlying processes of T2 decay and field inhomogeneities of the main magnetic field. The loss of phase coherence due to the T2 process cannot be recovered because it is an expression of the system's entropy. However, it is possible to undo the phase dispersion due to inhomogeneities of the main magnetic field. This can be achieved by generation of a "spin echo." Consider a collection of spins dephasing in the presence of a magnetic gradient. Physically, the spins are distributed throughout the selected slice and each spin experiences the additional dephasing effect of the inhomogeneous magnetic field. If after a time T, the spins are flipped like a pancake, then they find themselves in a position in which the applied gradient (which has not been reversed) continues to evolve their phase, but in this instance, they evolve to undo the phase differences accumulated during the time interval T, thus forming an echo at time $2T$ (Fig. 14). The spin echo process relies on flipping the spins like a pancake at time T that can be accomplished by application of an RF pulse designed to flip the spins by 180° at the time point T. The elements of a spin echo are:

- excitation of spins by application of an RF pulse at time $t = 0$,
- application of a 180° RF pulse at time $t = T$,
- sampling of the echo signal centered on time $t = 2T$.

Stimulated Echo

Although to form an echo with the gradient echo sequence requires one RF pulse and a spin echo requires two RF pulses, a stimulated echo requires application of three RF pulses. The sequence of events is:

- the first pulse brings M_0 into the transverse plane where it evolves in-phase in the presence of a gradient for a time T_{S1},
- a second RF pulse sends the magnetization back along the B_0-axis, at which point, the T2 relaxation process ceases to exert any influence on spin dephasing,
- after a time delay of T_{S2}, a third pulse brings the magnetization back into the transverse plane, where a refocusing gradient is applied to "undo" the phase evolution formed during the initial period T_{S1}. An echo forms after a further time interval equal to T_{S1},
- thus, an echo is formed at time $T_{S1} + T_{S2} + T_{S1}$,
- during the time interval T_{S2}, while spins are unaffected by T2 relaxation, T1 relaxation continues to operate and influences contrast.

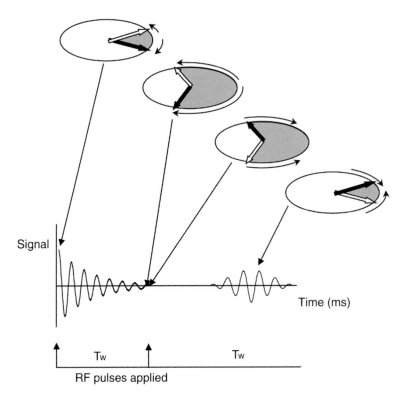

Figure 14 The elements of the spin echo sequence are shown. An initial RF pulse is applied and spins dephase as represented by the black and white arrows, continuously rotating away from each other. This dephasing continues for a time T_w at which point, a 180° RF pulse is applied. Note the effect that "flipping" the spins has, i.e., the black and white arrows are flipped like a pancake. Each arrow continues to evolve in the same direction, which will eventually rephase the spins at a further time T_w. However, the spins will not perfectly rephase, due to T2 dephasing, which cannot be rephased. *Abbreviation*: RF, radiofrequency.

Thus, it can be appreciated that a stimulated echo is affected directly by the T1 and T2 processes (Fig. 15).

Moving Blood and Echoes

One of the most important features of cardiovascular magnetic resonance (CMR) is the ability to distinguish cardiac chamber blood from myocardium. Each mechanism of echo formation affects the blood/myocardium contrast in a different way.

Gradient Echo: As gradient echoes can be applied in rapid succession, it is possible to partially suppress (i.e., partially "saturate") static tissue,

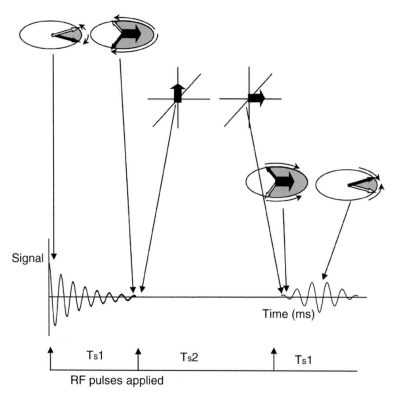

Figure 15 The stimulated echo sequence is illustrated. It requires the application of three RF pulses at the times indicated. The first RF pulse brings spins into the *x–y*-plane during which time they start to dephase, represented by the thin black and white arrows. At the end of the T_{S1} period, the net magnetization (represented by the thick black arrow) is put back along the *Z*-axis by application of a second RF pulse. During the next period, T_{S2}, the T1 process continues to relax the spins. Following this period, a third RF pulse is applied to bring the net magnetization into the *x–y*-plane. However, the spins retain a "memory" of their relative phase prior to being put along the *Z*-axis, but the phase of the spins is reversed (as indicated by reversal of the positions of the thin black and white arrows). During the next T_{S1} interval, the spins proceed to rephase in the manner of a spin echo, forming an echo at time T_{S1} following the third RF pulse. *Abbreviation*: RF, radiofrequency.

because this tissue experiences a number of RF pulses and cannot fully relax via the T1 process. However, moving blood may refresh the slice being imaged and contribute a "fresh" signal each time and thus contribute a bright signal. This is referred to as the "flow refreshment" phenomenon, and is the main mechanism for producing bright blood signal in gradient echo imaging sequences.

Spin Echo: The time interval between two pulses required for a typical spin echo sequence is on the order of tens of milliseconds. During this interval, it is possible that moving blood could have exited the plane being imaged. Thus, blood may not experience the two pulses necessary to form a spin echo and appear as a signal void. Commonly, spin echo sequences are referred to as "dark blood" sequences.

Steady-State Echo

During rapid and uniform application of a series of RF pulses, a steady-state signal can be established. In the steady-state, all three echo types are generated, i.e., gradient echo, spin echo, and stimulated echo signals, the time interval between successive pulses is on the order of 4 msec.

As all the three echoes contribute to one signal, the signal to noise ratio (SNR) is superior to any one echo method considered individually. Steady-state free precession (SSFP) sequences have found a widespread application in cardiovascular imaging due to the excellent contrast between blood and myocardium in addition to the good signal-to-noise characteristics. There are several commonly used sequences that fall into the SSFP category:

- true FISP (true fast imaging with steady precession),
- balanced FFE [balanced (gradient) fast field echo],
- FIESTA (fast imaging employing steady-state acquisition).

IMAGING SEQUENCES

An imaging sequence is the set of RF and gradient waveforms that, together with the data processing routines, are required for image formation. Different pulse sequences can be used to highlight a variety of features concerning the cardiovascular system including blood, myocardium, fluids, and masses. A common feature of most cardiovascular imaging systems is that images are acquired in a cardiac-triggered mode. To accomplish this, the ECG signal "R" wave signal is used to initiate each pass of the imaging sequence. To obtain data resolved over the cardiac cycle, it is necessary to repeat the basic imaging sequence at several regularly spaced points through each cardiac cycle (Fig. 16). Typically, over a series of several cycles, a complete cardiac image data set is acquired at a series of the points through the "composite" cardiac cycle, such that when displayed in a series, the beating motion of the heart can be appreciated. In principle, any of the basic imaging sequences can be applied in a cardiac-triggered mode. In practice, some are better suited to generation of cine data sets (i.e., movies of the CV system), whereas others are better suited to generation of "static" images, which are nevertheless triggered to a certain point in the cardiac cycle. However, it can be appreciated that if only one line of k-space was acquired at each point in each cardiac cycle, then to build up a series of images would require as

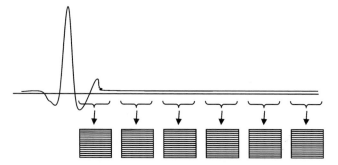

Figure 16 The cardiac imaging sequence is triggered to the ECG R-wave and several k-space data sets are generated, spanning the cardiac cycle.

many cardiac cycles as there were k-space lines in each image, typically 128 or 256 cycles (i.e., 2–4 min). To speed up this process, the concept of "segmentation" of k-space was introduced. Segmentation is the process by which several lines (typically 10–20) are acquired in a compact group within each cycle and assigned to an individual k-space set (8). Consequently, segmentation speeds up the imaging process by factors of 10–20, thereby bringing the scan time down to within a comfortable breath-hold time period (10–20 sec). The segmentation approach has its limitations, in that if a very high segmentation level is used, then excessive temporal blurring can occur. Typically, the segmentation value is set such that each seg mentation duration does not exceed 50 msec. The combination of high-performance scanner systems and imaging sequences designed to address cardiac imaging issues have led to the development of a viable environment for performing CMR.

Contrast Pulses

Each of the basic CMR imaging sequences can be applied with a "contrast pulse" designed to either highlight or suppress some specific features (e.g., blood, fat, and muscle). The term "pulse" refers to the short duration of the RF pulse that is applied prior to activation of the imaging sequence. One of the basic contrast pulses is the "inversion recovery" pulse (Fig. 17). This pulse inverts the magnetization vector M_0, which then "recovers" towards the equilibrium condition by the T1 relaxation process. Pulses can be applied in singles or in multiples (e.g., double and triple inversion pulses). Each of these variations is designed to suppress a tissue with a different characteristic T1 value. One characteristic of inversion pulses is that they are applied several tens or even hundreds of milliseconds prior to acquiring image data and thus, they typically do not allow for acquisitions that are time-resolved throughout the cardiac cycle. Another contrast pulse is provided by the "saturation pulse," which can be used to suppress tissue

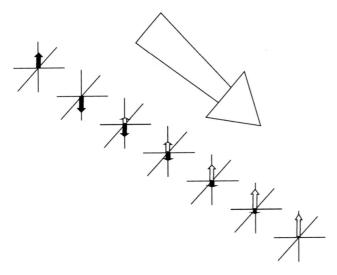

Figure 17   The inversion recovery contrast mechanism is illustrated. The large arrow indicates the passage of time, with the top frame representing time $t = 0$ with the net magnetization vector, $\mathbf{M_0}$, is aligned along the positive Z-axis. In the second panel, the effects of an inversion (i.e. 180° radio frequency pulse) are indicated whereby the $\mathbf{M_0}$ vector is initially aligned along the negative Z-axis. As time progresses, the $\mathbf{M_0}$ vector relaxes "through the origin" towards the positive Z-axis. Note that at one point, there is an equal positive and negative contribution to $\mathbf{M_0}$. If imaging were applied at this time, then no signal would be seen from these spins, this is the "null point."

signal (e.g., muscle or blood) by applying a 90° RF pulse which brings the magnetization into the transverse plane, where it is rapidly dephased by application of "dephasing" gradients. In this case, signal is destroyed by the $T2^*$ process. One characteristic of saturation pulses is that they are applied in close proximity to the imaging sequence and typically can be used in a cardiac cine mode. A commonly applied pulse is a fat or lipid suppression pulse. This relies on the fat and water signals having slightly different resonant frequencies (i.e., the Larmor frequency) due to differences in the gyromagnetic ratio, γ, between fat and water. Magnetization transfer contrast (MTC) exploits the fact that chemical transport of spins occurs in some materials (e.g., muscle) and not in others (e.g., blood or fat). Where the transport of spins occurs, they may move from one chemical environment to another, and may also move from one local magnetic environment (e.g., magnetically shielded by electron clouds) to another and consequently experience different resonance conditions in each environment. If spins are subjected to a train of saturation pulses while in one environment (i.e., at one resonant condition), they will not be affected by those pulses when they move to the new environment (i.e., due to differences in resonant frequencies). Thus MTC can help differentiate material based on the chemical transport mechanisms and the mobility of their protons by actively suppressing signal from these spins.

Gated Spin Echo Imaging

Gated spin echo is typically employed in a manner that uses segmentation in the form of recalling multiple echoes. Thus, gated spin echo utilizes a long train of echoes (e.g., 16–30). This long echo train may occupy 80–200 msec in the cardiac cycle, and thus time-resolved data sets are not commonly acquired. Gated spin echo sequences are commonly employed with an inversion pulse to enhance the appearance of either muscle or fat (e.g., for the visualization of fat infiltration in patients with right ventricular arrhythmia displasia). As is common to all spin echo sequences, moving blood appears as a region of signal void. Static or slow moving blood can appear as bright regions in SE images and these signals may be confused with other materials such as fat. When this happens, a specific contrast pulse may be employed to further differentiate regions.

Gated Gradient Echo Imaging

Gradient echo sequences are typically employed in a segmented manner. Segmentation can be accomplished by applying the basic imaging sequence in rapid succession or by rapidly recalling a number of echoes, or a combination of both approaches. The typical performance time to obtain one line of k-space is less than 10 msec, and if multiple echoes are performed (e.g., four) then times of 12 msec are typical for the set of echoes. Thus, it can be appreciated that 5–20 segments can be acquired using gradient echo approaches during cardiac-triggered imaging. Gradient echo approaches are typically applied to acquire cine images, with 15–20 images evenly distributed throughout the cardiac cycle (9).

Gated Steady-State Imaging

Recently, a number of imaging approaches have been developed that employ the SSFP signal. Importantly, the SSFP signal is derived from all the three echo types, and under conditions of uniformly spaced RF pulses, it is possible for all the three echoes to coincide. This requires careful control of the imaging sequences and also that the basic pulse separation be relatively short (e.g., 5 msec). The advantage of this approach is that significantly higher SNR can be achieved for blood (10). Thus, blood is seen with an intensity that is almost independent of its motion. This has the advantage that in views, where the blood remains in the imaging plane for relatively long intervals (e.g., for long axis views), the blood signal will be clearly seen and the myocardial boundary well-delineated (Fig. 18) (11,12).

(A)

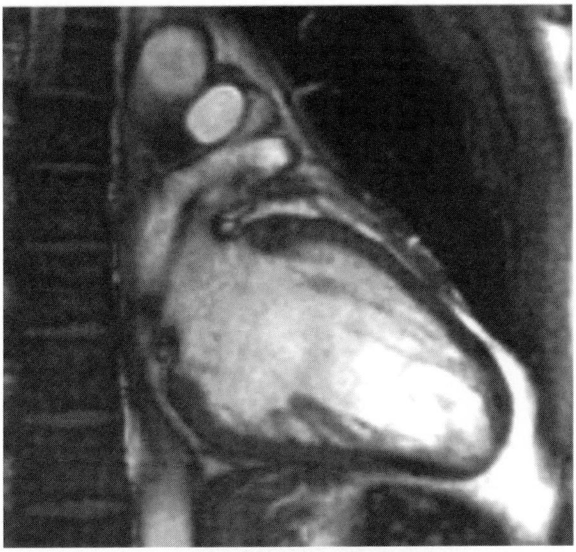

(B)

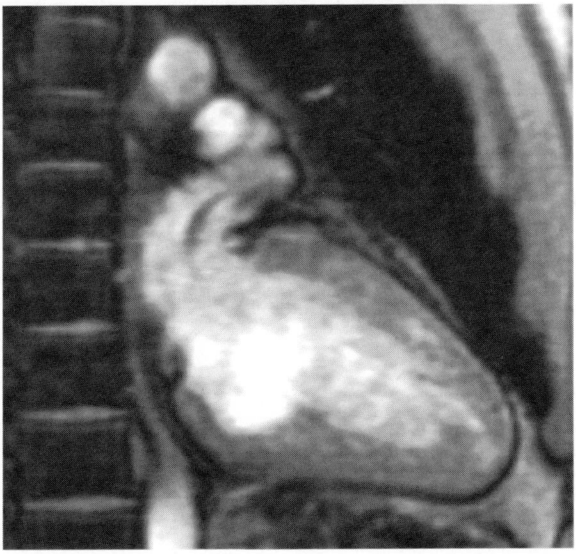

Figure 18 End-diastolic images of same volunteer, obtained with (**A**) an FIESTA and (**B**) a conventional cine imaging method. Note the higher blood-myocardial contrast in the SSFP image. *Abbreviations*: FIESTA, fast imaging employing steady-state acquisition; SSFP, steady-state free precession.

RAPID CARDIAC IMAGING

One of the key development areas in CMR over the past decade has been the development of rapid cardiac imaging approaches. It is noteworthy that while steady improvement in scanner technology has allowed cardiovascular scans to be acquired either with increased resolution or decreased scan time, the option has overwhelmingly been exercised to reduce the scan time. As indicated above, the segmentation approach to cardiac-triggered scans allowed scan times of the order of a breath hold to be achieved. Shorter scan times are now sought to achieve even shorter breath-hold times, or eventually real-time CMR. There are several approaches to reducing the scan time, and it is possible to combine many of these to achieve further reductions in scan time.

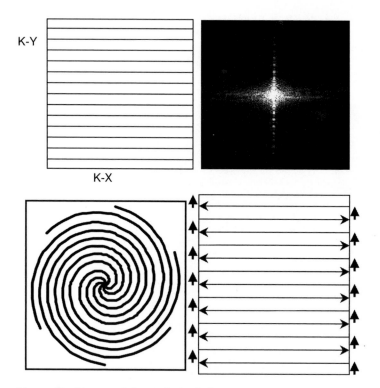

Figure 19 Top panel shows the basic form of k-space (*right*), typically acquired as a series separate parallel lines (*left*). The lower panel indicates the manner in which k-space is acquired in the spiral (*left*) and echo planar (*right*) sequences. In the spiral sequence, curved lines of k-space are rapidly acquired and in the EPI sequence, a series of lines are rapidly acquired as one long acquisition, indicated by the arrows showing the direction in which data are acquired. *Abbreviation*: EPI, Echo Planar Imaging.

Inherently Fast Sequences

Commonly, the k-space matrix required to form each image is acquired as a series of individual lines of data. However, it is possible to more rapidly acquire k-space data using inherently rapid approaches of Echo Planar Imaging (EPI) and spiral imaging (Fig. 19). These approaches are achieved by appropriate application of rapidly generated gradations. They broadly fall into the gradient echo category, but not exclusively so. Each of these inherently rapid approaches (capable of generating a complete image in under a 100 msec) has certain sensitivities to $T2^*$ effects and tend to be employed in specialized sequences, such as performing coronary artery imaging and myocardial perfusion imaging.

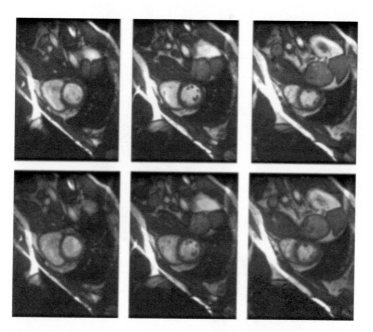

Figure 20 Top panel shows end-systolic frames from three short axis slices. Images for each slice position were acquired using the SSFP acquisition approach, and acquired in a breath-hold time of 13 sec per slice, requiring application of three breath-hold scans. The lower panel shows the corresponding images obtained with the rapid BRISK imaging approach. Data for all the three BRISK images were acquired in a single breath-hold of 16 sec duration, i.e., approximately three times faster than the conventional data, all other parameters being similar. *Abbreviations*: SSFP, steady-state free precession; BRISK, Block Regional Interpolation Scheme for k-space.

Rapid Data Sampling

Application of the segmentation data acquisition approach to cardiac-triggered imaging was primarily responsible for allowing breath-hold scans to be acquired. As indicated above, one limitation of the segmentation approach is that if too high a segmentation value is used, dynamic cardiac features in images could become excessively blurred. An approach that effectively allows increased segmentation values to be used is BRISK (Block Regional Interpolation Scheme for k-space). The BRISK approach employs a dynamically distributed data sampling pattern, which attempts to match

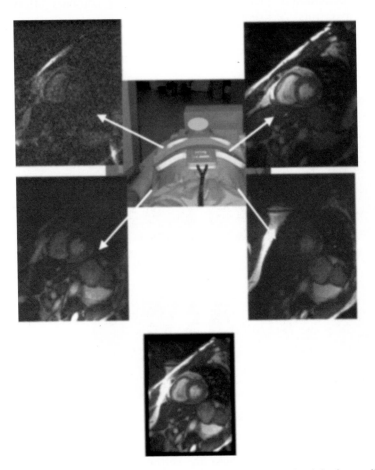

Figure 21　Illustration of the sub-images formed by each of the four coils comprising a single phased-array cardiac receiver coil. The four separate images are combined to form the single composite that is typically seen. Note that due to the physical location of each element of the phased-array coil, separate image features are seen with different SNR by each coil. *Abbreviation*: SNR, signal-to-noise ratio.

the segmentation level to the dynamic content of the data. BRISK can be employed to reduce the scan time for a time-resolved cardiac image set by factors of 2–4 (Fig. 20).

Parallel Imaging

An approach to reduce the scan time exploits the distributed nature of MRI signal reception. Typically, a phased-array surface coil is used to acquire the magnetic resonance images. Each element of the phased-array coil can effectively be used to acquire an image highlighting the image region closest to the position of the coil (Fig. 21). This feature can be used to effectively split the acquisition between each coil element, thereby reducing the scan time. This is referred to as the parallel imaging approach and scan time reduction factors of 2–4 are common (Fig. 22). Common acronyms for parallel imaging include:

- SMASH (SiMultaneous Acquisition of Spatial Harmonics),
- SENSE (SENSitivity Encoding scheme),
- ASSET (Array Spatial and Sensitivity Encoding Technique).

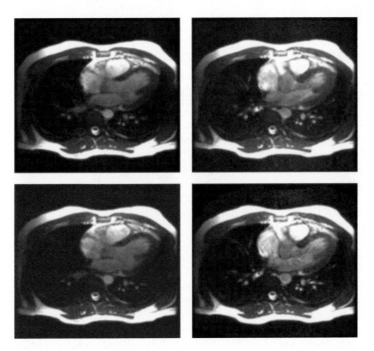

Figure 22 The top panel illustrates a 20-sec conventional acquisition, with frames shown at end-diastole and at end-systole. The lower panel illustrates corresponding frames acquired in 11 sec using the parallel imaging approach (images courtesy of Yi Wang, MR Research Center, University of Pittsburgh Medical Center, Presbyterian, Pittsburgh, Pennsylvania, U.S.A.).

SUMMARY

The process of generating images using the principles of MRI is really one of mapping the water distribution within the body. The application of magnetic gradients imposes an order on the spin system to allow the spatial distribution of spins to be determined. MRI data are acquired in the "time domain" and require transforming via the Fourier transform into the image domain. This allows MRI a freedom not enjoyed by any other major imaging modalities i.e., that image orientation is dissociated from the orientation of the receiver system. This allows MRI to generate images in arbitrary orientation within the body (i.e., not just axial, but oblique planes). Further, the exact geometric relationship between slices is known allowing extraction of 3D information such as volumes. When cardiac triggering is introduced, MRI can acquire data in four dimensions, i.e., space and time, allowing cardiac dynamics to be viewed and quantified. There are many parameters that can be exploited in MRI to distinguish physiologic formations. Chiefly, the appearance of static fluid such as effusions and moving fluids such as blood can be distinguished. Technology is sufficiently advanced to allow cardiovascular magnetic resonance (CMR) examinations to be routinely performed in under an hour, even for difficult cases.

REFERENCES

1. Bloch R, Hensen WW, Packard ME. Nuclear induction. Phys Rev 1946; 69:127.
2. Purcell EM, Torrey HC, Pound RV. Resonance absorption by nuclear magnetic moments in a solid. Phys Rev 1946; 69:37–38.
3. Lauterbur PC. Image formation by induced local interactions: examples employing nuclear magnetic resonance. Nature 1973; 242:190–191.
4. Mansfield P, Grannell PK. NMR diffraction in solids? J Phys C: Solid State Phys 1973; 6:1422.
5. Blackwell G, Doyle M, Cranney G. Cardiovascular MRI techniques In: Blackwell GG, Cranney GB, Pohost GM, eds. MRI: Cardiovascular System. New York: Gower Medical Publishing, 1992.
6. Twieg DB. The k-trajectory formulation of the NMR imaging process with applications in analysis and synthesis of imaging methods. Med Phys 1983; 10(5):610–621.
7. Edelstein WA, Hutchison JM, Johnson G, Redpath T. Spin warp NMR imaging and applications to human whole-body imaging. Phys Med Biol 1980; 25(4):751–756.
8. Riederer SJ, Tasciyan T, Farzaneh F, Lee JN, Wright RC, Herfkens RJ. MR fluoroscopy: technical feasibility. Magn Reson Med 1988; 8(1):1–15.
9. Hernandez RJ, Aisen AM, Foo TK, Beekman RH. Thoracic cardiovascular anomalies in children: evaluation with a fast gradient-recalled-echo sequence with cardiac-triggered segmented acquisition. Radiology 1993; 188(3):775–780.
10. Pereles FS, Kapoor V, Carr JC, et al. Usefulness of segmented trueFISP cardiac pulse sequence in evaluation of congenital and acquired adult cardiac abnormalities. Am J Roentgenol 2001; 177(5):1155–1160.

11. Thiele H, Nagel E, Paetsch I, et al. Functional cardiac MR imaging with steady-state free precession (SSFP) significantly improves endocardial border delineation without contrast agents. J Magn Reson Imaging 200; 14(4):362–367.
12. Plein S, Bloomer TN, Ridgway JP, Jones TR, Bainbridge GJ, Sivananthan MU. Steady-state free precession magnetic resonance imaging of the heart: comparison with segmented k-space gradient-echo imaging. J Magn Reson Imaging 2001; 14(3):230–236.

2

Cardiovascular Magnetic Resonance Instrumentation: What Equipment Do You Need for CMR?

Edward Walsh

Department of Neuroscience, Brown University,
Providence, Rhode Island, U.S.A.

INTRODUCTION

The instrumentation needed for cardiovascular magnetic resonance (CMR) consists of a standard clinical scanner with several notable enhancements. The physical principles governing image acquisition are essentially the same irrespective of the particular application. However, in cardiovascular applications, imaging a moving target, be it the myocardium or the blood (as in angiographic studies), requires certain enhancements to improve the acquisition speed, the image reconstruction speed, and the ability to minimize motion and susceptibility artifacts. We will treat each of these needs in the following descriptions of the relevant scanner components.

THE MAGNET

The central component of magnetic resonance (MR) imaging is the static magnetic field. It is this field that produces the "splitting" in the nuclear spin states that permit excitation [with the "radiofrequency (RF) magnetic field"] resulting in the production of a detectable signal. For CMR, the static field is generally produced using a superconducting magnet. The field strength if such magnets range from 0.5 to 3.0 T. Remember 1 T = 10,000 G and the magnetic field of the earth is approximately 0.5 G. Thus, the widely available 1.5 T magnet is 30,000 times the earth's magnetic field at the Tropic of Cancer or Capricorn. For research purposes, field strengths higher than 8 T have been produced. Superconducting magnets typically use a set of superconducting coils (usually niobium–titanium) immersed in liquid helium (boiling point 4.2°K). The niobium–titanium coils and liquid helium are contained in a dewar, within the main housing of the magnet (Fig. 1). The remaining space in the dewar is pumped out to produce a vacuum. This vacuum limits heat transfer to the cryogenic vessel and reduces the loss or "boil-off rate" of the liquid helium. As long as the superconducting material is kept below its critical temperature, it will conduct an electric current with effectively no resistance. Thus, once the current is introduced into the superconducting coil, it will continue conducting and produce the static magnetic field indefinitely with excellent stability (for practical purposes, less than 1 μT/hr actual field variation). Furthermore, this allows the magnetic field to be produced without the need for a continuous supply of electrical current (and resultant cost). This is one reason that conventional resistive electromagnets (usually consisting of wound copper wire) are not used in CMR. Another reason is that a resistive electromagnet of body size and suitable field strength would also generate considerable heat during operation, requiring a cooling system (and additional expense). Also contained with the main field coil is a set of the so-called shim coils. These superconducting shim coils are used to introduce slight variations in the main magnetic field distribution that accounts for manufacturing variations and metallic structures near the magnet that can have a slight effect on the uniformity of the main field within the magnet

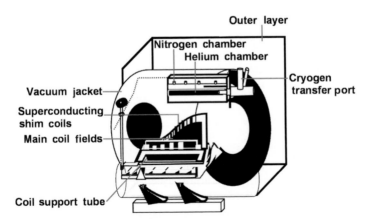

Figure 1 (*See color insert*) A cylindrical bore superconducting magnet showing the arrangement of main field, shim, and gradient coils within the cryostat housing. *Source*: Courtesy of Dr. Vicki Johnson.

bore at the imaging location. An alternative approach uses thin metal sheets arrayed in holders surrounding the bore, the arrangement of which modifies the static field in the desired fashion. A primary requirement for the imaging magnet (besides stability, which is excellent in the superconducting systems) is the need for considerable field uniformity. That is, the strength of the main field should not vary by more than a few parts per million over the entire imaging volume (up to 50-cm diameter spherical volume). To attain this level of uniformity, a single large solenoid field coil is not adequate. Instead, multiple coil sets are used. The diameter of the magnet bore is typically 1 m, with the direction of the main magnetic field aligned with the long axis of the bore. Effective diameters in clinical systems will be smaller because of the presence of the gradient coil(s) and RF coil(s).

One concern in the siting of MRI scanners is the fringe field. This is the extension of the main static magnetic field beyond the confines of the magnet into the surrounding space. All else being equal, the fringe field strength will vary linearly with the main field strength at a given location near the magnet. In the case of an unshielded 1 T magnet, the 5 G line will be located approximately 16 m from the ends of the bore and about 9 m from the sides of the magnet. Newer scanners incorporating active shielding can reduce these distances to about 3 and 2 m, respectively. Shielding can be accomplished by either active or passive means. In an actively shielded magnet, additional field coils of radius greater than that of the main field coils are used to establish a second field that tends to cancel the primary field outside the magnet. The additional fields have the potential to affect the main magnetic field. The effect of the secondary field inside the bore is taken into account by increasing the current of the main field coils over that necessary when active shielding is not employed. Active shielding increases the purchase cost of the magnet, but does not add to the operating costs because the shielding coils are also superconducting. Because the fringe field is smaller, it is possible that the additional cost of a shielded magnet can be offset by the less expensive easier siting requirements (the place or site where the magnet is located). In a passively shielded system, iron materials are incorporated into the magnet design to restrict the fringe field. The disadvantage of this approach is that the magnet becomes heavier, which can complicate siting and installation. Also, due to manufacturing variations, each magnet must be individually optimized. The fringe field is a concern that affects magnetically sensitive equipment (e.g., fluoroscopy equipment) and devices (e.g., pacemakers or implanted cardiovertor defibrillators). Fortunately, a wide array of MR-compatible medical equipment and devices are available.

THE GRADIENT SYSTEM

Recall that the spatial encoding of the magnetic resonance signals is accomplished through the use of linear magnetic field gradients. These linear gradient fields are superimposed on the static magnetic field and are switched on and off as necessary to accomplish image acquisition. The gradient system consists of two major components: the gradient field coils and the gradient amplifiers.

To provide three-dimensional spatial encoding, it is necessary to provide linear field gradients in the three directions corresponding to the orthogonal axes of the spatial reference frame. For MRI, these are defined as the z-direction (along the bore of the magnet), and the x, y directions (horizontal and vertical directions, respectively). For each of these directions, a set of field coils are provided that will produce a linear field gradient when current is passed through the coil (Fig. 2). These coils are resistive (not superconducting) and only produce their fields when current is sent through them. This is necessary because imaging sequences require that the gradients fluctuate quickly.

Gradient amplifiers are used to produce the large current pulses that are required to drive the gradient coils. These currents can exceed 100 A. Typical maximum gradient strengths range from 1 to 4 G/cm in clinical systems, and gradient slew rates are up to 20 G/(cm/msec). For a given gradient coil, the strength of the gradient field is linearly proportional to the current flowing through the coil. Gradient strength has implications with respect to speed of imaging. Another important factor, especially for cardiac imaging and angiography, is the slew rate (or ramp time) that is achievable in a given gradient system. The greater the maximum slew rate, the less time is required for the gradient field to reach its assigned strength (and to be switched off). Maximum slew rate is a function of the characteristics of both the gradient coils and of the amplifier performance. Any coil has an associated inductance (L) and as $V = L(dI/dt)$, where V is the amplifier output voltage and dI/dt the rate of current change (slew rate), it is seen that

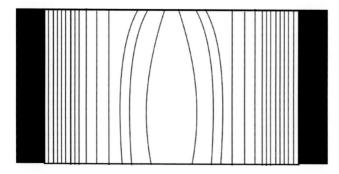

Figure 2 Diagram of the side view of a z-gradient coil. Gradient coils are placed on a cylindrical form which is sized to the bore of the magnet in which they are to be used. Coil windings are rigidly fixed to the form (sometimes embedded in epoxy) to prevent displacement due to forces experienced when current flows through the windings in the presence of the main magnetic field. *Source*: Courtesy of Dr. Vicki Johnson.

the greater the maximum output voltage of the amplifier, the greater the slew rate will be. Alternatively, minimizing the inductance of the gradient coil will also increase the slew rate. The greater the slew rate, the less time is needed to reach the desired gradient strength.

Increasing gradient slew rates allows reduction in the echo time (TE) of both gradient echo and spin echo acquisitions [not to mention echo planar (1,2) and spiral scan techniques (3,4)]. For cardiac imaging and angiography with gradient echo sequences, minimization of the TE provides a number of important benefits:

1. Greater immunity to motion artifacts,
2. Reduced artifacts arising from susceptibility gradients,
3. Reduced signal voids resulting from turbulent blood flow around stenoses,
4. Ability to reduce repetition time (TR) in rapid gradient echo imaging for reduced imaging time (important for first-pass myocardial perfusion techniques and for breath-hold imaging).

For a scanner intended for cardiovascular imaging applications, it is desirable to have a gradient system capable of at least 2.5 G/cm achievable with a ramp time of about 200 μsec. Although faster ramp times can be achieved with adequate gradient amplifier systems, concerns exist regarding neurostimulation that can result from currents induced in the body from the rapidly switching gradient field (a time-varying magnetic field will induce a current in a conductor). However, for the gradient switching rates available in clinical scanners, central nervous system stimulation is not an issue.

The rapidly switching gradient fields can also induce currents in other components of the magnet. These induced currents, in turn, will generate their own gradient fields that act to degrade image quality. As with the static magnetic field, these effects can be reduced through the use of active shielding in which additional coils are used to cancel the gradient field outside the gradient coil set. Such gradient sets involve greater purchase cost than unshielded gradient sets and require greater currents and drive voltages (owing to increased inductance). However, such gradient systems are essential for cardiovascular applications. The lifetime of induced currents in the magnet structure from unshielded gradients is typically longer than the desirable TE (TE < 2.5 msec) for gradient echo cardiovascular applications.

Another specification to consider for gradient systems is the linearity. A gradient coil set is intended to produce linear gradient fields on the three spatial axes. However, this linear portion of the gradient field does not cover the full extent of the magnet bore. As shown in Figure 3, the isocenter of the magnet is defined as the point where the magnetic field strength does not change when gradients are turned on. Slice offsets are defined with the isocenter as a reference (i.e., slice offset = 0 mm). For images to appear without geometric distortion, the gradient fields must be linear throughout the

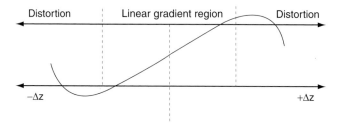

Figure 3 Variation in magnetic field strength when the gradient field is present. Outside the region of linearity, geometric distortion will result. *Abbreviation*: Δz, distance from the center. *Source*: Courtesy of Dr. Vicki Johnson.

region defined for the tomographic plane to be acquired. This must be considered when defining angiographic studies in particular. If the aortic arch and descending aorta are to be examined with a single acquisition, it is important that the patient be placed such that the full extent of the aorta to be examined is within the region of linearity for the gradient set. If this is not done, any anatomy outside the linear region of the gradient set will be spatially distorted. For clinical scanners, a typical linearity specification would permit the use of field-of-view (FOV) settings as large as 50 cm.

During operation, the gradient coil set produces a considerable sound level. When a current is passed through a conductor that is in a magnetic field, that conductor will experience a force. This principle is exploited in the design of electric motors. In a clinical scanner, the large static magnetic field, combined with the high currents used for the gradient pulses, results in large forces generated in the gradient conductors, with resulting sound. The characteristic sounds produced are a function of the type of imaging sequence, the TR and TE, number of slices, etc. Depending on the sound intensity produced by a given gradient system, it may be necessary to provide patients with hearing protection during studies. Typically, disposable earplugs are used.

THE RADIO FREQUENCY COIL

The Radio Frequency (RF) coil, sometimes referred to as a resonator, acts as the antenna for transmission of the RF excitation and for reception of the resulting MR signals. Although an antenna is typically thought of as a device intended to transmit an RF field away from the transmitter site, an RF coil for MR imaging is designed to confine the RF field to a specific volume. At the same time, this RF field is intended to be as uniform in intensity as possible over the imaging volume. Coils fall into two classes: volume coils and surface coils (with a further subdivision known as array coils). In all cases, the RF coils are resonant devices, intended for operation at a specific frequency (although some coils permit operation at two frequencies for spectroscopy). A resonant coil develops stronger transmit fields (for a given transmit power) and is capable of receiving weaker signal strengths than non-resonant structures. Additionally, the frequency selectivity (bandwidth) of the coil improves received signal-to-noise ratio (SNR) by imposing an additional degree of selectivity to the receiver system. For imaging, coils are resonant at the proton (^{1}H) frequency of the scanner. On a 1.5 T system, this is approximately 63 MHz. For spectroscopy, coils are made resonant at the frequencies of the nuclei to be examined. For ^{31}P at 1.5 T, the resonant frequency is approximately 25 MHz. For proton spectroscopy, the same coils that are used for imaging can be applied (with due regard for SNR for the specific study).

Most scanners are equipped with a large-volume coil (generally referred to as the body coil) that actually forms the innermost "layer" of the scanner bore (it is located inside the gradient set). This coil has a plastic inner lining and is not visible to the patient. A common configuration for volume coils is the "birdcage" configuration, an example of which is shown in Figure 4. In this design, one or two legs are driven, with the remainder acting as passive radiators such that a uniform RF field is produced within most of the volume

(A)   **(B)**

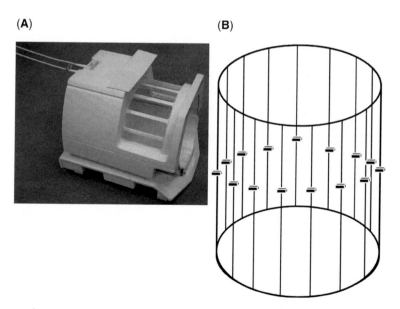

Figure 4   (**A**) A quadrature head coil suitable for use in cerebral angiography studies. The open construction of the coil allows the patient to see beyond the volume of the coil, which is helpful in reducing effects of claustrophobia. (**B**) Typical electrical layout for a birdcage coil showing the elements and capacitors. *Source*: Courtesy of Dr. Vicki Johnson.

of the coil. The inner diameter of the body coil actually defines the usable diameter of the scanner bore. Although a magnet may have a 90–100 cm bore, once the gradient and shim coil sets, and the body RF coil are inserted, the remaining diameter available to accommodate the patient will be on the order of 55–70 cm. The body coil is intended to produce an adequately uniform RF field over a range 40–50 cm in the x, y-plane (transverse to the axis of the bore) corresponding approximately to the linear region of the gradient set. The most basic mode of operation for the body coil is the one in which it is used for both transmission and reception. This is a convenient mode of operation, especially for scout imaging in which a large volume is to be imaged quickly for purposes of identifying the regions of interest and establishing tomographic planes for detailed study. The body coil is also suitable for use in extensive angiographic studies of the entire aorta where coverage on the order of 30–40 cm is desired. In general, the larger the coil, the greater the transmit power required to produce a given flip angle in the region of interest (ROI). Thus, the body coil requires more transmission power than the other coils used on a clinical scanner. For the 180° pulses required for spin echo imaging, several kilowatts peak power can be needed in order to permit the use of adequately short RF pulses.

The SNR of an image depends (among other factors) on the fill factor. The fill factor is defined as the ratio of the volume of tissues excited to the sensitive volume of the coil. Typically, the ratio of the volume of a tomographic slice to the sensitive volume of the body coil is very small. To improve the SNR for specific studies and to permit the use of smaller FOV settings, surface coils are employed. As the name suggests, a surface coil is placed on the body, as close as possible to the structure to be imaged. Surface coils may be used as transmitter/receiver antennas, or they may be used in a mode in which the body coil transmits the RF field, and the surface coil is used as the receiver antenna. The latter approach has the advantage of providing a uniform transmission field, effectively improving the intensity profile of the image. The reason for this is that a surface coil produces a non-uniform field when used as a transmission coil. The field intensity falls off with distance from the plane of the surface coil (Fig. 5). This same dependence applies to sensitivity for receiving the signal. Use of the body coil as the transmission antenna removes the spatial dependency of the transmitted RF field. The spatial dependence of the received profile can be exploited to improve the spatial resolution of images. If the FOV of the scanner in the phase-encoding direction is set smaller than the size of the subject, signal from outside the FOV will alias ("fold-over") into the image. As the surface coil will pick up signal only from its vicinity, the FOV can be set to smaller values, corresponding to the size of the surface coil without the possibility of fold-over because there is no signal arising from outside the ROI. As the FOV can be set smaller, for a given matrix size (e.g., 256 × 256) the pixel size will be smaller, and finer detail can be resolved.

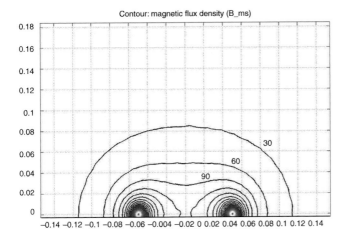

Figure 5 A calculated RF field intensity profile plot for a 10 cm surface coil. Horizontal and vertical distance scales are in meters. Contour lines for 30, 60, and 90° are shown for the case where a 90° pulse is established 3 cm from the plane of the coil. *Abbreviation*: RF, radiofrequency.

An important safety (and image artifact) concern is associated with the use of a surface coil as a receiver when the body coil is used for transmission. Consider that both coils are resonant at the same frequency. Thus, when the body coil transmits, the surface coil can act to receive the transmitted signal as it is being delivered. As the surface coil is resonant, a very high RF current will be induced in the coil. Simultaneously, the surface coil will transmit its own intense RF field as a result of the body coil excitation. This retransmitted field can result in significant tissue heating, or in an extreme case, RF burns. This action is prevented by a process known as decoupling. Each surface coil that is intended for use as a receiver coil (with body coil transmission) includes a circuit that acts to shift the resonant frequency of the coil on a momentary basis when activated by a control signal from the scanner (or on a passive basis in which the transmit RF signal forces the coil to decouple). During the imaging process, when the transmitter is activated, the decoupling circuit in the surface coil is also activated, shifting its resonant frequency. As the surface coil is now non-resonant at the transmission frequency, it does not receive and retransmit a signal. Upon termination of the body coil transmission signal, the decoupling circuit is deactivated and the resonant frequency of the surface coil returns to the proton frequency in order to receive the MR signal.

In many spectroscopic applications, particularly those where the nucleus under examination is not hydrogen, surface coils are used as both transmitters and receivers. One example is ^{31}P spectroscopy which is used to examine the concentrations of adenosine triphosphate, phosphocreatine, and inorganic phosphate in studies related to tissue ischemia. Another example is ^{13}C spectroscopy which is used in metabolic studies. Other nuclei such as ^{23}Na have been used in specific research applications. Of the non-hydrogen nuclei, ^{31}P has been the most extensively examined nucleus for cardiac spectroscopic studies.

A class of surface coils that is increasingly used in cardiovascular studies is the array coils. As the name indicates, such coils consist of multiple elements that are arranged in a single housing and connected in such a manner that they can be as simple to use as a single element surface coil. With some coil designs, the housing can be flexible such that the coil array can conform to the geometry of the patient (Fig. 6). The purpose of array coils is to attempt to combine the best aspects of surface coils and volume coils. Surface coils are intended to produce images of improved SNR over a specific region (when compared to the same images acquired with a body coil). Volume coils provide a more uniform RF field homogeneity to provide consistent intensity and contrast across the entire FOV. A phased-array receiver coil can provide receiver sensitivity over a larger area (as it consists of multiple coil elements) and can rely on the body coil for a uniform transmitting field. Use of array coils requires the ability to receive the individual element signals and combine them in the proper manner (e.g., phase relationships) to produce the composite receiver signal. This generally requires the use of multiple receiver channels on the scanner, with appropriate signal-processing capability. Although these capabilities add to the cost of the scanner, the results appear to justify the costs. Array coil capabilities have therefore become standard on scanners intended for cardiovascular applications. Although some variation of signal intensity characteristic of surface coils is seen in the array coil image, the difference in SNR is readily apparent. Performance improvements of this nature are important for the visualization of structures such as the coronary arteries. Improved SNR also improves the ability to quantify small contrast changes, which can prove helpful in

(A)   **(B)**

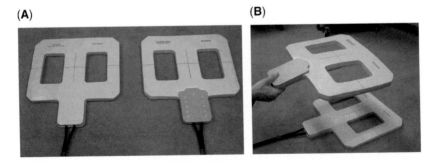

Figure 6 (A) An array coil for cardiac applications. This unit consists of two sections that are placed anterior and posterior. (B) The cables lead to a combiner for connection to the scanner. The housings are flexible and conform to the patient.

some first-pass myocardial perfusion imaging techniques. Larger array coils, essentially "whole body" receiver array coils, are available for use in angiographic studies. These coils have adequate coverage to permit first-pass angiographic studies using bolus contrast agent delivery in which the entire aorta, iliacs, and femorals (and even tibials for smaller patients) can be visualized in a single acquisition.

Array surface coils with multiple receivers permit the use of techniques to increase the speed of image acquisition. This class of parallel imaging acquisitions such as simultaneous acquisition of spatial harmonics (SMASH) (5), sensitivity encoding (SENSE) (6), and generalized autocalibrating partially parallel acquisitions (GRAPPA) (7) make use of the known sensitivity profile of an array coil set to simultaneously acquire information corresponding to more than one k-space line at a time. With the use of appropriate post processing to resolve the spatial harmonics in order to produce the complete k-space representations of the images, time savings on the order of two- to fourfold can be achieved. Such methods can be applied to most fast imaging methods, further multiplying the speed of these techniques without incurring a significant SNR penalty. These methods also go by several trade names as used by the various scanner manufacturers.

THE SPECTROMETER

The spectrometer (Fig. 7) is the system that generates the NMR transmit excitations, receives the NMR signals, and controls the gradient switching. A computer system contains the software that produces the pulse sequence

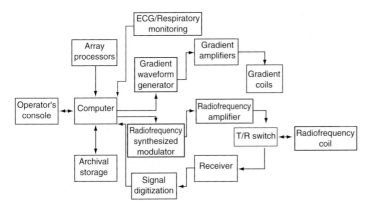

Figure 7   Block diagram illustrating the components common to most clinical MR scanners. These components will typically be divided over three rooms with the magnet in one room, the operators console in an adjacent room (with a view of the magnet), and most of the electronics in a separate temperature controlled room. *Abbreviation*: MR, magnetic resonance. *Source*: Courtesy of Dr. Vicki Johnson.

activity, performs the image reconstructions, provides viewing and analysis of the images, and provides a user interface to permit control of the scanner. These activities are controlled at the scanner console, which is the operating interface for the scanner, and is typically located just outside the magnet room, in front of a window that allows the operator to see the patient in the magnet.

A pulse sequence consists of three components: RF transmitter, signal receiver, and gradient switching. Programs controlling these functions are stored together on a disk drive and are called up according to selected protocols, e.g., spin echo, gradient echo, multi-slice 2D, 3D, etc. The operator then selects relevant parameters, such as flip angles, slice thickness, FOV, resolution, etc. Software interlocks prevent the operator from selecting parameters that could result in exceeding Food and Drug Administration limits for specific absorption rate (SAR) and gradient switching rates. Compiling of the pulse sequence results in the generation of RF and gradient waveforms that are downloaded to a pulse sequence generator. The pulse sequence generator produces signals that are sent to the RF modulator and gradient amplifiers to produce the RF transmit and gradient fields. The receiver is turned on at the appropriate times when the imaging sequence is run.

RF excitations begin with a software-controlled synthesizer set to the resonant frequency corresponding to the magnetic field strength. The low-level signals generated by the synthesizer are fed to a modulator where the appropriate pulse shape is produced (e.g., a sinc pulse for slice selection). Modulated RF pulses then are fed to an amplifier system which brings them up to the required transmission power (which can be kilowatts in the case of body coil transmission) for delivery to the resonator.

Gradient control signals produced in the pulse sequence generator are sent to the gradient amplifiers. There are three gradient signals, one signal for each gradient axis. Finally, there is a control signal to turn the receiver on and off, and to control the transmitter/receiver switch. All these signals are delivered in a synchronized fashion.

The operator's console also permits viewing of the images produced. Image reconstructions are performed on the scanner computer and can involve various filtering mechanisms in addition to the basic Fourier transform image reconstruction. Various tools for image analysis are typically provided to allow the operator to determine distances, areas, and intensities from image data sets (e.g., ventricular volume across the cardiac cycle, myocardial intensity during first-pass bolus perfusion studies, blood flow velocities, etc.). Scanner software is periodically updated by the scanner manufacturer to provide new capabilities and variations on pulse sequences and analysis tools.

PHYSIOLOGICAL MONITORING

The most obvious monitoring requirement in CMR imaging is for the electrocardiogram (ECG). ECG monitoring is needed both for assessment of the patient's condition and to provide the synchronization (gating) for image data acquisition. For cardiac image acquisitions that require more than one cardiac cycle to complete, it is necessary to acquire data at reproducible points in the cardiac cycle. Otherwise, the heart will appear blurred in the resulting images. Remember the three golden rules for high-quality cardiac imaging: triggering, triggering, and triggering. Cine imaging of the heart (to assess mechanical function) requires the generation of multiple image frames, each frame corresponding to a specific time point in the cardiac cycle. Such a data set, when played as a cine loop, allows visualization of the myocardial contraction and displacement across the cardiac cycle. To provide this time referencing, image data acquisition is synchronized to the peak of the ventricular depolarization wave of the electrocardiogram (ECG) R-wave.

In preparing the patient for scanning, the technician will apply (MR-compatible) ECG electrodes. The electrode placement may differ from the typical 3-lead placement. The reason for this is that the static magnetic field produces a distortion in the ECG as the result of magnetohydrodynamic effects. A typical manifestation of this effect is a greatly enlarged ventricular depolarization wave of the electrocardiogram (T-wave), which can be erroneously interpreted as an R-wave by amplitude or derivative threshold circuits (or algorithms if digital signal processing is used). ECG lead placements will be made in an attempt to attenuate these flow artifacts. Another source of difficulties in obtaining the ECG during imaging arises from gradient switching and RF transmission signals. These two processes can induce their own signals in the ECG lead system and confound identification of the R-wave for triggering purposes. Important safety concerns are also associated with the interaction between the RF/gradient systems and the ECG lead system. For the gradient system, the rapidly switching gradient fields can induce currents in the ECG leads. This, of course, is undesirable. ECG monitors approved for clinical use meet specifications for leakage currents at the lead inputs, which are periodically measured during the service life of the monitor to ensure that the specification is met whenever the device is used on patients. To ensure that physiologically significant currents are not generated in the ECG lead system, lead placement is such that loops in the cables are not present and cable lengths are minimized. To eliminate the possibility of RF burns, the cables are kept as short as possible, they are prevented from forming loops, and they are placed away from the resonators. ECG cable assemblies on current scanners are also heavily shielded to minimize induced currents. In general, as scanner field strength increases, so do the difficulties in obtaining an adequate ECG for triggering purposes. This field dependence results from the generation of electrical currents by moving blood. As blood contains ions, moving blood constitutes a moving conductor in a magnetic field resulting in induced currents that can be detected by the ECG system. In particular, there can exist a large flow artifact at the time of the T-wave. Depending on the overall quality of the ECG signal, such a T-wave flow signal can be mistaken for the R-wave as was mentioned earlier. This could potentially cause an error in gating. However, use of digital signal processing techniques, along with improvements in cable shielding and lead placement, has made obtaining an adequate ECG nearly routine for main field strengths up to 3 T.

Monitoring of respiratory activity is another concern that relates both the condition of the patient and image quality. As the heart can translate over a range 2–3 cm in the superior–inferior direction and 1 cm in the anterior–posterior direction, correction for respiratory motion is necessary in imaging sequences that cannot be performed during breath holds. Basic monitoring of respiratory rate can often be accomplished by using a low-frequency component derived from the ECG baseline. Some scanners have employed a pneumatic or stress transducer mechanism worn as a belt around the abdomen to provide an indication of gross respiratory motion for scanner gating purposes. Methods employing navigator echoes are also used to provide information on the location of the diaphragm or ventricular blood pool to effect data correction during acquisition and reconstruction.

Blood pressure can be monitored using approved automated monitors designed for use in the MRI environment. These systems will pressurize a cuff at preset time intervals and display systolic/diastolic blood pressure measurements so that they can be seen by the technician and attending physicians during the course of image acquisition.

Arterial blood oxygen saturation (SaO_2) is monitored using a pulse oximeter. As pulse oximeters rely on an optical technique for assessment of arterial oxygen saturation, MRI compatibility is not difficult to achieve. Pulse oximeter capability is often incorporated into MR physiologic monitoring systems, with the SaO_2 displayed along with the blood pressure and pulse rate during the image acquisition.

SITING REQUIREMENTS

A clinical MRI scanner is a large and complex system that places certain demands on the environment in which it is to be operated. Factors to be taken into account when selecting a location for installation include: total floor area, weight-bearing ability of the floor for the magnet, electrical service capacity, nearby structural elements, heating/AC, traffic within the fringe field, RF shielding, floor plan, etc. Depending on the nature of the building in which the scanner is to be located (unless new construction is planned), it is possible that modifications to an existing building can run as high as $500,000. Scanner manufacturers provide siting requirements and planning assistance for their customers.

THE MAGNET

A superconducting 1.5 or 3 T magnet can weigh as much as 13,000 lb (5900 kg). Magnets therefore are generally located on a ground floor (or basement) with a concrete floor of adequate strength. Certainly important is a provision for an adequate opening so that the magnet can be placed in the room. Other concerns include the presence of metal structural members (these should be adequately far from the magnet so as not to affect field homogeneity), provisions for cryogen delivery (and recovery if the magnet is so equipped), nearby activity (preferably, the magnet should not be sitting against the wall on the side of a road where moving traffic can affect the field homogeneity), and adequate ceiling height to accommodate the cryogen fittings on the top of the magnet. Shielded magnet designs are easier to locate owing to their smaller fringe fields.

ADDITIONAL HARDWARE

The floor plan must provide a location for the operator's console, scanner computer, spectrometer, and RF and gradient amplifiers. Provisions also must be made for patient reception and waiting areas, and for a properly equipped examination/preparation room. The spectrometer and amplifiers are typically located in a room adjacent to the magnet room in order to minimize cable lengths between the electronics and the magnet (gradients and resonators). Provisions are typically made to pass cabling under the floor between the magnet and hardware rooms. If liquid cooling is required for the gradient system, the cooling unit will be located in the hardware room and water lines run under the floor to their connections on the gradient set.

AIR CONDITIONING AND HEATING

MR scanner components have environmental limits that must be maintained for reliable operation. In particular, the electronic systems all generate heat that must be removed in order to maintain a constant temperature within the manufacturer's defined limits. Individual components, such as the computer, RF amplifier, etc., typically have individual blowers to provide forced air cooling for high dissipation components. For adequate cooling, however, it is necessary to maintain the room temperature within specified limits. A typical specification is 55–70°F (13–21°C) with relative humidity of 30–60% (non-condensing). The air conditioning system must be capable of maintaining the temperature in the hardware room with all systems producing heat on the order of 70,000 btu (17,640 kcal).

POWER

The peak power requirement for a clinical MRI scanner can be on the order of the total electrical capacity of four single-family homes. The primary power feed will typically be a 440 V line (50–60 Hz) with at least 100 A current capacity (continuous). The peak power demand for a complete scanner system can be as high as 62 kW. The majority of the power is required by the gradient amplifiers, the RF power amplifier, and gradient cooling system. Specifications will also be provided by the scanner manufacturer for line voltage regulation (voltage variation with varying current demand), phase variation, wire gauges, circuit breaker capacities, etc.

TERMINOLOGY

Acquisition time—The total time required to obtain all the image information in a given scan. It is a function of the image resolution, number of slices, TR, and number of averages.

Angiography—The visualization of blood vessel patency. In MR imaging, this is accomplished by enhancing the contrast of flowing blood through suppression of stationary tissue signal.

Array processor—A device in the scanner computer which performs certain frequently needed operations (such as the Fourier transform for image reconstruction) in hardware rather than in software to provide a substantial increase in speed (i.e., reduction in image reconstruction time).

Artifact—A defect in an image that can obscure diagnostic information. Artifacts can arise from subject motion, cardiac motion, pulsatile flow as well as from incorrect scanner parameter settings or hardware difficulties.

Averaging—The process of acquiring the same image data more than once. This is done to improve SNR and to reduce motion artifacts.

Cine—Applies to imaging techniques in which reconstructed images are intended to be viewed as a movie loop permitting visualization of dynamic activity such as ventricular function or contrast agent arrival.

Cryostat—The physical magnet including the superconducting coils, cryogen containers, and housing.

Effective TR—The actual repetition rate for cardiac gated data acquisition taking into account the R–R interval occurring during the scan.

Fourier transforms—The mathematical operation that converts the scanner's raw k-space data into viewable images. It may be thought of as the operation that converts between the spatial domain and the spatial frequency domain. When applied to an audio signal, the Fourier transform shows the pitch content of the sound.

Fringe field—The extension of the static magnetic field beyond the bore of the magnet into the surrounding space. Shielded magnets have reduced fringe fields compared to conventional magnets.

Gating—The process of synchronizing image data acquisition to the electrocardiogram and/or position in the respiratory cycle. Gating is necessary for the production of time-resolved images as used for ventricular function assessment.

Gradients—Magnetic field gradients superimposed on the static (main) magnetic field to produce spatial encoding in the MR signals. Also applied to the physical coil set used to produce the gradient fields.

Inversion recovery (IR)—A technique for generating T_1 contrast by inversion of magnetization followed by a delay (inversion time) prior to image acquisition. The inversion time is set to maximize signal differences between different tissues in the FOV in order to provide optimum contrast.

k-space—This is essentially the frequency space (Fourier transform) representation of an image. A scanner acquires information in frequency space and carries out a Fourier transform in order to reconstruct an image which can be read. A 256×256 image acquisition will involve the acquisition of 256 k-space lines (phase encode lines) in which each line consists of 256 points (read encode points).

Oblique planes—Image planes that are angled from the three orthogonal image planes corresponding to the axes of the magnet (i.e., axial, sagittal, and coronal). Oblique planes are produced using linear combinations of x, y, and z gradients for the slice select, phase encode, and read gradient functions, respectively.

Orthogonal—Perpendicular. The axial, sagittal, and coronal slice orientations are mutually orthogonal.

Parallel processors—Data processing units that are designed to operate at the same time. A typical PC has one processor. Use of multiple processors (including array processors) permits multiple functions to take place at the same time. For example, image reconstructions and display can take place as image data is being acquired to permit real-time imaging of catheter placement.

Partial volume effect—Inclusion of anatomic features or artifacts as the result of image slices being too thick.

Peripheral gating—Gating of the scanner by monitoring pulsatile blood flow. This is used primarily to reduce cerebrospinal pulsatility artifacts in head imaging.

Phase—(1) Applied to signals indicating the relative magnitudes of the real and imaginary components. Signal phase can be made to correspond to flow velocity for phase velocity mapping angiography techniques. Phase—(2) A specific point in the cardiac cycle corresponding to an image acquisition (e.g., a 20-phase ventricular function scan contains 20 images corresponding to 20 different time points in the cardiac cycle). Phase—(3) Phase encode applied to spatial encoding represents encoding of one of the in-plane dimensions (the other being read or frequency encoding).

Read—Usually applied to one of the in-plane directions encoded by the gradient which is turned on while echoes are collected (read gradient).

Resonator—Another name for an RF coil. This term is sometimes used as RF coils are tuned to resonate at the operating frequency of the scanner.

ROI—Usually refers to a subset of the imaged region on which some analyses will be performed, such as mean and standard deviation of the pixel intensities.

Segmentation—This term can be used in two different contexts: (1) The breaking up of image acquisition into a number of blocks. All of the k-space lines in a given block are acquired during one repetition interval. This provides more rapid image acquisition than a single k-space line per repetition interval and (2) identification and delineation of specific tissues or organs by some identifying characteristic (such as T_1, T_2, diffusion coefficient, etc.) from images in which contrast has been made dependent on the identifying characteristic.

Slice selection—Excitation of one tomographic plane of finite thickness accomplished by turning on a gradient while the RF excitation is delivered.

SNR, S/N—An important parameter which indicates the ratio of the MR signal to background noise. Noise results from both the patient and from the scanner electronics. Noise can also result from external causes if the RF shielding of the scanner room is inadequate.

Spatial resolution—The FOV divided by the number of pixels across the image. This is an indicator of the smallest features than can be visualized in a given scan.

Spectrometer—The scanner electronics (and operator's console) that execute the pulse sequences and receive the MR signals.

Surface coil—A (typically receive) coil placed on the surface of the patient to provide for enhanced SNR over a small region to be observed.

Temporal resolution—Typically refers to the phase interval in a ventricular function scan, but can also refer to the interval between image frames for a dynamic contrast agent study.

Trigger—Sometimes used interchangeably with gate. Specifically, a trigger is a signal issued to the scanner by the gating system to initiate image data acquisition given that the gating system has detected a valid gating event (such as an ECG R-wave).

Trigger delay—A user-introduced time interval which allows a specific period of time to elapse between the gating event, and initiation of image data acquisition.

Trigger window—Term used in two opposite senses, referring to a period of time during which triggers will be accepted, or when triggers will not be accepted. Trigger windows are often applied when both cardiac and respiratory gating are used in the same scan.

Volume coil—A coil that encloses the subject to be examined. These include body coils, head coils, and extremity coils. Volume coils can be used both in the receiving/transmitting mode, or can be used for transmission with surface coil receiver.

Volume imaging—Usually refers to 3D imaging techniques in which individual slices are not discreetly acquired. Rather, the slice-select direction is phase encoded. These methods allow for isotropic resolution imaging (i.e., slice thickness is the same as the in-plane voxel size) with high SNR. Slice thickness in the resulting data set is typically thinner than would be permitted using conventional gradient slice selection.

SUMMARY

This chapter provides an understanding of the basic instrumenttion and siting requirements for a CMR laboratory. Cardiovascular applications are among the most demanding, and require the latest technology for optimum results. This includes high-speed gradients, customized RF coil arrays, and high-field strengths. CMR also requires special equipment for real-time physiological monitoring. All of these are described in the present chapter.

CONCLUSIONS

This chapter provides an understanding of the basic instrumentation and siting requirements for a CMR laboratory. Cardiovascular applications are among the most demanding, and require the latest technology for optimum results. This includes high-speed gradients, customized RF coil arrays, and high-field strengths. CMR also requires special equipment for real-time physiological monitoring. All of these are described in the present chapter.

REFERENCES

1. Mansfield P, Maudsley AA, Baines T. Fast scan proton density imaging by NMR. J Phys E Scient Instrum 1976; 9:271–278.
2. Cohen MS, Weisskoff RM. Ultra-fast imaging. Magn Res Imaging 1991; 9:1–37.
3. Ahn CB, Kim JH, Cho ZH. High speed spiral-scan echo planar imaging. IEEE Trans Med Imaging 1986; MI-5:2–7.
4. Meyer CH, Hu BS, Nishimura DG, et al. Fast spiral coronary artery imaging. Magn Reson Med 1992; 28:202–213.
5. Sodickson DK, Manning WJ. Simultaneous acquisition of spatial harmonics (SMASH): fast imaging with radiofrequency coil arrays. Magn Reson Med 1997; 38:591–603.
6. Pruessmann KP, Weiger M, Scheidegger MB, et al. SENSE: sensitivity encoding for fast MRI. Magn Reson Med 1999; 42:952–962.
7. Griswold MA, Jakob PM, Heidemann RM, et al. Generalized autocalibrating partially parallel acquisitions (GRAPPA). Magn Reson Med. 2002; 47:1202–1210.

3

The Cardiac Magnetic Resonance Examination: Basic Considerations

Luigi Natale

Department of Radiology, Cardiovascular Magnetic Resonance Unit, Catholic University of Rome, Rome, Italy

Gerald M. Pohost

Department of Medicine, Division of Cardiovascular Medicine, Keck School of Medicine, University of Southern California, Los Angeles, California, U.S.A.

INTRODUCTION

In the early days of cardiovascular magnetic resonance (CMR) imaging, the methodology was appropriately called nuclear magnetic resonance (NMR) imaging since there are other types of magnetic resonance applied to spectroscopic approaches including electron spin resonance and Mössbauer magnetic resonance. However, in the late 1980s the "nuclear" in medical NMR was dropped and the name changed to the non-specific name magnetic resonance imaging so as not to confuse it with nuclear medicine and so that the public would not think the methodology was in any way associated with ionizing radiation. The first "NMR" examinations of the heart were performed in the early 1980s. Goldman et al. evaluated myocardial perfusion in excised canine models of coronary artery occlusion using the paramagnetic contrast agent manganese chloride ($MnCl_2$) administered prior to sacrifice (1). Due to the high toxicity of the intravenously administered manganese compound, it could not be used as a clinical agent. Shortly after the administration of the agent the dogs died and hearts excised and imaged in an 5-inch bore, 1.4 T superconducting magnet. Studies were performed in vivo in 1984 with the addition of gating; however, the images were low resolution acquired in a 0.1 T system in Aberdeen, Scotland (2). Many technical problems were evident, including relatively poor image quality resembling radionuclide studies and long acquisition times of greater than 10 minutes. Cardiac MR imaging represented a challenge for physicians and manufacturers. The assessment of morphology and function was essential initially. The challenge was to identify the appropriate pulse sequence to generate diagnostically adequate resolution and contrast and to improve upon two-dimensional (2D) echocardiography and relatively low-resolution radionuclide imaging. Other applications of CMR were clear from previous work including assessment of myocardial perfusion (3). The application of CMR for detection of diseases of the aorta and peripheral arterial vasculature suggested the use of CMR for non-invasive coronary angiography (4).

Such approaches require optimization of field and gradient strengths, hardware and software configurations. This meant development of new scanner strategies including innovative methods to construct radiofrequency (RF) coils. Ultimately, due to the specialized approaches required by the imaging of the heart in all of its facets cardiac-dedicated systems were introduced in the late 1990s.

The first step in a CMR examination is to precisely define the clinical question. The optimal diagnosis under most circumstances is generated through a close collaboration between radiology and cardiology. A CMR team should be organized to include a CMR cardiologist, a CMR radiologist, and preferably a CMR technologist. The team should meet on a daily basis prior to CMR study to determine the most appropriate imaging approach to optimally evaluate the question being asked. Interpretation should be undertaken at sessions involving both radiologist and cardiologist, sometimes with the help of the technologist. A given CMR session should be undertaken to address a specific question. For example, what is there myocardial scar? how much? and what is its distribution? Or, what is the distribution of the pulmonary arteries in a patient with congenital heart disease?

Prior to any CMR examination it is essential to obtain an accurate history of any potential contraindication such as the presence of a magnetic- or RF-sensitive device such as an implantable cardiac defibrillator. In this chapter, the most important aspects of CMR will be discussed and will focus on patient preparation, cardiac gating, optimal pulse sequence(s), scan planes, and post processing.

PATIENT PREPARATION

Patient cooperation is essential in performing a CMR examination. Before scanning, the importance of his/her cooperation must be explained and emphasized. Appropriate patient understanding prior to the examination can reduce the severity of claustrophobia and suggest the need for a sedative. In addition, the patient should be instructed in quiet and regular respiration and the need for lying still within the magnet during the time of the imaging study. This is to avoid motion artifacts that would degrade image quality making it inadequate for diagnosis. With ultra-fast acquisition approaches, the patient must be instructed on deep-inspired breath-holding during deep inspiration or partial exhalation, depending on the protocol. Finally, when contrast agents must be injected the details (for example, the use of a power injector) and the safety of the injected contrast agent must be explained. It is essential to monitor the vital signs including the pulse rate, the blood pressure and the respiratory rate, before, during, and after the examination. Pulse oximetry and/or electrocardiography (ECG) are used to monitor the heart rate and to provide signals for gating. The appearance of the ECG is changed due to the magnetohydrodynamic effects and RF interference. Accordingly, within a CMR system, the ECG cannot be used for diagnostic purposes (i.e., the appearance of the ST and T waves make them of no diagnostic value). Thus, the ECG is only useful for heart rate monitoring and for providing the QRS signal for gating. Lead positioning can be difficult for the uninitiated. The ECG leads must be positioned so as to obtain the best QRS complex conspicuity. Recent external monitoring systems and developments in cable manufacturing can improve the quality of the QRS portion of the ECG, improving ECG gating. When pharmacological agents such as dobutamine or adenosine are to be infused, such as for wall motion studies and perfusion studies, ECG and hemodynamic (i.e., blood pressure) monitoring before, during, and after such infusions is mandatory. CMR laboratories must be equipped with resuscitation equipment and all medical personnel certified in resuscitation methods.

CARDIAC GATING

Cardiac gating (or synchronization) is necessary to "freeze" cardiac motion, to avoid artifacts related to cardiac and blood pool motion, and to generate images to evaluate atrial ventricular and function. Most scanners are provided with two types of cardiac gating devices, the peripheral approach using finger plethysmograph and the central approach using the QRS complex of the ECG. The ECG approach is optimal for cardiac imaging since it is more precisely related to ventricular contractile function.

Electrocardiographic synchronization is based on the recorded ECG during the examination. The usual approach to gating is prospective, where the QRS complex is identified and the scanner generates an RF pulse sequence applied after a delay time as determined by the operator. Gating is implemented either prospectively or much less commonly, retrospectively. The less common "retrospective gating" approach involves ECG recorded with imaging excitations and measurements delivered in continuous succession. CMR imaging data are acquired continuously throughout the cardiac cycle representing all phases of the cardiac cycle. This allows post-acquisition synchronization of the imaging data with the ECG. This allows substantial flexibility in the generation of a cinematic display.

Proper positioning of the ECG electrodes is important, to minimize the artifacts induced on the ECG tracing by the switching of the gradients; different manufacturers suggest individual positioning systems, based on the gating approach used. In general, when a three-lead approach is used, two leads are placed on the upper chest, in the right and the left anterior axillary lines and the third is placed over the cardiac apex; when a four-lead system is used, the fourth lead is positioned on the sternum, midway between the right arm lead and the apex lead.

Another approach uses the electrodes positioned on the back, since there is less respiratory motion (and consequently artifact), but generally this approach generates reduced QRS amplitude and ECG quality with sometimes suboptimal unpredictable synchronization.

The larger the dipole (i.e., the further apart each pair of electrodes), the larger the amplitude of the ECG signal. However, the larger dipoles lead to the increase in the amplitude of artifacts, especially those resulting from the magnetic field and the gradients. For adequate gating, the QRS complex must have amplitude substantially higher than the baseline noise. Another noteworthy problem is when the T wave approaches the R wave amplitude. When this pattern is observed, the position of the electrodes must be modified and the distance between electrodes reduced. In such cases ECG setup time can be considerable, but this is crucial for an optimal examination.

Another manufacturer has introduced a new gating system, based on the use of one electrode containing four leads. This electrode is usually positioned on the precordium.

Vectorcardiographic gating is a robust approach for CMR image acquisition. Vectors are generated throughout the cardiac cycle indicating the maximal magnitude of the QRS determined from multiple ECG electrodes using real-time processing. This approach automatically adjusts to the actual electrical axis of the patient's heart and to the specific multi-dimensional QRS waveform, resulting in reduction of ECG setup time, since the result is much less dependent on the position of the chest electrodes. This technique is also more robust in the presence of the magnetohydrodynamic effects, making it suitable for cardiac gating at high field strengths (≥ 3 Tesla).

PULSE SEQUENCES

Basic cardiac pulse sequences include (i) spin echo (SE) for "black blood" imaging (Fig. 1), (ii) gradient echo (GRE) for "white blood" imaging (Fig. 2), and (iii) inversion recovery (IR) which optimizes contrast and steady-state free precession (SSFP) which allows high-speed acquisitions.

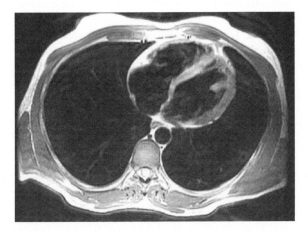

Figure 1 Axial FSE image of the heart; black blood imaging allows clear differentiation between myocardium and blood pool. *Abbreviation*: FSE, fast spin echo.

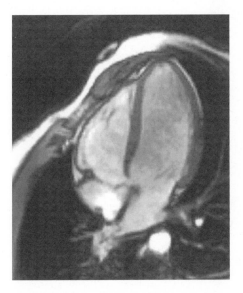

Figure 2 Four-chamber SSFP image of the heart; bright blood imaging permits good definition of endocardial borders. *Abbreviations*: SSFP, steady-state free precession.

The SE pulse sequence (5) uses a 90° followed by a 180° RF pulse. This pulse sequence has been used to evaluate cardiac morphology as a multi-slice, single-phase approach, i.e., acquisition of a tomographic slice through the heart in a given cardiac phase. Of course, no functional information can be obtained from such an imaging approach. Acquisition time is relatively long since averaging is necessary; for this reason the old approach of using the SE pulse sequence, per se, is no longer used. This approach generated multiple slices in multiple phases of the cardiac cycle, in order to obtain "black blood" images of each slice throughout the cardiac cycle. SE images can be weighted for longitudinal relaxation time (T1), transverse relaxation time (T2), or proton density (PD). T2-weighted SE imaging is more difficult, due to artifacts, but newer approaches have solved this problem (Fig. 3). With the SE pulse sequence, the repetition time (TR) is generally equivalent to the R–R interval or a percent of that interval, to prevent premature heart beats; for example, in a patient with a cardiac heart rate of 60 bpm, TR would be lower than one second (1000 msec). Basically, as the patient's heart rate decreases, T1 weighting shifts to proton density weighting, because of the increase in TR. This weighting can be modified by changing the timing of the RF pulses. The so-called delay time is the time between the R wave and the RF pulse that can be modified by the operator to obtain images in a desired phase of the cardiac cycle.

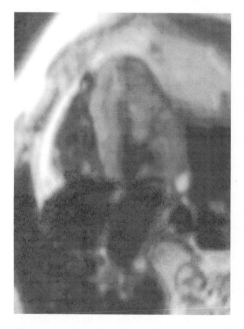

Figure 3 Four-chamber T2-weighted FSE image. *Abbreviation*: FSE, fast spin echo.

Echo time (TE) can be chosen between 6 and 40 msec; the lower the value the more the signal related to slowing of blood flow, whereas the highest values can decrease signal intensity from thin structures, like the valves or the interatrial septum. Unfortunately, conventional SE imaging is time-consuming and is affected by motion and flow, which can lead to artifacts. The long acquisition time precludes high-resolution imaging. Newer pulse sequences have improved spatial and contrast resolution by using segmented *k*-space approaches coupled with double inversion recovery pulse preparation which nulls the blood pool signal, resulting in "black blood" imaging. In this double inversion recovery pulse preparation approach, the second inversion pulse is used to select the slice: consequently stationary spins are refocused and provide signal, while flowing spins are not refocused by the second pre-pulse. A third inversion pre-pulse can be added to cancel "bright" fat tissue signal. Finally, rapid acquisition with such segmentation of *k*-space allowing generation of high-resolution images ($\geq 256 \times 256$).

Gradient-recalled echo sequences are used for imaging of function, since they generate cine images in which the blood appears as bright and the myocardium as dark (5,6). Conventional cine-CMR imaging is based on single-slice, multi-phase acquisition and is less time consuming than spin echo imaging. Spatial resolution is low to moderate because of the need for averaging. Recent developments introduced *k*-space segmented cine-CMR, allowing the acquisition of a cine run during a 20- to 30-second breath-hold acquisition. The most important advantages of this technique are the absence of respiratory motion artifacts and full coverage of the ventricles, with the possibility of real three-dimensional (3D) measurement of volumes and ejection fraction. The ability to generate 3D images of both ventricles has made CMR imaging the gold standard for assessment of global and regional ventricular function. For determination of the volumes of the left ventricle, no geometric assumptions are necessary. This is particularly important in diseased ventricles, where shape is distorted and the area–length method is imprecise. For the right ventricle, no geometric formulae are needed. Only 3D methods, as are obtained using CMR imaging allow assessment of global function.

With segmented *k*-space techniques, temporal resolution is better than in conventional cine CMR. Repetition time is very short and view sharing software is able to improve the effective temporal resolution. The most important disadvantage of methods using breath-holding is poor differentiation between the endocardial interface and the blood pool (Fig. 4A, B). Furthermore, the intensity of the signal arising from flowing blood is particularly high only if the flow is perpendicular to the imaging plane. Blood flow across the imaging plane will result in poor signal intensity. First, breath-hold sequences employed very short TEs, 3 to 4 msec, eliminating the flow voids that provide evidence of turbulence as is the case in valvular stenosis or regurgitation. Improved sequences are able to increase TE up to 10 to 12 msec, avoiding this problem.

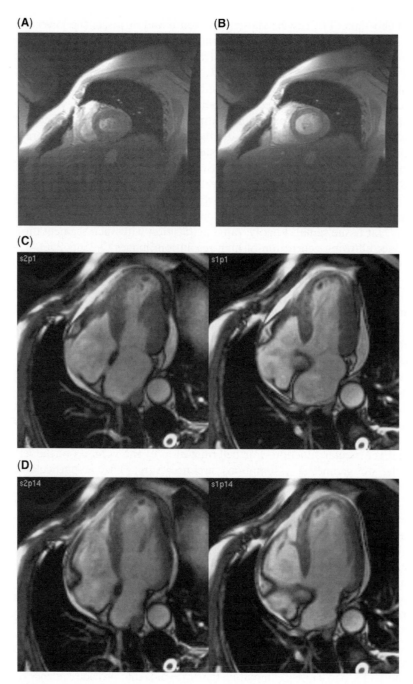

Figure 4 (*Caption on facing page*)

The ideal approach for cine imaging to assess heart function is the use of an SSFP technique (known commercially as FIESTA, True-FISP, and Balanced FFE). This approach basically uses a continuous signal where intensity depends on the T2/T1 ratio and not on flow. Images demonstrate optimal differentiation between myocardium and blood pool. Regional and global function are superbly assessed with this technique (Fig. 4C,D), with very short TR and TE, resulting in further reduction of acquisition time. In summary, morphology and function are assessed by black blood and white blood imaging approaches, respectively. For black blood, a spin echo technique is used; for white blood a gradient echo or now, preferably, an SSFP technique is used.

Perfusion and viability are assessed by an inversion recovery pulse sequence in combination with injection of a paramagnetic contrast agent, usually using a gadolinium chelate. Using the appropriate timing between the initial RF pulse and the inversion (180°) pulse, the myocardium can be nulled, i.e., the signal from the myocardium approaches zero. When the contrast agent is injected intravenously, using a non-magnetic power injector, the first-pass of contrast through the myocardium produces a bright signal in territories that are normally perfused. However, there is reduced signal in territories that have abnormally reduced perfusion: the greater the reduction in perfusion, the lower the signal intensity. Such images resemble radionuclide perfusion scans, but have substantially higher resolution.

Flow can be quantified using a cine phase-contrast pulse sequence in which the phase shift in spins is proportional to spin velocity (7). This approach was previously performed during free breathing (with acquisition lasting minutes and using respiratory gating) and is now performed in "real time" during breath-holding. The flow images that are obtained are coded in gray scale, where flow is black or white depending on its direction. Generally, flow is bright when it is oriented toward the observer. This approach is similar to the color-Doppler echocardiography only in monochrome (Fig. 5A, B). It is possible to color code flow with CMR also. From the phase-shift calculation and the cross-sectional area of the blood vessel, flow velocity and volumes can be derived. Some applications of this flow determination technique include quantification of shunts by measurement of aortic and pulmonic flows (8), the quantification of pressure gradients across a stenotic vessel or valve, and the assessment of ventricular diastolic function.

Figure 4 (*Facing page*) Cine-MRI: (**A**, **B**) end-systolic and end-diastolic short axis frames with segmented *k*-space GRE ("Fastcard"); (**C**, **D**) end-systolic and end-diastolic horizontal long axis frames with SSFP sequence. Endocardial and epicardial borders are more readily defined using such SSFP pulse sequences. *Abbreviations*: MRI, magnetic resonance imaging; SSFP, steady-state free precession.

(A) **(B)**

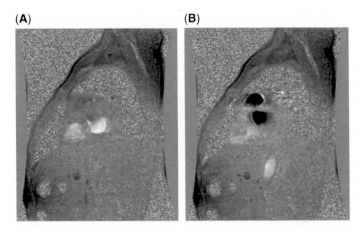

Figure 5 Cine-phase contrast, short axis: **(A)** diastolic frame, **(B)** systolic frame, showing flow through mitral valve and aortic root and right pulmonary artery, respectively.

High-performance gradients are necessary for full coverage of the left ventricle allowing perfusion imaging of the first-pass of contrast agent. Short axis images are preferred to assess the coronary artery territories, with at least 4 to 6 base-to-apex slices are necessary for optimal evaluation of myocardial perfusion (Fig. 6) (9,10).

Detection of delayed enhancement of contrast agent distribution (11) should follow imaging of first-pass perfusion evaluation. Delayed enhancement

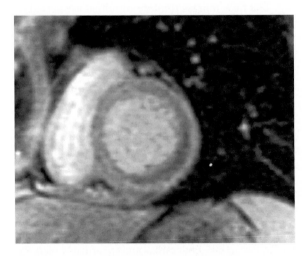

Figure 6 Frame from a first-pass perfusion study with IR-prep fast-GRE sequence: sub-endocardial perfusion defect is clearly evident in the infero-lateral left ventricle wall.

is observed in inflammation, necrosis and fibrosis, but not in healthy tissue. A number of different readout methods can be used based on k-space-segmented gradient-echo techniques, or recently on hybrid echo–planar sequences. For this kind of assessment, inversion recovery-prepared k-space-segmented 2D or 3D gradient-echo sequences are employed (12); correct choice of inversion time (TI) is crucial for correct and complete nulling (substantially reducing signal intensity in healthy myocardium and other tissues), so that contrast is maximized and enhanced regions are clearly depicted (Fig. 7A–C).

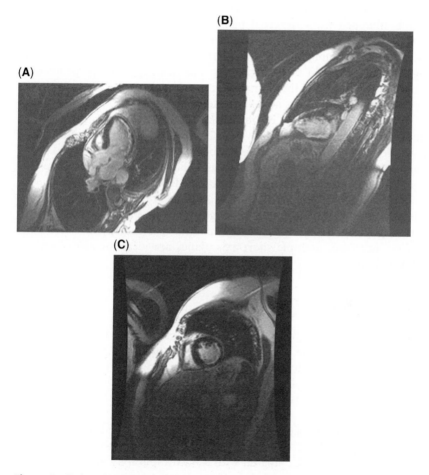

Figure 7 Delayed enhancement study with IR-prep fast-GRE sequence: (**A**) horizontal long axis, (**B**) vertical long axis, (**C**) short axis show sub-endocardial hyper-enhancement in the inferior and lateral basal, mid and apical left ventricle walls (same case as in Fig. 6).

SCAN PLANES

One of the most important advantages of CMR is its ability to image multiple planes during a single examination. The CMR system allows imaging in the axial planes (i.e., coronal, sagittal, and transverse) commonly used for the study of the central nervous, musculoskeletal, gastrointestinal, and urogenital systems, but not as useful for cardiac imaging. Nevertheless, axial imaging is frequently used for the evaluation of congenital heart diseases. In the assessment of cardiomyopathies (13,14), valvular diseases and ischemic heart disease, the single oblique and double oblique planes are most useful.

The true cardiac axes are represented by the vertical long axis, the horizontal long axis, and the short axis (Fig. 8A–F). The vertical long axis image is obtained from the axial plane, with a line parallel to the interventricular septum and represents the so-called two-chamber view, since it depicts the left atrium and the left ventricle (15). The horizontal long axis image is obtained from the vertical long axis, tracing a line perpendicular to the inferior leaflet of the mitral valve to the left ventricular apex (16). The short axis view is perpendicular to either of the long axis views.

Many other planes can be obtained, based on the cardiac structure or chamber to be evaluated, with any possible single or double obliquity (17). The left ventricular outflow tract can be best imaged in a semi-coronal plane obtained from the axial plane or in an oblique plane derived from the coronal plane (Fig. 9). The right ventricular (RV) outflow tract is imaged in a semi-sagittal plane obtained from the coronal plane (Fig. 10). Special planes are used to study the complex geometry and volume of the right ventricle (RV), particularly for the evaluation of tricuspid valve function. However, here too, multiple short axis planes are ideal for assessment of the RV volume.

POST PROCESSING

The evaluation of function, perfusion, and viability can be initially assessed qualitatively, but another advantage of CMR is the ability to quantify ventricular volumes, the extent of perfusion abnormalities, and the extent of scar making the results less operator dependent and more reproducible. The 3D nature of CMR is one reason that it provides accurate quantitative results (6).

Cardiac analysis packages were developed in the last few years, for complete analysis of global and regional function of both ventricles and for flow quantification. Compared with echocardiography and echocardiographic software packages, CMR software provides more reliable results. Furthermore automated contour evaluation is now possible, although occasional manual correction is sometimes required. Analysis of myocardial perfusion is more complicated and only more recently developed

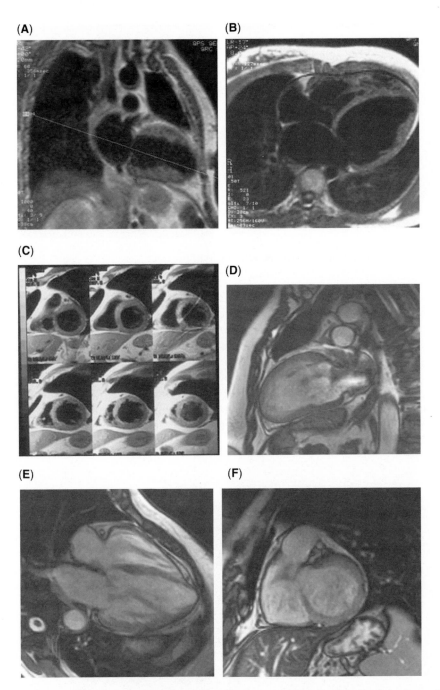

Figure 8 Scan plane through cardiac axes: (A–C) black blood vertical, horizontal and short axes images; (D–F) bright blood vertical, horizontal and short axes images.

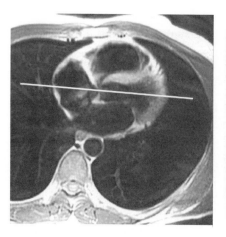
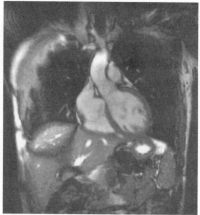

Figure 9   Scan plane through left ventricle outflow tract.

post processing software allows more accurate quantization. In addition, derivation of myocardial perfusion from signal intensity/time curves is easily performed (Fig. 11A,B). Perfusion and function data can be displayed using a bull's eye method (Fig. 12), a familiar tool in nuclear cardiology.

Flow and velocity curves are now easily obtained from many types of software, including the processing of phase-contrast flow data. However, manual contouring of the vessel or the chamber to be imaged is still required. More sophisticated evaluation can be derived using tagging techniques (16).

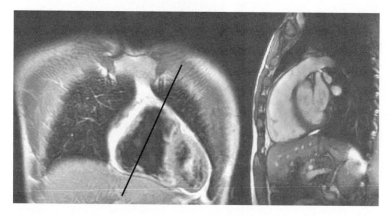

Figure 10   Scan plane through right ventricle outflow tract.

(A) **(B)**

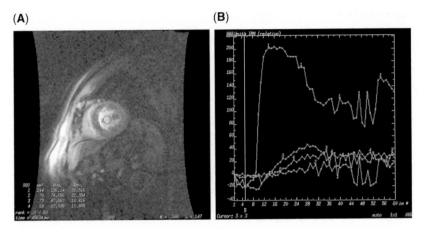

Figure 11 First-pass perfusion study (**A**, single frame) with signal intensity versus time curve (**B**), showing wide transmural perfusion defect in anterior acute myocardial infarction.

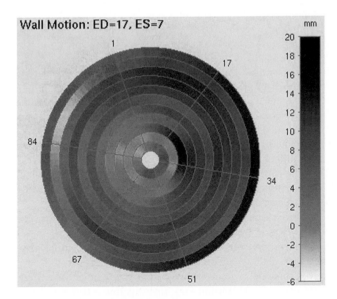

Figure 12 (*See color insert*) Bull's eye display of left ventricle wall motion, showing reduced function at the apex.

CONCLUSIONS

This chapter provides a general overview of the CMR study. Concepts of patient preparation, gating and most commonly employed pulse sequences have been introduced, providing the basis for a more complete and detailed evaluation in the chapters that follow.

REFERENCES

1. Goldman MR, Brady TJ, Pykell IL, et al. Quantification of experimental myocardial infarction using nuclear magnetic resonance imaging with paramagnetic ion constrast enhancement in excised canine hearts. Circulation 1982; 66:1012–1016.
2. Smith FW, Mallard JR, Hutchison JM, et al. Clinical application of nuclear magnetic resonance. Lancet 1981; 10(1):78–79.
3. Lorenz CH, Flacke S, Fischer SE. Noninvasive modalities. Cardiac MR imaging. Cardiol Clin 2000; 18(3):557–570.
4. Gatehouse PD, Firmin DN. The cardiovascular magnetic resonance machine: hardware and software requirements. Herz 2000; 25(4):317–330.
5. Firmin DN. Magnetic resonance imaging formation. In: Underwood R, Firmin DN, eds. MRI of the Cardiovascular System. Oxford: Blackwell, 1991:11–25.
6. Natale L, Meduri A, Caltavuturo C, Palladino F, Marano P. MRI assessment of ventricular function. Rays 2001; 26(1):35–44.
7. Lotz J, Meier C, Leppert A, Galanski M. Cardiovascular flow measurement with phase-contrast MR imaging: basic facts and implementation. Radiographics 2002; 22:651–671.
8. Glockner JF, Johnston DL, McGee KP. Evaluation of cardiac valvular disease with MR imaging: qualitative and quantitative techniques. Radiographics 2003; 23(1):e9.
9. Villa A, Meloni G, Montagna C, Sammarchi L, Campani R. Magnetic resonance imaging in the study of ischemic heart disease. Rays 1999; 24(1):33–45.
10. Nagel E, al-Saadi N, Fleck E. Cardiovascular magnetic resonance: myocardial perfusion. Herz 2000; 25(4):409–416.
11. Judd RM, Kim RJ. Imaging time after Gd-DTPA injection is critical in using delayed enhancement to determine infarct size accurately with magnetic resonance imaging. Circulation 2002; 106(2):e6.
12. Smith HJ. Contrast-enhanced MR imaging in the diagnosis and preservation of cardiac viability. Acta Radiol 2001; 42(6):539.
13. Di Cesare E. MRI of the cardiomyopathies. Eur J Radiol 2001; 38(3):179–184.
14. Friedrich MG. Magnetic resonance imaging in cardiomyopathies. J Cardiovasc Magn Reson 2000; 2(1):67–82.
15. Boxt LM. Primer on cardiac magnetic resonance imaging: how to perform the examination. Top Magn Reson Imaging 2000; 11(6):331–347.
16. Meduri A, Natale L, Lauro L, Ruggiero M, Cavallo T, Marano P. Cardiac magnetic resonance imaging: technique and anatomy. Rays 1999; 24(1):4–18.
17. Boxt LM. Cardiac MR imaging: a guide for the beginner. Radiographics 1999.
18. Masood S, Yang GZ, Pennnell DJ, Firmin DN. Investigating intrinsic myocardial mechanics: the role of MR tagging, velocity phase mapping, and diffusion imaging. J Magn Reson Imaging 2000; 12(6):873–883.

4

Magnetic Resonance and the Morphology of the Heart

Benigno Soto

Department of Radiology and Medicine, Cardiovascular MRI Laboratory, University of Alabama, Birmingham, Alabama, U.S.A.

Vikas K. Rathi

Division of Cardiology, Cardiovascular MRI Lab, Allegheny General Hospital, Drexel University College of Medicine, Philadelphia, Pennsylvania, U.S.A.

GENERAL FEATURES OF THE HEART

The heart is a mediastinal structure that lies within the pericardial sack, such that one-third of its bulk is to the right of the midline. The cardiac long axis has oblique orientation in relation to the sagittal plane of the body, with the base in right superior location and the apex extending anterior inferior and to the left in a position called levocardia. Rarely, a normal heart is located in the right hemi-thorax and the cardiac apex anterior and to the right in a position called dextrocardia.

The heart is formed by two atria and two ventricles, which are positioned around the central fibrous body. The atria are in posterior–superior location and the ventricles located anterior and to the left. Heart receives the systemic and pulmonary veins as they connect to the right and left atrium, respectively. The cardiac outlet is through the aorta and pulmonary artery (1).

The cardiovascular system is composed of three segments: atria, ventricles, and great arteries. They are connected in a sequential manner.

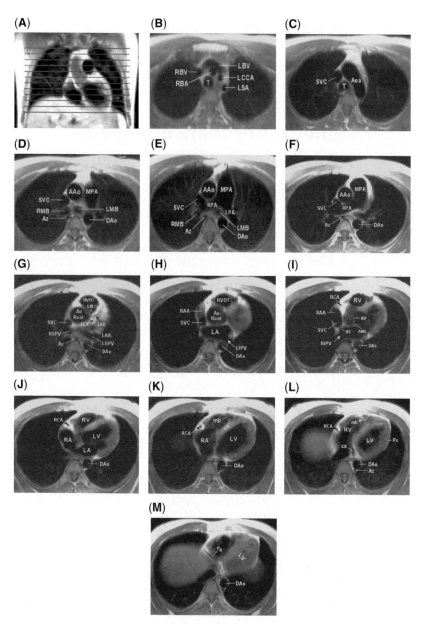

Figure 1   (*Caption on Facing Page*)

Atrium joins the ventricles through the atrioventricular valves. The ventricles connect to the great arteries by the arterial valves (2).

Cardiovascular magnetic resonance imaging (CMR) shows the cardiovascular morphology through a series of slices obtained from different planes (3). The following are the standard planes used: (i) transverse axial (Fig. 1B–1M), (ii) coronal (Fig. 2A–2G and 6), (iii) two-chamber long axis (Figs. 3 and 4), (iv) four-chamber long axis (Fig. 5), (v) left ventricular outflow tract (Figs. 6 and 7), and (vi) short axis (Fig. 8B–8D). Special plane sections are needed for visualizing specific areas of the heart, such as the aortic valve/right ventricular outlet view through the crista supraventricularis (4). The morphology of the cardiovascular system will be described through images acquired using the described sections.

Images were acquired by using standard techniques. The spin echo (SE) images also called as black blood technique and the gradient–recalled echo (GRE) or steady-state free precession (SSFP) images also referred as white blood technique are displayed to demonstrate the anatomy.

THE ATRIA

The atrial chambers are called right and left atria according to their morphology. Each atrium has a main chamber, inlet, outlet, and atrial appendage.

Figure 1 (*Facing Page*) (**A**) The plane centered on coronal section for obtaining spin echo (SE) or steady-state free precession (SSFP) multislice transverse axial images. Each line indicates one slice through that plane (**A**). The slice thickness is user dependent. SE transaxial images are represented cranio-caudally in sequential manner. Image (**B**) is the slice obtained at the level of origin of great vessels, (**C**) is at the level of aortic arch, (**D**) is at the level of carina, (**E**) is at the level of left pulmonary artery, (**F**) is at the level of right pulmonary artery, (**G**) is at the level of aortic root, (**H**) is at the level of left atrium, (**I**) is at left ventricular outflow tract level, (**J**) is at the level of left ventricle, (**K**) is at the level of right atrium, and (**L**) and (**M**) are at the level of inferior venae cava and inferior wall of the left ventricle. *Abbreviations*: Aoa, aortic arch; Ao Root, aortic root; AAo, ascending aorta; AV, aortic valve; AS, atrial septum; Az, azygous vein; CS, coronary sinus; DAo, descending aorta; LAD, left anterior descending; LA, left atrium; LAA, left atrial appendage; LBV, left brachiocephalic vein; LCCA, left common carotid artery; LCX, left circumflex; LM, left main coronary; LMB, left main bronchus; LIPV, left inferior pulmonary vein; LPA, left pulmonary artery; LSA, left subclavian artery; LSPV, left superior pulmonary vein; LV, left ventricle; MPA, main pulmonary artery; mb, moderator band; Pc, pericardium; RA, right atrium; RAA, right atrial appendage; RBA, right brachiocephalic artery; RBV, right brachiocephalic vein; RCA, right coronary artery; RMB, right main bronchus; RPA, right pulmonary artery; RIPV, right inferior pulmonary vein; RSPV, right superior pulmonary vein; RV, right ventricle; RVOT, right ventricular outflow tract; SVC, superior venae cava; VS, ventricular septum; T, trachea.

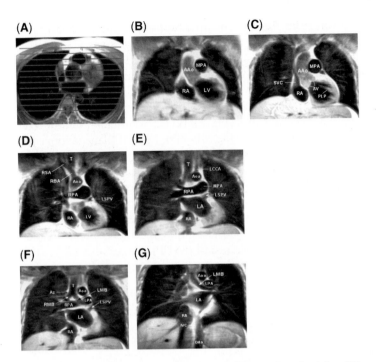

Figure 2 (A) The plane centered on axial image for obtaining SE or GRE/SSFP multislice coronal images. Figures (B–G): Spin echo coronal images represented anterior to posteriorly. Figures (B) and (C) are anterior coronal images at the level of aortic root, (D) and (E) are at the level of aortic arch and right pulmonary artery, (F) and (G) are at the level of carina and descending aorta posteriorly. *Abbreviations*: Aoa, aortic arch; Ao Root, aortic root; AAo, ascending aorta; AV, aortic valve; Az, azygous vein; DAo, descending aorta; GRE, gradient–recalled echo; LA, left atrium; LCCA, left common carotid artery; LMB, left main bronchus; LPA, left pulmonary artery; LSPV, left superior pulmonary vein; LV, left ventricle; MPA, main pulmonary artery; PLP, posterolateral papillary muscle; RA, right atrium; RBA, right brachiocephalic artery; RMB, right main bronchus; RPA, right pulmonary artery; RV, right ventricle; SE, spin echo; SSFP, steady-state free precession; SVC, superior venae cava; T, trachea.

The right atrium forms the superior and right aspect of the heart. The inlet is by the entrance of the superior and inferior caval veins, located on the posterior atrial wall. The entrance of the inferior vena cava has a rudimentary Eustachian valve. The coronary sinus enters the right atrium through an opening located in the space between the entrance of the inferior vena cava and the tricuspid valve. The outlet is through the tricuspid valve located in the anterior and inferior aspect. The right atrial appendage is a triangular cavity with a wide connection to the superior aspect of the atrial wall, in an area located to the right of the superior vena caval entrance. The atrial septum forms the posterior left atrial aspect (Figs. 1I–1K, 2E, 2F, and 5).

The left atrium forms the superior and left aspect of the heart. The inlet is by the entrance of four pulmonary veins at the superior–posterior aspect. The outlet is through the mitral valve, a part of the anterior–inferior atrial wall. The atrial septum forms the anterior and right aspect of the left atrium. The left atrial appendage is a long tubular structure, which connect to the main chamber by a narrow opening in the superior and anterior wall. It courses anterior and to the left of the aorta and pulmonary artery. The

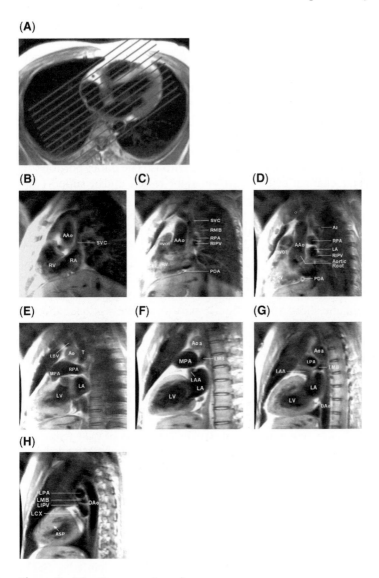

Figure 3 (*Caption on next page*)

right and left atrial appendages are seen well in transverse sections as cavities to the right and left of the great arteries (Fig. 1G and 1H). The left atrial appendage is best shown in two-chamber section through the left cardiac chambers (Figs. 3F and 4).

THE VENTRICLES

The right and left ventricles are composed of thick myocardial walls and form the ventricular segment. The ventricles are recognized by their morphology. They lie aside the ventricular septum in such a manner that morphologically right ventricle is anterior and to the right of the septum and the left ventricle is posterior and to the left aspect of the septum. Each ventricle has three components: (i) the inlet, related to the atrioventricular valve, (ii) the trabecular forming the apical part, and (iii) the outlet, related to the outflow and arterial valves.

The right ventricle is shown on CMR images using transverse sections, showing its inlet portion in lower slices, its trabecular portion in the middle sections, and its outlet portion in cephalic slices (Fig 1G–1M). The inlet portion is related to the tricuspid valve and its environs. The outlet portion is a tubular muscular channel extending from right to left and it support the pulmonary valve. The tricuspid and pulmonary valves are not in fibrous continuity; they are separated by a muscular structure called crista supraventricularis, a part of the right ventricular outlet. The trabecular part of right ventricle has coarse trabeculations, moderator band, and in some hearts the septo-parietal band. The anterior papillary muscle is a prominent muscular structure of this ventricle.

The right ventricle is shown in CMR, on transverse sections, showing its outlet in cephalic slices, the trabecular part in middle sections, and the inlet part in lower slices (Fig. 1G–1M). In these slices, the entire muscular wall of the outlet is well seen. The right ventricular outlet is best visualized through slices passing the right and left ventricular outlets. The aortic valve

---

Figure 3 (*Figure on previous page*) The plane centered on axial image for obtaining SE or GRE/SSFP multislice vertical long axis images (**A**). Figure (**B**) is anterolaterally at the level of right ventricle, (**C**) and (**D**) are at the level of right ventricular outflow tract and ascending aorta, (**E**) and (**F**) are at the level of main pulmonary artery and aortic arch, (**G**) and (**H**) are at the level of descending aorta. *Abbreviations*: Aoa, aortic arch; Ao Root, aortic root; AAo, ascending aorta; AV, aortic valve; ASP, anteroseptal papillary muscle; Az, azygous vein; DAo, descending aorta; GRE, gradient–recalled echo; IVC, inferior venae cava; LA, left atrium; LAA, left atrial appendage; LBV, left brachiocephalic vein; LIPV, left inferior pulmonary vein; LMB, left main bronchus; LPA, left pulmonary artery; LV, left ventricle; MPA, main pulmonary artery; PLP, posterolateral papillary muscle; RA, right atrium; RIPV, right inferior pulmonary vein; RV, right ventricle; SE, spin echo; SSFP, steady-state free precession; SVC, superior venae cava.

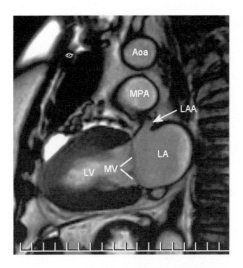

Figure 4 Two-chamber left ventricle long axis SSFP echo image. *Abbreviations*: Aoa, aortic arch; LA, left atrium; LAA, left atrial appendage; LV, left ventricle; MV, mitral valve; SSFP, steady-state free precession.

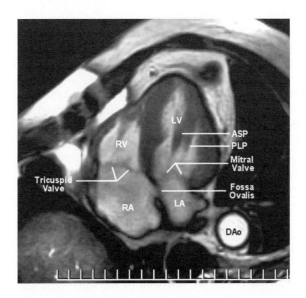

Figure 5 SSFP long axis four-chamber image. *Abbreviations*: ASP, anteroseptal papillary muscle; DAo, descending aorta; LA, left ventricle; LV, left ventricle; PLP, posterolateral papillary muscle; RA, right atrium; RV, right ventricle; SSFP, steady-state free precession.

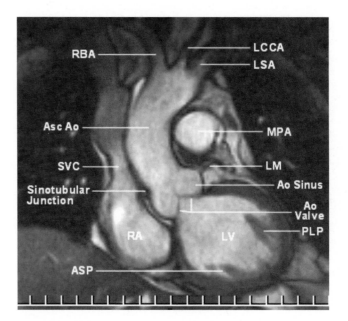

Figure 6 SSFP coronal left ventricular outflow tract image. *Abbreviations*: Asc Ao, ascending aorta; Ao Valve, aortic valve; Ao Sinus, aortic sinus; ASP, anteroseptal papillary muscle; LM, left main; LCCA, left common carotid artery; LSA, left subclavian artery; LV, left ventricle; MPA, main pulmonary artery; PLP, posterolateral papillary muscle; RA, right atrium; RBA, right brachiocephalic artery; SSFP, steady-state free precession; SVC, superior venae cava.

is seen face up showing the three cusps (Fig. 9). The infundibular septum is seen covering the right cusp of the aortic valve and forming the posterior wall of the right ventricular outlet and the pulmonary valve. In short axial sections, the right ventricle shows different shapes according to the level of sections. At the inlet/outlet sections, an area close to the atrioventricular valve, the right ventricle is presented as an asymmetric truncated pyramid (Fig. 9 and 10G). The plane of the tricuspid valve and crista supraventricularis forms the right posterior border of the ventricle. The posterior and left lateral borders of the ventricle are formed by the ventricular septum, which is convex toward the center of the ventricular cavity. The anterior free wall of the ventricle, measures 0.5 ± 0.1 cm at end-diastole. The thickness of the right ventricular free wall is maximum at the base and progressively decreases as it approaches the apex. The inferior wall of the right ventricle is flat and rests on the diaphragm. The inlet of the right ventricle is by the tricuspid valve. The annulus normally measures 11.9 ± 0.9 cm in circumference and is guarded by three leaflets: anterior, inferior, and medial or septal.

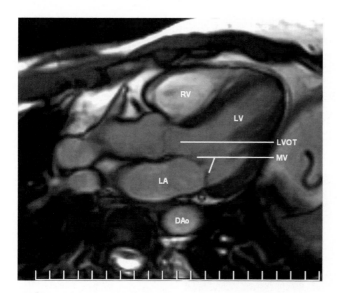

Figure 7 SSFP four-chamber left ventricular outflow tract (LVOT) image. *Abbreviations*: DAo, descending aorta; LA, left atrium; LV, left ventricle; RV, right ventricle; SSFP, steady-state free precession.

The left ventricle is a conical-shaped cavity with the base in posterior and right and the apex projecting anterior, inferior, and to the left. The ventricular walls are: the right anterior formed by the ventricular septum and the left posterior by the free wall myocardium. The inlet and outlet part of the left ventricle forms the posterior–superior wall of this chamber (Fig. 7).

The left ventricle comprises an inlet portion, containing the mitral valve and its tension apparatus; an apical trabecular zone characterized by fine trabeculations and an outlet zone supporting the aortic valve, which is incomplete posteriorly by the aortico-mitral fibrous continuity (Fig. 10G). Two papillary muscles support the mitral valve leaflets in the left ventricle; the antero-lateral also known as anteroseptal and the postero-lateral; each one supports the corresponding commissural chordae tendinae of the mitral valve (Fig. 5). The papillary muscles have a conical shape implanted in the middle of the ventricle. The papillary tip is usually one; but two heads are common in the normal population.

Complete assessment of the left ventricle on CMR is through multiple sections using transverse, four chambers, two chambers, short axis, and left ventricular outflow tract. Each section shows different portions of this chamber. The left ventricular size and wall thickness is measured on short axis sections with only one drawback, that the apical wall is somewhat tilted and is not perpendicular to the parallel short axis images, creating some partial volume effect and overestimation which can be compensated by

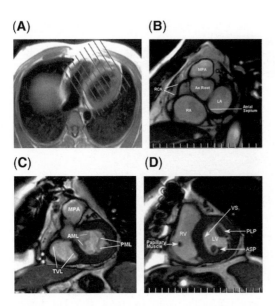

Figure 8 The plane centered on axial image for obtaining SE or SSFP multislice short axis images (**A**). The images are displayed in order from base toward apex. Figure (**B**) is basal SSFP short axis image, Figure (**C**) is at the tip of the mitral leaflets and Figure (**D**) is the midventricular short axis image. *Abbreviations*: Ao, aorta; AML, anterior mitral leaflet; ASP, anteroseptal papillary muscle; LA, left atrium; LV, left ventricle; MPA, main pulmonary artery; PLP, posterolateral papillary muscle; PML, posterior mitral leaflet; RCA, right coronary artery; RA, right pulmonary artery; RV, right ventricle; RVOT, right ventricular outflow tract; SE, spin echo; SSFP, steady-state free precession; TVL, tricuspid valve leaflet; VS, ventricular septum.

3D reconstruction. Proper images in short axis allow good delineation of the epicardial and endocardial borders which allow to analyze the mean wall thickness values, myocardial mass, percent wall thickening, and end-systolic and end-diastolic volumes. Normally the left ventricle is measured on short axis at the level of the tip of the papillary muscles, where the chordae tendinae start.

The inlet of the left ventricle is by the mitral valve. The valve annulus is located at the left atrioventricular junction. The mitral annulus is in fibrous continuity with the aortic valve at the central fibrous body (Fig. 10G). The mitral valve orifice is guarded by two leaflets: the anterior also called septal and the posterior or mural. Gradient echo on short axis sections usually show the annulus and the mitral leaflets. The diastolic frame delimitates the actual functional mitral orifice. In systolic frames it is possible to see the posterior leaflet with three scallops and the long anterior septal leaflet.

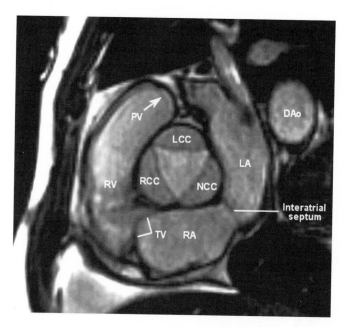

Figure 9 SSFP short axis aortic valve image. *Abbreviations*: DAo, descending aorta; LA, left atrium; LCC, left coronary cusp; NCC, non-coronary cusp; RA, right atrium; RCC, right coronary cusp; RV, right ventricle; PV, pulmonary valve; SSFP, steady-state free precession; TV, tricuspid valve.

The outlet of the left ventricle is formed by the muscular septum anterior and to the right and by the anterior leaflet of the mitral valve which is posterior and to the left of the outflow track. The outlet of the left ventricle is best seen in left ventricular outlet section (Fig. 7). The outlet is crowned by the three leaflet aortic valve. The anterior is the right coronary cusp, the posterior left is the left coronary cusp and the posterior right is the non-coronary cusp (Fig. 9).

THE CARDIAC SEPTATION

The atrial and ventricular chambers are separated by three septal structures: the atrial, the ventricular, and the atrioventricular septum. The atrial septum is a thin-walled structure, which separates the right and left atrium (Figs 1I, 1K, 10E, 8B, and 5). It is formed by the fossa ovalis and the limbus. The inferior border of the septum joins the sinus septum posteriorly and the atrioventricular septum anteriorly. In its superior border, it fuses with the infolding of the atrial wall and the wall of the sinus venosus.

In cardiovascular magnetic resonance (CMR) imaging transverse sections of the heart, the atrial septum is shown as a membrane starting at the middle part

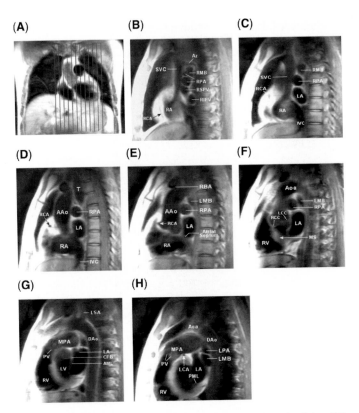

Figure 10 The plane centered on coronal image for obtaining SE or SSFP multislice sagittal images (**A**). The images are in chronological order from right to left. Figures (**B**, **C**, and **D**) are at the level of right atrium and ascending aorta. Figures (**E**, **F**, and **G**) represent images through aortic root and right ventricular outflow tract. Figure (**H**) is through left atrium. *Abbreviations*: AAo, ascending aorta; Aoa, aortic arch; Ao Root, aortic root; AML, anterior mitral leaflet; AV, aortic valve; AS, atrial septum; Az, azygous vein; CFB, central fibrous body; DAo, descending aorta; IVC, inferior venae cava; LA, left atrium; LCA, left coronary artery; LCC, left coronary cusp; LMB, left main bronchus; LPA, left pulmonary artery; LSA, left subclavian artery; MPA, main pulmonary artery; MS, muscular interventricular septum; PV, pulmonary valve; PML, posterior mitral leaflet; RA, right atrium; RCA, right coronary artery; RCC, right coronary cusp; RIPV, right inferior pulmonary vein; RSPV, right superior pulmonary vein; RV, right ventricle; SE, spin echo; SSFP, steady-state free precession; SVC, superior venae cava.

of the non-coronary cusp of the aortic valve (Fig. 9) and coursing posterior and to the right 10° to 15° relative to the sagittal plane (Fig. 1I). In four-chamber sections, passing through the inlet muscular septum, the atrial septum appears as a line from the left ventricular–right atrium junction, coursing posterior and to the right (Fig. 5). This structure is usually interrupted at its middle segment, due to a very thin septum secundum. It is important to consider this fact as an anatomical variation and not as atrial septal defect. In short axis sections of the normal heart, the atrial septum is seen on slides through atrial level as a thin structure, with swelling borders, in between the atrial chambers. The imaging sequence is very useful to detect small atrial septal defect (Fig. 8B).

THE VENTRICULAR SEPTUM

The normal ventricular septum has two portions: the muscular and the membranous. The membranous septum is a 5-mm fibrous structure as a part of the central fibrous body, located in the left ventricular outlet, beneath the aortic valve (underneath the right and non-coronary cusps' commissure). The right side of the membranous ventricular septum merges with the anterior and medial portions of the atrioventricular septum. It is divided in two parts by the insertion of the septal leaflets of the tricuspid valve.

The normal membranous septum is rarely seen on SE or SSFP, CMR images. In some individuals, the septum is large enough to be identified on CMR. It is seen as a short line on top of the muscular septum, covered by the septal leaflet of the tricuspid valve, on four-chamber sections.

The muscular portion of the ventricular septum has three segments: the inlet, trabecular, and the outlet. The inlet part supports the septal leaflet of the tricuspid valve on the right side, and a short segment of the septal leaflet of the mitral valve on the left side. The aortic valve joins the majority of the anterior superior edges of the ventricular septum. Sections of the heart through four-chamber plane will show the inlet muscular septum.

The trabecular muscular septum forms the major part of this structure. The apical part is characterized by fine trabeculations on the left side and with coarse trabeculations on the right. The trabeculations are best showed on sections passing through the apical septum. The majority of the left septal aspect of normal heart is smooth without trabeculations.

The outlet part of the septum makes a turn from the right to the left and anteriorly, around the left ventricle-aorta exit. The right-sided aspect is very short and it is located underneath the aortic valve. The majority of this septum is formed by a sleeve of left ventricular myocardium. Transverse CMR sections of the heart from the inlet up to the arterial valves will show the outlet septum in detail. A sagittal section of the heart through the aortic valve and right ventricular outlet will show the relationship of the right coronary cusp of the valve with the infundibular septum in the posterior wall of the right ventricular outlet (Fig. 10F and 10G).

The ventricular septum is also visualized on short axis sections through multiple slides. It shows the semicircular shape, with its concave surface toward the left ventricle and the convex aspect toward the right ventricle. The normal muscular septum measures 10 mm ± 2 mm in width. The most cephalic part of the ventricular septum forms part of the left ventricular outflow tract.

The aorto-pulmonary septum is short fibrous structure, which separate the aorta and pulmonary artery at their proximal segments. It extends up to 3 to 6 mm above the arterial valves. Transverse section of the heart will demonstrate this structure as a short line immediately above the valve leaflets (5–7).

THE ATRIOVENTRICULAR SEPTUM

The atrioventricular septum is a fibro-muscular structure, which in the normal heart separates the right atrium from the left ventricle. It is composed of a muscular and membranous part. The muscular component is the largest, it lies in between the atrial septum, the sinus septum, and the muscular inlet ventricular septum (this part is delimited by the insertion of the septal leaflet of the tricuspid valve). On the left ventricular aspect, the atrioventricular septum extends from the crux cordis up to the subaortic part of the left ventricular outlet; where it becomes a membranous structure. It forms the superior limit of the left ventricle with the insertion of the septal leaflet of the mitral valve. The membranous portion of the atrioventricular septum is a short fibrous structure located beneath the non-coronary cusp of the aortic valve; it continues inferiorly as membranous interventricular septum.

SSFP and SE images demonstrate the atrioventricular septum as linear image, extending from the medial part of the tricuspid valve to the mitral valve insertion. The septum separates the left ventricular outlet from the right atrium inlet (Fig. 6) (7).

THE GREAT ARTERIES

The aorta originates from the left ventricle, it courses anterior, superior, and to the right in the anterior mediastinum, the segment called ascending aorta. In this segment the aorta runs to the left of the superior vena cava and to the right of the pulmonary trunk also called main pulmonary artery. The right pulmonary artery is posterior to the ascending aorta as it courses transversally. The upper part of the ascending aorta courses posterior and to the left to reach the posterior mediastinum. This segment is called aortic arch, it extends from the origin of the right brachiocephalic artery and ends at the level of the ligament arteriosus. The left main bronchus is medial to the aortic arch while the left pulmonary artery is inferior (Fig. 2F). The superior or convex wall of the aortic arch gives off the brachiocephalic arteries, starting anteriorly with the right brachiocephalic artery, then the left common carotid artery and, lastly and most posteriorly, the left subclavian artery (Fig. 1B). The descending thoracic aorta courses to the left of the spine in the posterior mediastinum. It passes behind the left atrium and it continuous downward into the abdomen.

The main pulmonary artery originates in the right ventricular outlet anterior and to the left of the aorta. It continues upward and divides in right and left pulmonary arteries (Fig. 1E). The right pulmonary artery arises from the pulmonary trunk toward the right, in a right-angled fashion. It courses behind the ascending aorta and in front of the right main bronchus in its proximal course and beneath the right main bronchus distally (Figs. 1E, 2E, 3C, 3D, 10B, 10C, and 10D). The left pulmonary artery originates from the pulmonary trunk as a continuous branch (Fig. 1E); it courses posterior and to the left above the left main bronchus (Figs. 2G and 3H). The location, size, and course of the great arteries are seen on SE and GRE/SSFP images in transverse, left anterior oblique, coronal, and sagittal planes.

THE GREAT VEINS

At the base of the heart there are two great systemic veins descending and ascending anteriorly and to the right to enter the right atrium. The intrathoracic segment of the inferior vena cava is short, ascending from the liver and enters the inferior wall of the right atrium (Fig. 2G). The superior vena cava is a long channel, being formed by the union of the right and the left brachiocephalic veins (Fig. 1B), before descending to the right of the aorta (Fig. 1C–1I), receiving the azygous vein en route to reach the upper border of the right atrium (Figs 2F, 3C, and 3D).

THE TRACHEOBRONCHIAL TREE

Extending down into the thorax behind the head and neck arteries is the trachea (Fig. 1B), which bifurcates into the right and left bronchi at the level of the aortic arch (Fig. 1D). The two bronchi run down toward the lung hila, curling beneath the branches of the pulmonary arteries. The right main bronchus gives off its main branch (the eparterial bronchus) to the upper lobe of the right lung before it is crossed by the right pulmonary artery extending into the lung to supply the middle and the lower lobes. In contrast to this arrangement, the left main pulmonary artery crosses over the left main bronchus before it divides into upper and lower lobe bronchi. The bronchus to the left upper lobe is consequently a hyparterial (below the artery) bronchus. This bronchial arrangement provides considerable information in children with congenital heart disease (8).

CONCLUSIONS

CMR assessment of cardiac morphology is performed mainly using a combination of "black-blood" and "bright-blood" pulse sequences. The advantage of CMR is that it can image the cardiac chambers the great vessels, and the valves in three dimensions, with high spatial resolution and without the need for ionizing radiation.

REFERENCES

1. Anderson RH, Becker AE. Cardiac Anatomy. New York: Grover Medical Publishing Ltd, 1980.
2. McAlpine WA. Heart and Coronary Arteries. New York: Springer-Verlag, 1975.
3. Pohost GM, O'Rourke Principles and Practice of Cardiovascular Imaging. 1st ed. Little, Brown and Company June 1991.
4. Blackwell GG, Cranney GB, Pohost GM. MRI: Cardiovascular System. : Gower Medical Publishing, 1992.
5. Fletcher BD, Jacobstein MD. Magnetic Resonance Imaging of Congenital Heart Disease: Anatomic, Angiographic, and Echocardiographic Correlations. St. Louis, MO: Mosby Co., 1988.
6. Anderson RH, Ho SY. Diagnosis and naming of congenital malformed heart. In: McCartney FJ, ed. Congenital Heart Disease. Boston; MTP Press Ltd, 1986:1–34.
7. Anderson RH, Becker AE, Lucchese F, Soto B. Morphology of Congenital Heart Disease. Turdbridge Wells, Kent, U.K.: Castle House Publications Ltd, 1983.
8. Partridge JB, Scott O, Deverall PB, Macartney FJ. Visualization and measurement of the main bronchi by tomography as an objective indicator of thoracic situs in congenital heart disease. Circulation 1975; 51(1):188–196.

5

Assessment of Left Ventricular Function

Hakki Bolukoglu, Mark Doyle, and Robert W. W. Biederman
Division of Cardiology, Cardiovascular MRI Laboratory, Allegheny General Hospital, Pittsburgh, Pennsylvania, U.S.A.

INTRODUCTION

Currently, several modalities exist for imaging the heart and the cardiovascular system. Since all modalities have their inherent advantages and disadvantages, the choice of imaging tool dictates the type of information obtained, its quality, and its accuracy. A general cardiac survey, in which only gross data are required, may be accomplished with an imaging modality of relatively low accuracy, recognizing the need to balance the information obtained with the machine's capabilities, expense and the time available. In today's environment, time and expense dominate the choice of modality. The obligate tradeoff is that time and expense are traded with accuracy and reproducibility, thus the acquired data are typically of lower than optimal caliber. Ideally, there would exist an amalgam in which little compromise was required; such a device would have attributes of speed, accuracy, and reproducibility, all at an acceptable cost. Cost calculations are complicated by the fact that they are not simply limited to performance of the examination. Often costs are tied in with accurate diagnosis which results in reduced resource utilization and eliminates the need for further evaluation by treating the correct disease process. In the long run, a more accurate diagnostic modality, though expensive up-front, may be more cost effective than seemingly less expensive alternatives (1).

Cardiovascular magnetic resonance (CMR) imaging has emerged as having many of the desired attributes of an ideal imaging instrument. The inherent three-dimensional (3D) nature of its data, the exquisite spatial resolution, accuracy and reproducibility, have all contributed to the consensus that CMR is the "gold standard" for evaluating many aspects of the cardiovascular system. The focus of this chapter will be ventricular structure and function for which CMR is the undisputed modality of choice for the determination of right ventricle (RV)/left ventricle (LV) ejection fraction (EF) and mass.

Accurate measurement of left ventricular function and structure has significant impact on:

1. Detection of systolic function
2. Prediction of functional recovery and prognosis in the post-myocardial infarction period
3. Measuring the change in left ventricular function in the congestive heart failure patient post-manipulation (pharmacologic or interventional)
4. Evaluation of valve function and the degree of dysfunction, including the influence on the size and function of the heart
5. Congenital heart disease
6. Cardiomyopathies: diseases of the heart, such as dilated, infiltrative or restrictive heart diseases such as sarcoidosis, amyloidosis, and hypertrophic cardiomyopathy
7. Extent of viable (alive) heart muscle before interventions such as angioplasty or bypass (CABG)
8. Evaluation of the pressure gradient across stenotic valves
9. Detection and measurement of intracardiac shunts
10. Detection of anomalous coronary arteries and their potential for surgical correction
11. Evaluation of heart function before and after chemotherapy

Emerging uses, and the focus of research funded at the level of the National Institute of Health, American Heart Association, by us and others include: rapid imaging techniques (complete cardiac assessment in 4–5 seconds), non-invasive imaging of the coronary arteries, qualitative and quantitative calculation of mechanical properties of the heart before and after surgeries (including aortic valve replacement, bypass, LV surgical reconstruction, i.e., Dor procedure) (2), and evaluation of new medicinal treatments of heart disease (1,3).

Cardiac magnetic resonance (CMR) is one of the most accurate imaging techniques, and increasingly plays a crucial role in the management of patients. The ability of CMR to image in any oblique orientation remains a principle advantage over most imaging modalities. Its high spatial and temporal resolution, combined with the lack of signal attenuation, inter-reader reliability, and lack of the requirement for an ideal "window" has allowed CMR to become the gold standard for measuring cardiac volumes and mass (4,5).

The validation of cardiac mass measured by CMR has been well documented by autopsy, cardiac casts, and cardiac catheterization studies. The majority of these were performed in non-pathologic states where geometric assumptions of symmetry could be employed reliably (4,5).

Currently, the diagnosis and prognosis of cardiovascular disease is critically dependent upon the reliable assessment of global left ventricular chamber function. In clinical settings, the EF has traditionally dominated as a measure of systolic ventricular function, but several studies suggest that end systolic volume, mass, and wall stress may be more reliable indicators (6). The dominance of EF as a global indicator is likely more related to its ease of determination (by multiple modalities) than its intrinsic value, since it is known to be dependent on loading conditions and heart rate. While echocardiography and radionuclide cineangiography are both capable of assessing global left ventricular function, they have important limitations when compared with CMR. The ability to obtain information on anatomy, dimensions, vasculature, perfusion and viability in one setting, in a shorter time period (the "One-Stop-Shop") is a key advantage of CMR over other imaging modalities. However, CMR has its inherited limitations, which will be elaborated later in the chapter.

In the following, the authors' goal is not to compare other imaging modalities with CMR, but rather to summarize the techniques and protocols that are used in CMR for the assessment of left ventricular function. Described below is a standard, nearly step-by-step outline of the routine and even non-standard imaging considerations that have evolved to describe the current CMR imaging protocol at our institution. The information summarized in this chapter is presented to be of value to a wide range of medical personnel, including technologist, cardiovascular fellows as well as attending physicians. Where appropriate, we insert our experience ("Pearls"). We have included material that is applicable in exasperating instances.

PATIENT SELECTION AND SCREENING

It is important to select and screen the patient for the CMR procedure. Table 1 describes the absolute and relative contraindications. Note that certain prosthetic heart valves and stents, even hours after placement, are safe to scan (7–9). There is also mounting evidence that scanning patients with pacemakers may be safe if they are not pacer-dependent. Regardless of the known hazards of subjecting a patient with a cardiac pacemaker to the MR environment, numerous patients (more than 200) have undergone CMR imaging during purposeful, monitored procedures that were performed in order to conduct necessary diagnostic examinations. These

Table 1 Absolute and Relative Contraindications

Absolute contraindications (patients cannot have CMR scans)
Pre-1994 cerebral aneurysm clips unless known to be CMR compatible, with
documentation from the physician including make and model of the device. At
our institution we do not image patients with these devices, unless the clip has
been demonstrated to have never been autoclave sterilized, a process that can
anneal the metal, inducing partial ferromagnetism
Cochlear implant
Neurostimulator
Metal shrapnel in the body
Metal fragments on the optic nerve
Inability to perform CPR in CMR facility and lack of personnel to perform CPR
Recalcitrant claustrophobia

Relative contraindications (if benefit outweigh the risk)
Pacemaker or cardiac defibrillator
Pregnancy
Claustrophobia
Allergic reaction to gadolinium
Inability to give consents or follow commands
Nursing mothers that require i.v. gadolinium need not to feed the infant for 24 to 48
hr (a routine left ventricular function study does not require contrast agent use,
unless the study is combined with another CMR protocol)
Metal fragments in or around the eyes, or broken pacemaker lead on or around the
heart after bypass surgery, depending upon the location and the nature of the
metal. This is at the discretion of the physician responsible for the CMR scan

Abbreviations: CMR, cardiovascular magnetic resonance; CPR, cardiopulmonary resuscitation.

patients were safely and successfully imaged using MR systems operating at
static magnetic fields ranging from 0.35 to 1.5 T without any clinically
adverse events (7–9).

Recently, two studies have addressed MR safety for cardiac pacemakers. A laboratory investigation conducted by Roguin et al. (10) studied
the effects of MR performed at 1.5 T on "modern" cardiac pacemakers.
MR-related heating, magnetic field interactions, image artifacts, and the
effects of MR on the functional aspects of the pacemakers were evaluated.
The investigators concluded that modern cardiac pacemakers manufactured after 2000 may be MR-safe since they are smaller in size and
have less magnetic material and have improved electromagnetic interference protection.

This is a highly dynamic and controversial topic and not meant as a
statement of the safe usage of pacemakers in the scanner, only that in specialized situations where the benefit outweighs the risk, pacemaker patients
can be considered for MR imaging.

In a recently published study by Martin et al. (11), one of the largest non-pacemaker-dependent patient populations with permanent cardiac pacemakers underwent MR procedures at 1.5 T. In order to examine potential risks in the broadest possible population, no restrictions were placed on the anatomy that underwent imaging, the type of pulse sequence or conditions used, or the type of pacemakers present in these patients. Only pacemaker-dependent patients were excluded to eliminate problems if pacing was inhibited during the MR procedure. The findings in the study by Martin et al. indicated that patient symptoms were mild and transient and did not lead to discontinuation of the MR examinations. Significant alteration of the pacing threshold was found in a small number of leads tested. These threshold changes required a programmed output change in only two leads and were of no clinical consequence. Martin et al. concluded that, because of the infinite possibilities of pacing systems, cardiac and lead geometry, and variable static, gradient, and radio frequency (RF) electromagnetic fields and conditions used for MR procedures, the absolute safety of pacemaker and MR interactions presently cannot be assured. However, given appropriate patient selection as well as continuous monitoring and preparedness for resuscitation efforts with ACLS-trained personnel in attendance, performance of MR procedures in non-pacemaker-dependent patients may be achieved with reasonable safety even at static magnetic field strengths of 1.5 T with an acceptable risk/benefit profile.

Despite all these findings, the physician should do the risk–benefit evaluation for each patient, and should always refer to the manufacturer's manual and instructions (7,8). This step is ideally performed prior to any CMR request in duplicate at our hospital.

TRIGGERING

After the screening process, including in-depth questioning concerning absolute and relative contraindications, the patient will be escorted to the CMR suite and placed on the scanner table after a brief description of the equipment is given.

In CMR, triggering is one of the most important prerequisites. No detailed cardiac image will be produced without triggering. Triggering is not possible without a clean and strong electrocardiography (ECG) signal. Table 2 summarizes the patient preparation required for triggering and Table 3 details techniques of accurate ECG lead placement.

Even under normal circumstances ECG signal morphology is distorted, thus, one cannot make clinical decisions using aspects of the ECG other than rate. The distorted, elevated "T" wave is the result of rapidly moving conducting fluid (blood) in the presence of a magnetic field (magnetohydrodynamic effect). Distortions take many forms and it is often possible to trigger with such waveforms. A key feature to look for is that the R wave

Table 2 Patient Preparation

Place and position the patient on the scanner table, typically feet first
Place ECG leads, respiratory gating device, anterior surface receiving coil and blood
  pressure cuff. Posterior surface receiving coil may be imbedded in the scanner table
Connect ECG leads
Establish two (ideally) working i.v. sites to administer contrast media and/or
  medications for imaging protocols and/or in case of emergency resuscitation
Connect pulse oxymeter to monitor blood oxygenation
Supplemental oxygen may be administered depending on the patient's medical
  condition. We typically use a standard 2 L/min flow rate for most patients

Abbreviations: ECG, electrocardiogram; i.v., intravenous.

is higher and sharper than any other wave feature. A weak ECG signal often
suffers from "respiratory motion break-through." In this case, the baseline
ECG drifts up and down with the respiratory cycle. Changing the lead that
is used for triggering at the monitor rarely remedies the problem. When

Table 3 Techniques of Accurate ECG Lead Placement

To establish a clean ECG signal, good contact between the skin and the ECG
  electrodes is essential
Shave body hair if necessary
Abrade the skin for effective contact
Use a contact gel
Use the best and same brand dedicated CMR electrodes consistently
Let the patient wear loose clothing to prevent build up of sweat, which may
  destroys skin contact as the study progresses
Spend time prior to scanning to obtain a good ECG signal. If the signal is weak or
  otherwise poor, change the reference lead or reposition the leads
Consider positioning the leads on the patient's back over the heart region (if not
  contraindicated by the scanner manufacturer)
Consider the conditions that may weaken the ECG signal such as known
  myocardial infarction or pericardial effusion. If possible, position the leads
  toward the side of the heart where the most function is (if location of
  myocardial infarction is known)
If signal is weak, rather than changing the signal lead at the scanner interface,
  enter the scanner room and reposition the leads. Have extra pads available in
  anticipation to allow easier repositioning of leads
Formally, electrodes could be positioned at widely separated points on the chest.
  However, high-performance gradients and RF can induce currents in leads that
  form a loop configuration and can result in burning the patient. Keeping the
  electrode wires short and away from resonators is imperative to preventing burns.
  Today, a tight configuration of electrodes is optimal for safety (see Fig. 1 for
  correct placement of electrodes)

Abbreviations: CMR, cardiovascular magnetic resonance; ECG, electrocardiogram; RF, radio
frequency.

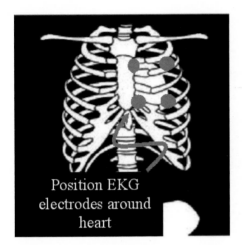

Figure 1 The correct placement of ECG leads around the heart. *Abbreviation*: ECG, electrocardiogram.

this is present, consider repositioning or re-attaching leads. Sometimes, an inverted R wave can be seen. Normally, the R wave should be upright and used for triggering to capture the first phase in end-diastole. Triggering on a wave other that R wave may result in missing the end-diastolic period. To remedy this problem, one can invert the signal at the console; also one can change the lead position at the patient.

If ECG triggering is problematic, most vendors have the option to use peripheral pulse gating permitting triggering via sensing the change in oxygen saturation in the nail bed or ear lobe. Importantly, the lag in detection of the freshly oxygenated signal will usually define a mid-systolic phase, requiring correction in interpretation of end-diastole.

Once the patient is on the scanner table and a strong ECG signal is established, the patient should be "centered" on the mid line of the chest, about 3 inches above the xyphoid notch (Fig. 2). Obtain vital signs and record.

BREATH-HOLDING

Many CMR scans are recorded under breath-holding conditions. During breath-holding, it is important to note that the heart may be in a different position compared with that of normal breathing. Reproducible breath holding will result in reproducible slice selection as well as optimal image quality. Most importantly, accuracy of volumetric calculations is, in part, dependent upon reproducible breathholds. Elderly or sicker patients may tire easily, thus the technologist should pace the frequency of breath-hold

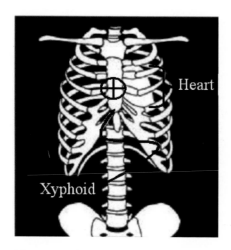

Figure 2 The patient should be "centered" on the mid line of the chest, about 3 inches above the xyphoid notch.

episodes for each individual. It is imperative that breath-holding instructions should be reviewed with the patient before placing them on the scanner table. To be well prepared, one can time the patient to determine their maximum comfortable breath-hold duration prior to starting scanning. The duration of a breath-hold will be pivotal in planning the durations of the scans and may require reducing and/or adjusting the scan times (the means of performing this is reviewed later in the chapter).

If the patient cannot perform an adequate breath-hold either in duration or consistency, the patient can be given supplemental oxygen or instructed to hyperventilate for a total of 10 to 15 seconds prior to each breath-hold. The rationale behind this maneuver is to reduce the carbon dioxide level in the blood, which in return reduces the respiratory drive. Occasionally, asking the patient to simply stop breathing may work. Further, simply scanning through the breathing may sometimes work, depending on the amplitude and frequency of respiration.

More reproducible results are achieved using scans obtained under the same breath-hold strategy. Breathing half way out is more reproducible than total exhalation due to the ease of finding a common comfortable diaphragmatic position.

For consistency in the breath-hold position and to maximize compliance, the following instructions may be given to the patient after all "prep" scan procedures are complete and the image acquisition scan is ready to proceed. A sample set of instructions used at our center follows:

- "Take a deep breath in."
- "Blow it out halfway."

- "Do not breathe" (start scan).

Upon scan completion, instruct patient to breathe.

Pearl: Occasionally asking the patient to simply stop breathing may work. Counterintuitively, simply scanning through the breathing periodically may work, if amplitude of respiration is low.

IMAGE ACQUISITION

After placement of the patient in the scanner, the next task is to obtain images. For optimal image quality, certain parameters have to be met. There are modifiable and non-modifiable parameters that have to be considered.

Nonmodifiable Parameters

Nonmodifiable parameters are parameters that cannot significantly be modified regardless of how sophisticated the equipment. These are:

1. Heart rhythm and rate.
2. Patient's ability to hold breath.
3. Body habitus.

Pearl: Attention to patient comfort and recognition of their apprehension prior to placing them in the scanner are crucial. A few minutes of time spent explaining the procedure and relieving patient anxiety will pay dividends during the scan.

Heart Rhythm and Rate

Patients with an irregular heart rhythm present one of the most important obstacles to CMR. Most recent scanners can handle high heart rates and some irregular rhythms with the arrhythmia recognition programs. Triggering algorithms will skip premature beats during image acquisition. However, atrial fibrillation presents a bigger problem for CMR. During atrial fibrillation, atrioventricular synchrony is lost. Thus, triggering and defining the beginning of diastole is not easily achieved, so that calculating scan-parameters such as the views-per-segment maybe challenging. In addition, scan time per slice will be longer and patients may not be able tolerate the longer scanning times. Efforts directed toward ventricular rate control are clearly beneficial pre-scan activities.

Patient's Ability to Hold Breath and Duration of Breath-Hold

Patient may be too sick or weak to be able to understand or follow commands. Sometimes, due to claustrophobia, patients may be sedated, limiting their understanding and ability to follow commands and especially impairing their breath-holding abilities. A partial solution to improving their ability to breath-hold is to apply a period of "hyperventilation" prior to breath-holding. This maneuver may double the time of a breath-hold, however, it is unlikely that the procedure could be repeated throughout a protracted scan session and should be reserved for key views. Patients with significant left ventricular dysfunction, decompensated heart failure, or pulmonary disease may not be able to hold their breath for more than five seconds. Under these circumstances, the scan duration may be truncated by changing the scanning parameters or an option termed "respiratory compensation" and/or "respiratory gating/triggering" may be used including use of navigator sequences if it is a machine option.

Modifiable Parameters

Modifiable parameters are parameters that are used during the image acquisition that affect temporal (shorter scans) and spatial (detailed and good quality images) resolution of the scans. These are:

1. Manner in which k-space is sampled
2. Matrix size
3. Field of view (FOV)
4. Views per segment (VPS)

k-space

k-space is the "raw data" format for CMR. The data acquired by the scanner are assembled and arranged internally into individual k-space arrays. Individual images are derived from a single k-space matrix. For example; for one cine series acquired at one slice of the heart and comprising 20 cardiac phases, there are $20\,k$-space arrays.

Matrix Size

Matrix size is an imaging parameter that, when considered along with FOV, is directly proportional to image resolution. In general, larger matrices result in higher spatial resolution (i.e., image detail). One drawback of larger matrices is that they are associated with longer scan durations, as a greater number of k-space lines are required. The matrix can be square or rectangular depending on the region of interest and body size. Typical matrices vary between 128^2 and 512^2. The axes of matrix are X and Y, conventionally referred to as frequency and phase, respectively. The phase axis can be reduced to achieve a shorter scan time. The smallest matrix for adequate image resolution should typically not be less than 128 × 128. The data in the matrix fill "*k*-space", typically one line at a time along the frequency encoding direction. Thus, reducing the size of the phase encoding axis has a direct impact on scan time. However, there is relatively little time penalty for altering the frequency dimension of the matrix, leading to rectangular matrices such as 256 × 128.

Field of View

Field of view (V) is the area chosen to be viewed or scanned. This is directly proportional to the body's dimensions. While the heart is small compared with the body, acquiring a reduced FOV may generate high levels of artifact which may interfere with the image region containing the heart. Peripheral body regions that may be required to be excluded from the image (by reducing the FOV) could "fold in" to overlay the image of the heart; such an artifact is often termed a "fold over" artifact. Typically, the largest selectable FOV in most scanners is approximately 50 by 50 cm while the typical effective FOV is 36 by 36 cm. The matrix and FOV are interlinked with each other in determining image resolution since they dictate the pixel size, which is ultimately responsible for the sharpness with which image features are detected.

Views per Segment

This is an important CMR parameter that influences scan time and image quality in cine series. Choice of VPS is also heart rate dependent as illustrated in Figure 3. Breath-hold and triggered cine images are acquired in a segmented manner within each R–R interval. In a typical series, each cardiac cycle will be represented by 20 cine images. In this example, if the heart rate is 60 beats/min, the R–R interval is 1 second or 1000 msec in duration. When divided by 20 (for the number of cine images) it is seen that the

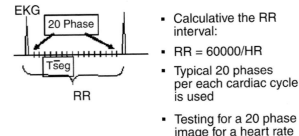

- Calculative the RR interval:
- RR = 60000/HR
- Typical 20 phases per each cardiac cycle is used
- Testing for a 20 phase image for a heart rate of 60 is 50 msec.

Figure 3 A representation of views per segment calculation. RR: interval between two R waves. T_{seg}: time for each segment is dependent upon the TR and the RR interval. For example: If the heart rate is 60 beats/min and if we are using 20 phases, T_{seg} is 50 msec and if our TR is between 3.5 and 4.0 msec, the views per segment will be between 12 and 14.

duration for each cardiac phase is 50 msec. Thus, during each 50-msec interval for each "cardiac phase," several lines of k-space or segments, can be acquired. The number of lines or "views" acquired during each segment interval depends on the repetition time of the gradients (TR). Typically the TR lies between 3 and 10 msec. Taking the TR as 4 msec and dividing this into the 50-msec interval yields that the number of VPS required is 12.5. Thus, in this example, selecting VPS in the range 12 to 14 yields images with a temporal resolution of about 50 msec within the cardiac cycle. Some scanners use "view sharing" to achieve better temporal resolution within the cycle. With this option the "scanner" will generate intermediate cine frame phases between each "acquired" segment, i.e., interpolating between two acquired phases to generate intermediate images, thus improving temporal resolution and allowing increased VPS values, which further reduce scan duration. Multiple interpolation schemas can be implemented.

After considering all the aforementioned modifiable and non-modifiable parameters, a typical scan prescription is as follows for cine imaging:

1. FOV: 30 by 30 cm
2. Matrix: 224 × 192
3. Slice thickness: 8 mm
4. Slice gap: 0 mm
5. VPS: depending on the heart rate and imaging sequence (between 10 and 24)
6. Cardiac phases: 20
7. Type of sequence: include gradient echo and steady-state free precession sequences

OBTAINING IMAGES

An initial image termed a "scout image" enables identification of the location and orientation of the heart:

1. The initial image sequence may be, but is not restricted to, a non-breath hold and non-triggered sagittal, axial (transverse), and coronal scout images (Fig. 4). Typically, seven images per axis are acquired, for a total of 21 images. Although these images are typically blurred, and too poor for identifying fine anatomic features, their main function is to enable the planning of and definition of further views.
2. Next, plan a set of about 12 to 18 transverse slices from the initial non-breath hold and non-triggered coronal scout images. These scans can usually be triggered and obtained in a non-breath hold manner (Fig. 5). We obtain black-blood, double inversion recovery images for the definition of anatomic features as opposed to physiologic information.

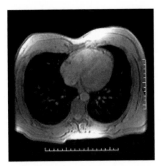

Figure 4   Non-triggered axial (transverse) scout.

3. From this set of scout images, it is possible to plan a two-chamber view, from which the four-chamber views is subsequently planned to obtain LV functional data. The next set of images is a cine series, preferably obtained with a steady-state free precession sequence, such as FIESTA, Balanced FFE, or True FISP.

4. Select the slice in which the left ventricle (LV) is seen in its largest view. Plan three slices (with zero gap) with the central slice passing through the LV apex and LV base (line is typically parallel to septum) and perform cardiac triggered gradient echo cine with breath holding. Ideally, the central slice acquired should be the desired two-chamber view. Although one of the slices on either side may be the required view, review all three slices to decide which is the best two-chamber view (Fig. 6). Important points to note in two-chamber view are: left atria should be seen throughout cardiac cycle and apex of LV should be clearly identifiable (Fig. 7). From the two-chamber view plan the four-chamber view by the same three-slice method. The central slice should pass through LV apex and bisect the valve plane at the base (Fig. 8). Ideally, the central slice acquired should be the desired four-chamber view; however, one of the slices on either side may be the required view.

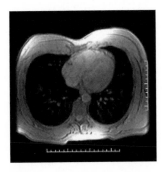

Figure 5   Triggered axial (transverse) scout.

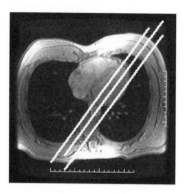

Figure 6 Planning of two-chamber view: three-slice method.

Therefore, all three slices should be carefully reviewed to select the best four-chamber view. Important points to note in the four-chamber view are: left and right atria should be seen throughout the cardiac cycle, apex of LV and right ventricle (RV) should be seen clearly, and ideally, RV and LV apex should come close to one point (Fig. 9).

Pearl: While it may seem to be an inefficient time management scheme to obtain three rather than one scan, the added time required to prescribe additional scans is usually well worth the additional data acquired that can be easily culled through to arrive at the optimized two- and four-chamber views.

Using the end-diastolic four-chamber view, plan short-axis slices perpendicular to the septum that extends beyond the mitral valve plane at the base and below the apex (Fig. 10). To ensure that the heart is fully imaged, it is important that the most apical slice does not contain any myocardium, i.e., image beyond the apex and the most basal slice should be positioned to be above the level of the mitral valve plane at end diastole (for ideal images see Figs. 11–13).

Obtaining high-resolution images is only part of the study. Although, it may seem simple, in patients with an ischemic cardiomyopathy,

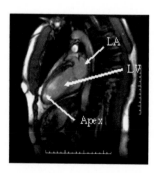

Figure 7 An ideal two-chamber view.

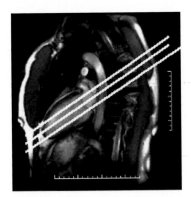

Figure 8   From the two-chamber view plan four-chamber view by three-slice method.

tomographic assessment of myocardial wall motion can be misleading. Areas of dysfunctional myocardium that are connected to normal myocardium may give the appearance of having intrinsic function, whereas in reality they are merely moving due to tethering. Conversely, due to the tethering phenomena, areas of moderately hypokinetic myocardium may be misrepresented as akinetic. To overcome this problem an assessment of wall translation as well as wall thickening must be performed. This is possible using CMR tagging or phase velocity imaging.

CMR tagging typically involves applying a set of parallel lines or a grid of orthogonal lines at the time of the ECG R wave. Once applied, these lines or grid move with the heart to highlight motion. Naturally, since the lines or grid are composed of tagged signal regions, they cannot interfere with cardiac function.

Numerous studies have been performed describing the utility of CMR to accurately identify regional wall motion (12–23). The tag signal is applied to each slice at the start of the ECG R wave. Such RF tagging allows quantification of cardiac function on a regional basis (Fig. 14).

Analysis of cine-tagged images can reveal the adequacy or deficiency of each of three function components separately: radial, circumferential,

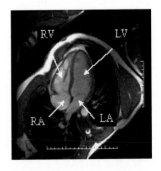

Figure 9   Ideal four-chamber view.

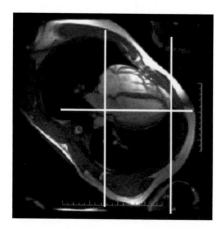

Figure 10 Planning of short axis views from four-chamber views.

and longitudinal. Interrogating the tag vertices, mechanical deformation can be quantified throughout the cardiac cycle allowing accurate insight into the mechanical properties of the heart. As part of left ventricular assessment, a phase velocity-encoded cine series of the chambers and vasculature can be performed. The phase velocity scan may be several minutes long and cannot typically be performed during a breath-hold unless acquired in only one plane, thus respiratory compensation/gating should be used. A view through the ascending aorta (AA) can be used to assess cardiac output. A gated sagittal scout can be chosen from viewing a transverse scout scan that best identifies the LV and descending aorta (DA) (Fig. 15). Then, eight sagittal slices centered slightly to the patient's right of the DA are planned

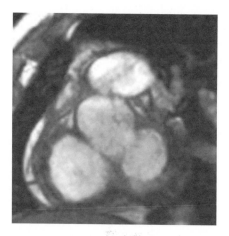

Figure 11 Most basal short axis view shows above mitral valve plane.

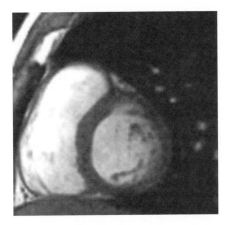

Figure 12 Mid ventricular slice shows left ventricular and right ventricular myocardium.

and a triggered gradient echo series obtained. Of the eight sagittal scouts, one plane should contain the AA and pulmonary artery (PA) as shown in Figure 16. Either draw or imagine a line originating at the aortic valve and following the initial direction of blood flow. The scan plane is positioned to cut this line at right angles and typically bisects the circular PA (Fig. 16). The aim is to see the aorta in circular cross-section. The phase velocity cine scan requires setting velocity encoding parameters:

1. Set velocity encoding direction to through plane.
2. Set velocity sensitivity to $\pm 1\,\mathrm{m/s}$.
3. Set phase method to "difference" or "quantitative" (manufacturer dependent).

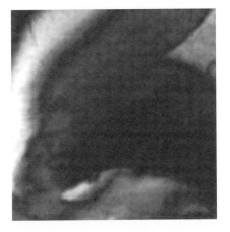

Figure 13 Most apical slice; no left ventricular myocardium is visible.

(A)   **(B)**

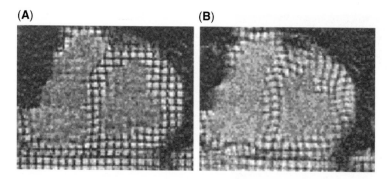

Figure 14 Tagged MR tomograms. (**A**) Depicts the application of set of parallel lines or a grid of orthogonal lines at the time of the ECG R wave, in diastole. (**B**) Once applied, these lines or grid then move with the heart to highlight motion. Naturally, since the lines or grid are composed of tagged signal regions, they cannot interfere with cardiac function. Such radio frequency tagging allows quantification of cardiac function on a regional basis. Note the distortion of the "grid lines" or "squares" during systole. *Abbreviations*: MR, magnetic resonance; ECG, electrocardiogram

After performing the velocity cine scan using respiratory gating/triggering, two sets of data are generated:

1. Magnitude images,
2. Phase/velocity images (Fig. 17).

A region of high intensity "bright" against a "dark" background, or vice versa, is usually a sign of signal aliasing. The velocity encoding limits being set too low causes aliasing. The remedy for this problem is to repeat

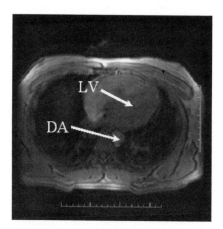

Figure 15 Gated axial scout. Select a transverse scout scan that best identifies the left ventricle and descending aorta. *Abbreviations*: LV, left ventricle; DA, descending aorta.

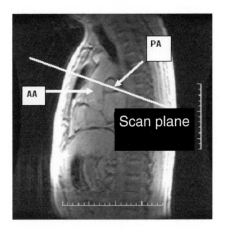

Figure 16 Of the eight sagittal scouts, one plane should contain the ascending aorta (AA) and pulmonary artery (PA) as shown here. Either draw or imagine, a line originating at the aortic valve and following the initial direction of blood flow. The scan plane is positioned to cut this line at right angles and bisects the circular PA. The aim is to see the aorta in circular cross-section.

the scan with the velocity limit increased, initially by 50%, until aliasing is no longer present.

Once completed, the images that are necessary to evaluate left ventricular function are complete. The next step is data analysis.

DATA ANALYSIS

As early as 1985, a means of determining ventricular volumes and ejection fraction (EF) was reported by Rehr et al., and consisted of a multislice spin echo approach (23). Presently, modifications of this original approach continue to

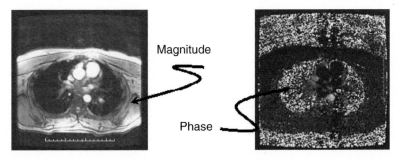

Figure 17 After performing the velocity cine scan using respiratory gating/triggering two sets of data are generated: magnitude and phase.

be used to calculate LV volumes and have been extensively validated (24–34). The major advance has been the incorporation of rapid cine CMR sequences, which possess excellent contrast and superior temporal resolution allowing acquisition of left ventricular volumes in clinically relevant scan times. After the acquisition of optimal quality images, data analysis can be performed on one of a number of proprietary software packages. In our facility it is performed on MEDIS® (MASS) software (Leiden, The Netherlands). Typically, each manufacturer has different software. The calculated parameters include: left ventricular mass, left ventricular end-diastolic and end-systolic and stroke volumes, cardiac output, and EF. Evaluation of diastolic function of the LV by CMR is in the early stages of application.

VENTRICULAR VOLUMES AND EF

"Short axis" tomograms orthogonal to the base to apex intrinsic LV axis are acquired and are stacked and summed using Simpson's rule. This approach is intrinsically the most accurate since it is independent of ventricular shape. Yet, it has limitations since meriodonal (longitudinal) shortening can be difficult to assess in the short axis view making identification of the basal plane difficult (35–37).

The endocardium and epicardium in diastole and endocardium in systole are outlined; this outlining process is repeated for every slice obtained. With knowledge of the slice thickness and any gap between slices (ideally no gap is used), the software will calculate the chamber volumes and mass, correcting for the specific gravity of myocardium (1.055). Care is taken to account for mitral valve plane motion and may be automatically accommodated in some algorithms (Fig. 18). Numerous studies have been performed describing the utility of CMR to accurately identify regional wall motion (12,17,38–46).

CARDIAC OUTPUT

For cardiovascular applications it is important to be able to assess flow across the aortic valve to determine forward cardiac output. Fortunately, this assessment can be accomplished by a CMR technique known as phase velocity mapping (47,48). Conventional CMR techniques produce an amplitude (modulus) image that is derived from a two-dimensional Fourier transformation of *k*-space data. Encoded within the raw data of the magnetic resonance signal is additional information concerning the phase angle of the magnetization vector. Stationary structures have similar phase angles, whereas moving spins (i.e., flowing blood) have markedly different phase angles that are dependent on the velocity of flow. Phase velocity maps can be produced in which pixel intensity is proportional to the velocity of flow

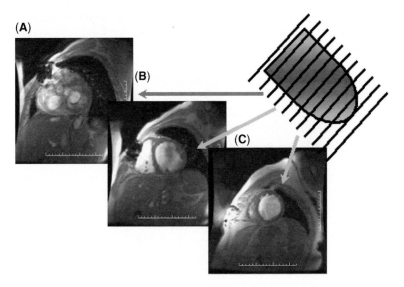

Figure 18 Ejection fraction was calculated using successive endocardial boundaries drawn on short axis images spanning base to apex and using Simpson's rule. (**A**) Base of left ventricle (LV), (**B**) middle segment of LV, (**C**) apical segment of LV.

in any pre-selected direction by modifying the standard gradient-echo pulse sequence and using appropriate processing. Accordingly, blood flow throughout the cardiac cycle can be determined.

An important feature of MR "phase velocity mapping" is that velocity can be encoded separately (and with equal accuracy) in all three spatial coordinate directions, allowing full 3D assessment to be made of flow. Typically flow quantitation is applied in association with cine acquisitions, and is sometimes referred to as "velocity encoded cine." A disadvantage of current implementations is that the scan time can be two to four times longer than conventional cine acquisitions, and thus breath-hold scans are less feasible (49–52). Data on flow patterns in the aorta, pulmonary, and coronary arteries have been presented (53–56).

REGIONAL VENTRICULAR FUNCTION

A number of CMR approaches have been developed to allow the detailed evaluation of regional wall function, thus making CMR ideally suited for evaluation of ischemic heart disease. The high contrast-to-noise ratio of CMR affords an unsurpassed view of the LV endocardium and its inherent 3D nature facilitates evaluation of myocardial and chamber function.

An obvious application of tomographic imaging techniques is direct evaluation of regional wall thickening during systole. Observation by CMR of diminished systolic thickening (<6.0 mm) or attainment of an absolute diastolic thickness of less than 5.5 mm has been correlated with radionuclide-defined non-viable myocardium (57). Additionally, observation of a systolic thickening of less than 1 mm correlates with non-viable myocardium (i.e., myocardium that does not benefit from subsequent revascularization, as assessed by radionuclide methodologies) (58).

In evaluating regional wall motion, the advantages of tomographic approaches are very apparent. However, it is true that even tomographic approaches may fail to successfully evaluate regions of hypokinesia if the heart is viewed in only one plane. Thus, it is important to view the myocardium in at least two orthogonal planes. Further, the acquisition time required to obtain this data has decreased dramatically in the last decade, and many studies have reported the ability of CMR to accurately assess regional wall motion. Indeed, it is the preferred modality.

While radial shortening of the myocardium is widely appreciated as making a major contribution to LV function, other aspects have received less attention, namely the base to apex (meridional) shortening and the torsion (or twisting) action of the heart. All three components are combined to effectively "wring" blood out of the LV cavity. However, these aspects are immediately apparent when viewing "tagged MR tomograms" (Fig. 14). An imaging sequence that can be used in conjunction with many of the above approaches is that of tagging (59–62).

In 1994 Palmon et al. reported on regional myocardial function in patients with mild left ventricular hypertrophy (LVH) (63). This was followed by a report from Kramer et al. (from the same institution) where tagging was used to describe ventricular remodeling after left anterior descending (LAD) occlusion (64). Young et al. have described the application of tagging to the disease state of hypertrophic cardiomyopathy, as have Nakatami who suggested that regional curvature within the ventricular septum may promote an aberrant loading condition, resulting in regional dysfunction (4). Recently, Curry et al. have reported the use of tagging to investigate resynchronization of the LV in patients with ischemic cardiomyopathy (65). The MR tagging technique offers the ability to gain unprecedented insight into the elaborate processes of regional myocardial motion. Currently, numerous clinical trials incorporate tagging to obtain precise indices of ventricular function.

VENTRICULAR MASS

The ability to quantitate both LV and RV mass with a high degree of accuracy is well established for CMR. Approaches have been developed that are suitable for both normal hearts and hearts deformed by acute myocardial infarction. In a landmark study, Bottini et al. (6) demonstrated the utility

(A)   (B)

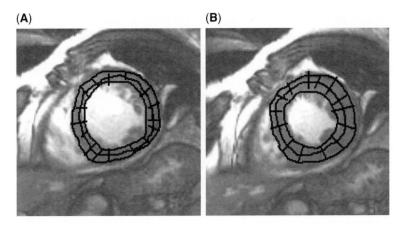

Figure 19 Wall thickening analysis: end-diastolic and end-systolic images were identified. The endocardial and epicardial boundaries were drawn. The centerline method was used to calculate. (**A**) Wall thickness at end-diastole. (**B**) Wall thickness at end-systole. Comparison of wall thickness at these time points was used to generate the wall thickening expressed as a percentage.

of high fidelity imaging when evaluating LV mass. The precision of LV mass measured with CMR (11 ± 8 g) was over twice that observed with echocardiography (26 ± 49 g) (Fig. 19). The implication of this for serial evaluation studies is impressive. In an example comparing the ability of CMR and echocardiography to determine LV mass, it was calculated that it would require 550 patients for echocardiography but only 17 patients for CMR to determine the mass within 10 g at a power of 80%. Similarly, Bellenger et al. (5) recently showed that, despite higher initial cost for CMR compared with echocardiography, the costs for a similarly powered study were half for CMR due to the need for fewer patients.

CONCLUSIONS

CMR imaging has emerged as having many of the desired attributes of an ideal imaging instrument. The inherent 3D nature of its data, the ability to image in any oblique orientation remains a principle advantage over most imaging modalities. Its high spatial and temporal resolution, combined with the lack of signal attenuation, inter-reader reliability, and lack of the requirement for an ideal "window" has allowed CMR to become the gold standard for measuring cardiac volume, mass and function.

However, two important issues remain to be addressed. First, with current relatively high costs of hardware coupled with software, the price tag of CMR becomes prohibitive to all but large academic centers and a few visionary private facilities. Secondly, while development costs are decreasing, the *tangible* costs still surpass the majority of traditional imaging modalities. However, as suggested in the monograph, the more *intangible* cost savings may trump those finite costs, since the ability to make the initial diagnosis correctly without patient morbidity or mortality is of direct value to patients and healthcare institutions.

REFERENCES

1. Pohost GM, Hung L, Doyle M. Clinical use of cardiovascular magnetic resonance. Circulation 2003; 108(6):647–653.
2. Dor V. The endoventricular circular patch plasty ("Dor procedure") in ischemic akinetic dilated ventricles. Heart Fail Rev 2001; 6(3):187–193.
3. Doyle M, Biederman RW. Future prospects in magnetic resonance imaging. Curr Cardiol Rep 2004; 6(1):70–75.
4. Young AA, Kramer CM, Ferrari VA, Axel L, Reichek N. Three-dimensional left ventricular deformation in hypertrophic cardiomyopathy. Circulation 1994; 90(2):854–867.
5. Bellenger NG, Davies LC, Francis, Pennel DJ. Sample sizes required by CMR to show a clinical change in volumes, ejection fraction and mass in patients with heart failure [abstr]. J Cardiovasc Magn Reson 1999; 1(4):309.
6. Bottini PB, Carr AA, Prisant LM, Flickinger FW, Allison JD, Gottdiener JS. Magnetic resonance imaging compared to echocardiography to assess left ventricular mass in the hypertensive patient. Am J Hypertens 1995; 8(3):221–228.
7. Shellock FG. Reference Manual for Magnetic Resonance Safety, Implants, and Devices. Los Angeles, CA: Biomedical Research Publications Group, 2004.
8. Shellock FG. Magnetic Resonance Procedures: Health Effects, Safety, and Patient Management. Boca Raton, FL: CRC Press, 2001.
9. Gerber TC, Fasseas P, Lennon RJ, et al. Clinical safety of magnetic resonance imaging early after coronary artery stent placement. J Am Coll Cardiol 2003; 42(7):1295–1298.
10. Roguin A, Zviman MM, Meininger GR, et al. Modern pacemaker and implantable cardioverter-defibrillator systems can be magnetic resonance imaging safe: in vitro and in vivo assessemnt of safety and function at 1.5T. Circulation 2004; 110(5):475–482.
11. Martin TE, Coman JA, Shellock FG, Pulling CC, Fair R, Jenkins K. Magnetic resonance imaging and cardiac pacemaker safety at 1.5 Tesla. J Am Coll Cardiol 2004; 43(7):1315–1324.
12. Arai AE, Gaither CC, Epstein FH, Balaban RS, Wolff SD. Myocardial velocity gradient imaging by phase contrast MRI with application to regional function in myocardial ischemia. Magn Reson Med 1999; 42(1):98–109.
13. Nagel E, Lehmkuhl HB, Bocksch W, et al. Noninvasive diagnosis of ischemia-induced wall motion abnormalities with the use of high-dose dobutamine stress MRI: comparison with dobutamine stress echocardiography. Circulation 1999; 99(6):763–770.
14. Anagnostopoulos C, Gunning MG, Davies G, Francis J, Underwood SR. Simultaneous biplane first-pass radionuclide ventriculography using 99Tcm-tetrofosmin: a comparison with magnetic resonance imaging. Nucl Med Commun 1998; 19(5):435–441.

15. Iwase M, Kondo T, Hasegawa K, et al. Three-dimensional echocardiography by semi-automatic border detection in assessment of left ventricular volume and ejection fraction: comparison with magnetic resonance imaging. J Cardiol 1997; 30(2):97–105.

16. van Rugge FP, van der Wall EE, Spanjersberg SJ, et al. Magnetic resonance imaging during dobutamine stress for detection and localization of coronary artery disease. Quantitative wall motion analysis using a modification of the centerline method. Circulation 1994; 90(1):127–138.

17. Kotlewski A, Kawanishi D, Rahimtoola SH. Management of valvular heart disease: an illustrative cases approach. Curr Probl Cardiol 1991; 16(1):1–88.

18. Meese RB, Spritzer CE, Negro-Vilar R, Bashore T, Herfkens RJ. Detection, characterization and functional assessment of reperfused Q-wave acute myocardial infarction by cine magnetic resonance imaging. Am J Cardiol 1990; 66(1): 1–9.

19. Akins EW, Brateman LF, Williams CM, Mietling SW, Franco EA. Improved detection of healed myocardial infarction by Fourier amplitude and phase imaging in two projections: validation with MRI. Radiographics 1989; 9(2):323–339.

20. Deutsch HJ, Smolorz J, Sechtem U, Hombach V, Schicha H, Hilger HH. Cardiac function by magnetic resonance imaging. Int J Card Imaging 1988; 3(1):3–11.

21. Sechtem U, Sommerhoff BA, Markiewicz W, White RD, Cheitlin MD, Higgins CB. Regional left ventricular wall thickening by magnetic resonance imaging: evaluation in normal persons and patients with global and regional dysfunction. Am J Cardiol 1987; 59(1):145–151.

22. Akins EW, Hill JA, Sievers KW, Conti CR. Assessment of left ventricular wall thickness in healed myocardial infarction by magnetic resonance imaging. Am J Cardiol 1987; 59(1):24–28.

23. Rehr RB, Malloy CR, Filipchuk NG, Peshock RM. Left ventricular volumes measured by MR imaging. Radiology 1985; 156:717–719.

24. Buckwalter KA, Aisen AM, Dilworth LR, Mancini GBJ, Buda AJ. Gated cardiac MRI: ejection-fraction determination using the right anterior oblique view. AJR Am J Roentgenol 1986; 147:33–77.

25. Dilworth LR, Aisen AM, Mancini J, Lande I, Buda AJ. Determination of left ventricular volumes and ejection fraction by nuclear magnetic resonance imaging. Am Heart J 1987; 113:24–32.

26. Underwood SR, Gill CR, Firmin DN, et al. Left ventricular volume measured rapidly by oblique magnetic resonance imaging. Br Heart J 1988; 60:188–195.

27. Stratemeier EJ, Thompson R, Brady TJ, et al. Ejection fraction determination by MR imaging: comparison with left ventricular angiography. Radiology 1986; 158:775–777.

28. Osbakken M, Yuschok T. Evaluation of ventricular function with gated cardiac magnetic resonance imaging. Catheter Cardiovasc Diagn 1986; 12:156–160.

29. van Rossum AC, Visser FC, van Eenige MJ, Valk J, Roos JP. Magnetic resonance imaging of the heart for determination of ejection fraction. Int J Cardiol 1988; 18:53–63.

30. van Rossum AC, Visser FC, Sprenger M, van Eenige MJ, Valk J, Roos JP. Evaluation of magnetic resonance imaging for determination of left ventricular ejection fraction and comparison with angiography. Am J Cardiol 1988; 62: 628–633.

31. Markiewicz W, Sechtem U, Kirby R, Derugin N, Caputo GC, Higgins CB. Measurement of ventricular volumes in the dog by nuclear magnetic resonance imaging. J Am Coll Cardiol 1987; 10:170–177.
32. Utz JA, Herfkens RJ, Heinsimer JA, et al. Cine NMR determination of left ventricular ejection fraction. Am J Roentgenol 1987; 148:839–843.
33. Sechtem U, Pflugfelder PW, Gould RG, Cassidy MM, Higgins CB. Measurement of right and left ventricular volumes in healthy individuals with cine MR imaging. Radiology 1987; 163:897–902.
34. Cranney GB, Lotan CS, Dean L, Baxley W, Bouchard A, Pohost GM. Left ventricular volume measurement using cardiac axis NMR imaging—validation by calibrated ventricular angiography. Circulation 1990; 82:154–163.
35. Buser PT, Auffermann W, Holt WW, et al. Noninvasive evaluation of global left ventricular function with use of cine nuclear magnetic resonance. J Am Coll Cardiol 1989; 13:1294–1300.
36. Semelka RC, Tomei E, Wagner S, et al. Normal left ventricular dimensions and function: interstudy reproducibility of measurements with cine MR imaging. Radiology 1990; 174:763–768.
37. Semelka RC, Tomei E, Wagner S, et al. Interstudy reproducibility of dimensional and functional measurements between cine magnetic resonance studies in the morphologically abnormal left ventricle. Am Heart J 1990; 119:1367–1373.
38. Nagel E, Lehmkuhl HB, Bocksch W, et al. Noninvasive diagnosis of ischemia-induced wall motion abnormalities with the use of high-dose dobutamine stress MRI: comparison with dobutamine stress echocardiography. Circulation 1999; 99(6):763–770.
39. Anagnostopoulos C, Gunning MG, Davies G, Francis J, Underwood SR. Simultaneous biplane first-pass radionuclide ventriculography using 99 Tcm-tetrofosmin: a comparison with magnetic resonance imaging. Nucl Med Commun 1998; 19(5):435–441.
40. Iwase M, Kondo T, Hasegawa K, et al. Three-dimensional echocardiography by semi-automatic border detection in assessment of left ventricular volume and ejection fraction: comparison with magnetic resonance imaging. J Cardiol 1997; 30(2):97–105.
41. van Rugge FP, van der Wall EE, Spanjersberg SJ, et al. Magnetic resonance imaging during dobutamine stress for detection and localization of coronary artery disease. Quantitative wall motion analysis using a modification of the centerline method. Circulation 1994; 90(1):127–138.
42. Meese RB, Spritzer CE, Negro-Vilar R, Bashore T, Herfkens RJ. Detection, characterization and functional assessment of reperfused Q-wave acute myocardial infarction by cine magnetic resonance imaging. Am J Cardiol 1990; 66(1):1–9.
43. Akins EW, Brateman LF, Williams CM, Mietling SW, Franco EA. Improved detection of healed myocardial infarction by Fourier amplitude and phase imaging in two projections: validation with MRI. Radiographics 1989; 9(2):323–339.
44. Deutsch HJ, Smolorz J, Sechtem U, Hombach V, Schicha H, Hilger HH. Cardiac function by magnetic resonance imaging. Int J Card Imaging 1988; 3(1):3–11.
45. Sechtem U, Sommerhoff BA, Markiewicz W, White RD, Cheitlin MD, Higgins CB. Regional left ventricular wall thickening by magnetic resonance imaging:

evaluation in normal persons and patients with global and regional dysfunction. Am J Cardiol 1987; 59(1):145–151.

46. Akins EW, Hill JA, Sievers KW, Conti CR. Assessment of left ventricular wall thickness in healed myocardial infarction by magnetic resonance imaging. Am J Cardiol 1987; 59(1):24–28.

47. Underwood SR, Firmin DN, Klipstein RH, Rees RS, Longmore DB. Magnetic resonance velocity mapping: clinical application of a new technique. Br Heart J 1987; 57:404–412.

48. Mostbeck GH, Caputo GR, Higgins CB. MR measurement of blood flow in the cardiovascular system. Am J Roentgenol 1992; 159:453–461.

49. van Rossum AC, Sprenger M, Visser FC, Peels KH, Valk J, Roos JP. An in vivo validation of quantitative blood flow imaging in arteries and veins using magnetic resonance phase-shift techniques. Eur Heart J 1991; 12:117–126.

50. Firmin DN, Nayler GL, Klipstein RH, Underwood SR, Rees RS, Longmore DB. In vivo validation of MR velocity imaging. J Comput Assist Tomogr 1987; 11:751–756.

51. Mohiaddin RH, Amanuma M, Kilner PJ, Pinnell DJ, Manzara C, Longmore DB. MR phase-shift velocity mapping of mitral and pulmonary venous flow. J Comput Assist Tomogr 1991; 15:237–243.

52. Kondo C, Caputo GR, Masui T, et al. Pulmonary hypertension: pulmonary flow quantification and flow profile analysis with velocity-encoded cine MR imaging. Radiology 1992; 183:751–758.

53. Kilner PJ, Yang GZ, Mohiaddin RH, Firmin DN, Longmore DB. Helical and retrograde secondary flow patterns in the aortic arch studied by three directional magnetic resonance velocity mapping. Circulation 1993; 88:2235–2247.

54. Bogren HG, Klipstein RH, Firmin DN, et al. Quantitation of antegrade and retrograde blood flow in the human aorta by magnetic resonance velocity mapping. Am Heart J 1989; 117:1214–1222.

55. Bogren HG, Mohiaddin RH, Klipstein RK, et al. The function of the aorta in ischemic heart disease: a magnetic resonance and angiographic study of aortic compliance and blood flow patterns. Am Heart J 1989; 118:234–247.

56. Bogren HG, Klipstein RH, Mohiaddin RH, et al. Pulmonary artery distensibility and blood flow patterns: a magnetic resonance study of normal subjects and of patients with pulmonary arterial hypertension. Am Heart J 1989; 118:990–999.

57. Bax JJ, de Roos A, van Der Wall EE. Assessment of myocardial viability by MRI. J Magn Reson Imaging 1999; 10(3):418–422.

58. Tadamura E, Kudoh T, Motooka M, et al. Use of technetium-99m sestamibi ECG-gated single-photon emission tomography for the evaluation of left ventricular function following coronary artery bypass graft: comparison with three-dimensional magnetic resonance imaging. Eur J Nucl Med 1999; 26(7):705–712.

59. Axel L, Dougherty L. Heart wall motion: improved method of spatial modulation of magnetization for MR imaging. Radiology 1989; 172(2):349–350.

60. Doyle M, Walsh EG, Foster RE, Pohost GM. Common k-space acquisition: a method to improve myocardial grid-tag contrast. Magn Reson Med 1997; 37(5):754–763.

61. Stuber M, Fischer SE, Scheidegger MB, Boesiger P. Toward high-resolution myocardial tagging. Magn Reson Med 1999; 41(3):639–643.

62. Denney TS Jr., McVeigh ER. Model-free reconstruction of three-dimensional myocardial strain from planar tagged MR images. J Magn Reson Imaging 1997; 7(5):799–810.
63. Palmon LC, Reichek N, Yeon SB, et al. Intramural myocardial shortening in hypertensive left ventricular hypertrophy with normal pump function. Circulation 1994; 89(1):122–131.
64. Kramer CM, Rogers WJ, Theobald TM, Power TP, Petruolo S, Reichek N. Remote noninfarcted region dysfunction soon after first anterior myocardial infarction. A magnetic resonance tagging study. Circulation 1996; 94(4):660–666.
65. Curry CW, Nelson SG, Wyman BT, et al. Mechanical dyssynchrony in dilated cardiomyopathy with intraventricular conduction delay as depicted by 3D tagged magnetic resonance imaging. Circulation 2000; 101:e2.

6

Magnetic Resonance Assessment of Valvular Heart Disease[†]

Agostino Meduri
Department of Radiology, Catholic University of Rome, Rome, Italy

Ronald M. Razmi
Cardiovascular MR/CT Center and Heart Center of Indiana, The Care Group, LLC, Indianapolis, Indiana, U.S.A.

INTRODUCTION

Diagnostic imaging is an important component of the management of the patients with valvular heart disease. Echocardiography and cardiac catherization are the methods traditionally used to evaluate valvular disease. Echocardiography allows quantitative techniques to assess stenotic valves by calculating transvalvular pressure gradient and valve areas from the increase in blood flow velocity caused by the stenotic orifice. Cardiac catherization allows direct measurement of pressures in the heart, as well as the connected vessels and thus continues to be the gold standard for accurate measurement of pressure gradients and valve areas in this patient population. Echocardiographic evaluation of valvular regurgitation is semiquantitative and relies more on the subjective visual assessment of the regurgitant jet with the use of color flow mapping. Color flow Doppler

---

[†] Editor's Note: To avoid confusion, the present chapter will use CMR (cardiovascular magnetic resonance) to indicate the imaging technology and will use MR (mitral regurgitation) to indicate one of the valvular pathologies.

111

images are more reflective of the velocity of flow rather than the volume of regurgitant jets. Cardiac catherization grading of regurgitant lesions is imprecise and depends on many factors such as catheter position, the amount and rate of injected contrast media, chamber size, etc. These cause significant overlap in a grading of valvular regurgitations. Also, X-ray angiographic methods to calculate regurgitant volumes involving angiographic, thermodilution, and Fick methods involve complex methodology and are less reliable at low or high cardiac outputs. Also, angiography, due to its invasive nature, is not suitable for long-term follow-up of these patients.

Cardiovascular magnetic resonance (CMR) offers a comprehensive method for evaluation of patients with valvular disease. Not only it offers accurate methods for morphological and hemodynamic assessment of valves, but also it allows reliable longitudinal evaluation of the associated complications. These include chamber dimensions, myocardial mass, function, etc. These parameters are increasingly important for a correct management of the patients with valvular heart disease to monitor therapy and select the timing when a valve replacement or repair would be beneficial (1,2). All valvular heart diseases result in heart chamber overload, which is initially tolerated, and then may lead to myocardial dysfunction, congestive heart failure and even sudden death (2).

CMR provides high soft tissue contrast for anatomical evaluation of the valves, allows visualization of stenotic and regurgitant jets as an area of signal void, and has the capability to encode velocity of motion, allowing for quantification of blood flow velocity and volume flow. Therefore, CMR imaging has the capability to provide an integrated, noninvasive approach for evaluation of patients with valvular heart disease.

METHODS

Spin Echo

With the introduction of the new steady-state free precession sequences, spin echo methods have fallen out of favor in assessment of valvular structure and integrity. They may still be of some value in evaluating for vegetations or abscesses but the new gradient echo methods offer excellent view of the valves, supporting structures such as chordae tendinae and surrounding structures. Information traditionally revealed with spin echo methods such as thickening of the leaflets or bicuspid valve can easily be seen in the steady-state free precession sequences.

Volume Measurements

Cine CMR sequences allow to acquire images during multiple phases of the cardiac cycle. Therefore, accurate measurements of ventricular volumes, their derived parameters [stroke volume and ejection fraction (EF)], and myocardial mass are possible (2).

Cine gradient echo (GRE) sequences or echo planar images have the necessary high temporal resolution to obtain precise end-systolic and end-diastolic images; the end-diastolic images are usually the first images after the R wave, while the end-systolic images show the smallest cavitary area (1).

While standard GRE sequences are often degraded by breathing and movement artifacts, fast gradient echo sequences can be acquired during a breath-hold or navigator-echo techniques can be applied so that artifacts caused by respiration are minimized.

Volume measurement can be obtained using the area–length method on images acquired along the horizontal and vertical long axes. More accurate measurements that do not rely on geometrical assumptions are obtained directly with the Simpson's rule. Contiguous short axis slices are obtained throughout the ventricle; ventricular volume is computed summing the cavity volume of each slice (cavity area × slice thickness). Similarly, myocardial mass is calculated by summation of myocardial section mass over the entire ventricle.

The right ventricular volumes, impossible to evaluate with geometrical assumptions for the complex shape of this cavity, are assessed accurately with this method. By acquiring images along the short axis plane, partial volume effects are reduced. The choice of this scanning plane makes it more difficult to determine the atrioventricular valve plane; this problem is overcome by starting the acquisition at the atrioventricular junction.

Volume measurements can be also used for the quantification of valvular insufficiency. A regurgitant volume can be calculated as the difference in left and right ventricular stroke volumes (2) (that in the absence of valvular insufficiency does not exceed 5%) while the regurgitant fraction is the ratio of regurgitant volume to stroke volume:

Regurgitant fraction
15–20% Mild
20–40% Moderate
> 40% Severe

The technique can be used for patients with a single insufficient valve; in combined mitral and aortic insufficiency it assesses the total regurgitation, while in the presence of a bilateral insufficient valve it underestimates the regurgitation and is meaningless.

Magnetic resonance and radionuclide measurements of ventricular EF and stroke volume ratio showed good correlation (1).

Signal Void Phenomena

In the gradient echo sequences the blood has bright signal due to the inflow effect. Turbulence and complex flow pattern cause dephasing of the blood spins with resulting cancellation of the signal (2). In dysfunctional valves the high-velocity stenotic and regurgitant jets appear as areas of diminished or absent signal persisting for most of the systole or diastole (2). Cine loop display of the gradient echo images allows a dynamic evaluation of the flow patterns (3). The extent of the signal void is highly dependent on several variables. Long Echo time TE cine sequences (TE > 12 msec) are more sensitive to lower turbulences therefore flow void is well demonstrated; by decreasing the TE the flow void becomes less evident (3).

Fast GRE sequences can acquire cine images during a single breath-hold, eliminating respiratory artifacts. While these sequences are well suited for evaluating wall motion abnormalities, the short TE do not show turbulent jets as well as GRE sequences with longer TE (Fig. 1). With an appropriate choice of parameters, TE of 7 to 9 msec can be achieved allowing the study of valvular function. Display parameters such as window width and level modify the appearance of signal void.

Hemodynamic parameters, including transvalvular pressure gradient, orifice size, and changes in volume and pressure of the receiving chamber also alter the conspicuity of the flow void. The jet is a three-dimensional structure often irregular, eccentric, and changing its shape during the cardiac phases; at least two imaging planes should be obtained to fully evaluate the extent of the flow void.

In mitral and tricuspid disease the turbulence is best studied along the horizontal and vertical long axis (Figs. 2 and 3); the aortic jets along the oblique axial and coronal planes (Figs. 4 and 5), pulmonary disease along the oblique sagittal and axial planes (Fig. 6). This method allows a semiquantitative study of valvular blood flow in concordance with color-Doppler and cardiac catheterization.

In the presence of valvular regurgitation a flow void can be seen also proximal to the valve where the blood accelerates before the incompetent orifice. In the aortic insufficiency the proximal acceleration area correlates better with the degree of regurgitation than the size of the distal regurgitant jet (2).

CMR can evaluate turbulence jet semi-quantitatively or qualitatively, with the same parameters used by echocardiography. The image on which the turbulence is larger is usually used for the measurements. In this case the sequence with the largest signal void is usually used for analysis. Several measurements have been used: the area or volume of the jet, its length, and the ratio of the signal void to the receiving chamber area (Fig. 7) (3).

Phase Contrast Velocity Mapping

Phase contrast (PC) methods are the most used for flow quantification expressed as velocity or volume per unit of time (4). A gradient is superimposed to the main magnetic field. Blood protons as they move along the gradient modify their precessional frequency. The gradient is then reversed

(A)

(B)

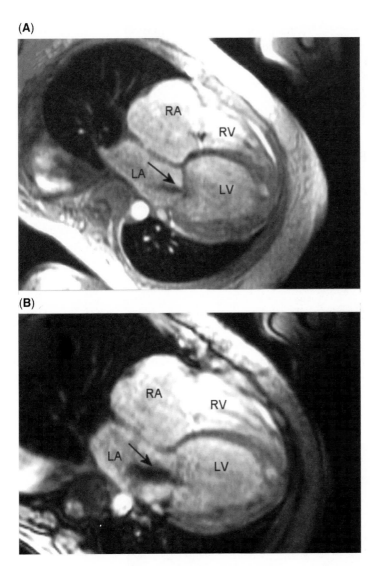

Figure 1 Axial four-chamber gradient echo acquisition with different echo times shows the difference in the extent of the signal void. (**A**) The echo time of 4 milliseconds shows a mild to moderate jet of mitral regurgitation (*arrow*). (**B**) The echo time of 8 milliseconds shows moderate to severe mitral regurgitation (MR) (*arrow*). *Abbreviations*: LV, left ventricle; LA, left atrium; RV, right ventricle; RA, right atrium.

so that the frequency returns to the original speed, but moving protons will have experienced a phase shift of their magnetic moments compared with stationary protons. In phase velocity imaging, at least two scans are

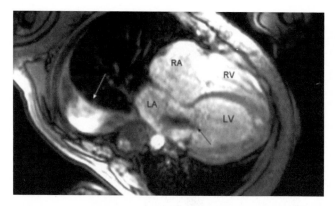

Figure 2 Axial four-chamber gradient echo acquisition shows mitral insufficiency jet (*black arrow*) from the LV into the LA. Note the right pleural effusion (*white arrow*). *Abbreviations*: RV, right ventricle; RA, right atrium; LV, left ventricle; LA, left atrium.

acquired simultaneously: a motion-compensated scan, in which there is no phase change owing to flow (magnitude images) and a velocity-encoded scan where a phase change is related to the flow velocity along the direction of the magnetic gradient (Fig. 8). Subtracting the two sets of images it is possible to calculate a phase shift proportional to velocity (5). Usually velocity is encoded along a direction perpendicular to the imaging plane. If velocity has to be encoded along more than one axis, additional sets of images are

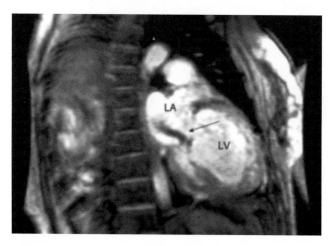

Figure 3 Sagittal right anterior oblique two-chamber view acquisition shows the mitral insufficiency jet from the LV into the LA (*arrow*). Note the peripheral direction of the jet to the posterior wall of LA. *Abbreviations*: LA, left atrium; LV, left ventricle.

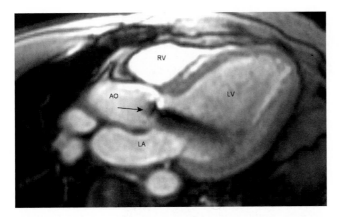

Figure 4   Axial gradient echo LVOT view showing the aortic insufficiency jet (*arrow*) from the AO into the LV. Note the area of flow convergence just distal to the aortic valve in the aorta. This is severe aortic insufficiency as the jet extends to the posterior wall of the LV. *Abbreviations*: LA, left atrium; RV, right ventricle.; AO, aorta; LV, left ventricle.

acquired using different gradient directions; images resulting from their vector sum will encode flow velocity along the different spatial planes.

On flow-encoded images, stationary tissues are represented as midgray areas; white or black areas code for flow toward opposite directions; more pronounced black/white levels correspond to higher velocities (5).

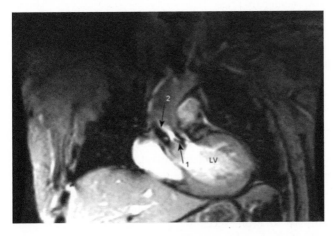

Figure 5   Coronary gradient echo view of the calcified aortic valve (*arrow 1*) and the high velocity aortic stenosis jet (*arrow 2*) of the aortic valve. Note the dark appearance of the aortic leaflets suggestive of the calcification of the valve. Also, note the two dark jets on either side of the central area of high velocity with the bright signal. *Abbreviation*: LV, left ventricle.

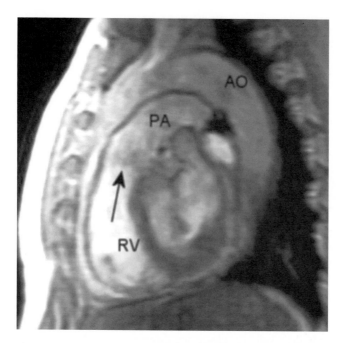

Figure 6   Sagittal gradient echo sequence shows the pulmonic valve (*arrow*). This is one of the best views for assessment of the right ventricular outflow tract and the valve. This is also the best plane to use to set up the PC sequence parallel or perpendicular to the direction of the flow through the valve. *Abbreviations*: RV, right ventricle; AO, aorta; PA, pulmonary artery.

A velocity window is chosen prescribing a velocity-encoded sequence; flow velocity should not exceed the window: velocities higher than the prescribed window will be coded as moving toward the opposite direction because of the phenomenon of aliasing (Fig. 9) (4). If the velocity window selected is too wide, the sensitivity to the flow will be low and this will also adversely affect the quality of the information (Fig. 10).

The imaging plane should be perpendicular to the flow direction to avoid misalignment errors. The relation between velocity and phase shift is linear; however, complex flow patterns may cause phase incoherence within the voxels and reduce the linearity the velocity/phase shift relation (4).

Data acquisition is synchronized to the cardiac cycle through retrospective gating usually 16 or more slices are obtained per cycle; irregular rhythm may diminish image quality (4). Fast imaging techniques allow data acquisition during a single breath-hold so that images are free from breathing artifacts.

A region of interest corresponding to the cross-sectional flow area is selected for each frame on the magnitude; in the flow analysis program it is transferred to the corresponding flow image to calculate the instantaneous

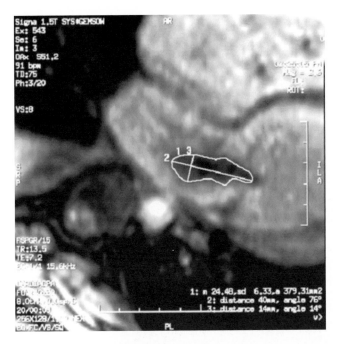

Figure 7   Mitral regurgitation jet analyzed by its area (1), length (2), and width (3). Each one of these parameters can be used to qualitatively analyze the severity of stenosis or regurgitation in the diseased valve.

average velocity and flow (average flow = average velocity × area). It is possible to draw flow curves by plotting instantaneous flow values against time. Where flow is retrograde, the flow curve will have negative values. Measuring the area under the curve, that is by integrating the instantaneous flow values, average flow per heartbeat is obtained.

In stenoses, velocity-encoded cine (VEC) allows measuring the increased velocity of the flow jet passing through the stenosis. This can be determined on a plane parallel or perpendicular to the jet. Using the through-plane approach it is possible to measure flow volume as the product of the average velocity and the flow area. It might be difficult to predict the exact position of the vena contracta (narrowest central flow region of a jet); however, the centerline velocity of the jet is usually constant over a distance of five times its width therefore allowing a certain margin to position the slice.

For stenoses the velocity-encoded window must be selected to encode velocities of 4 to 6 m/sec. The pressure gradient across the stenosis can be calculated with the modified Bernoulli equation:

$$\Delta P = 4 \times (V_{max})^2$$

where ΔP is the difference in pressure across the stenosis and V_{max} is the peak velocity.

(A)

(B)

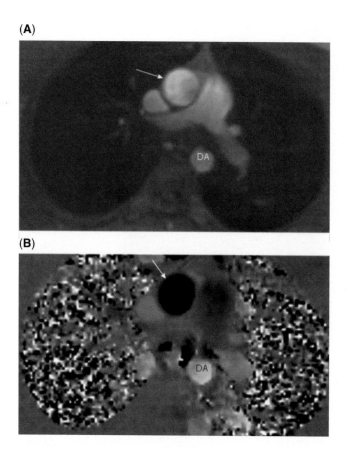

Figure 8 Transverse velocity-encoded sequence in the ascending aorta that shows the (**A**) magnitude image and (**B**) phase image. Note the blood traveling toward the gradient in the ascending aorta is dark (*arrow*) in the phase images while the blood going in the opposite direction in the DA is white. The area around the aorta is drawn in magnitude images and automatically applied to the phase images where flow information is produced. *Abbreviation*: DA, descending aorta.

Aortic Stenosis

Aortic stenosis is caused by different disorders affecting the cusps or annulus (3):

Causes of aortic stenosis
Congenital
Bicuspid
Monocuspid
Rheumatic
Degenerative

(A) (B)

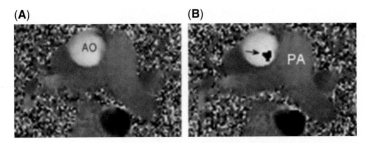

Figure 9 Transverse velocity-encoded sequences that show the phase images. (A) The Velcoity Encoding (VENC) is set at an appropriate level higher than the aortic (AO) peak velocity, hence there is no aliasing. (B) The VENC chosen is lower than the peak velocity in the aorta, hence there is aliasing (*arrow*). *Abbreviation*: PA, pulmonary artery.

More than 95% of patients with congenital aortic valve stenosis have a bicuspid or monocuspid valve. A monocuspid valve is the most frequent type in children with fatal aortic stenosis under 15 years of age. A bicuspid valve is present in 1% to 1.5% of live births. These patients may develop aortic stenosis or less commonly, infective endocarditis and/or aortic regurgitation. A bicuspid valve may have an anterior and a posterior leaflet or a left and right leaflet. In the first case the coronaries arise from the anterior leaflet; a false commissure (raphe) is usually in the anterior leaflet. In the second case the coronaries arise from the two different cusps while a raphe is located in the right cusp.

In rheumatic disease the leaflets are thickened, calcific deposits are present and the commissures may be fused. In degenerative aortic stenosis calcium is deposited on the aortic side of the leaflets, while the commissures are not fused.

Opening of the valve is restricted causing increase of transvalvular gradient. Studies have focused on the quantification of pressure gradient, but CMR can also measure orifice area and cardiac output that have great clinical impact.

The normal aortic valve area measures 2–3 cm^2. In clinically relevant stenoses valve area is restricted to less than 0.75–1.0 cm, producing a pressure gradient of 50 mmHg or more. The orifice size of bicuspid and degenerative valves is usually fixed; in calcific valves the obstruction is related to the leaflet stiffness and the orifice size may vary with the LV pressure.

Patients with severe aortic stenosis and low cardiac output often have relatively low pressure gradients, making it difficult to differentiate from mild/moderate stenosis.

Spin Echo Images

Spin echo images can provide the following information about the aortic valve (Fig. 11):

- Thickening or bulging of the cusps
- Areas of signal loss resulting from calcifications
- Fusion of the commissures

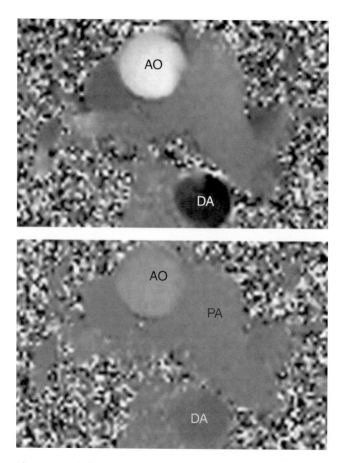

Figure 10 Transverse velocity-encoded sequences in the AO. (*Top*): The image shows appropriately selected VENC, higher than the peak velocity but not too high. (*Bottom*): The image shows the same sequence but with a VENC that is too high and the quality of this flow study is not as optima. Note the clear dark and white appearance in the AO and DA in the top image and the gray appearance of the same arteries in the lower image. When VENC exceeds the maximum velocity by significant amounts, the sensitivity to flow will decrease and the quality of the study deteriorates. *Abbreviations*: PA, pulmonary artery; AO, ascending aorta; DA, descending aorta.

- Poststenotic dilatation of the ascending aorta (mainly of the right border) more evident in patients with a bicuspid valve
- Concentric left ventricular hypertrophy (LVH) is the main mechanism to reduce LV wall stress, so that during early stages the EF is preserved
- Left ventricular dilatation in advanced or decompensated disease or when associated with aortic insufficiency.

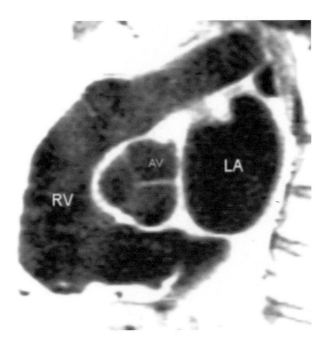

Figure 11 Spin echo acquisition in a plane parallel to the AV shows the morphology of the AV, including the number of leaflets and their contour. *Abbreviations*: RV, right ventricle; LA, left atrium; AV, aortic valve.

Cine GRE

Cine GRE acquisitions show a systolic jet from the aortic valve to the aortic root. Jet length and area correlate with the severity of the stenosis (6). With tight stenoses jets tend to be more horizontal. Patients with severe aortic stenosis and low cardiac output often have relatively low-pressure gradients; in this case it might be difficult to differentiate severe from mild/moderate stenosis.

A turbulence area proximal to the valve corresponds to the proximal acceleration area [proximal isovelocity surface area (PISA)] demonstrated by echocardiography. Optimal planes for the visualization of the jet are: the oblique coronal centered on LVOT and the oblique axial (Figs 3 and 4).

Recent studies have shown that gradient echo sequences can be used to directly measure aortic valve area using planimetry and have excellent correlation with transesophageal echocardiography and invasive methods (Fig. 12) (7,8).

Velocity Mapping

Phase velocity mapping allows calculation of the maximum velocity within the stenotic jet: it can be assessed on in-plane (parallel to the turbulence jet)

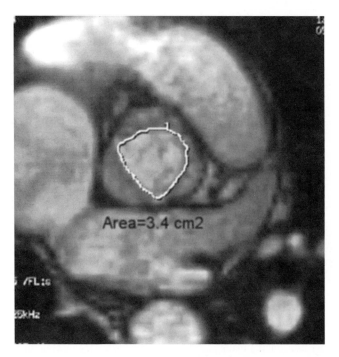

Figure 12   Oblique gradient echo acquisition parallel to the aortic valve provides an excellent view of the aortic valve. The valve area can be drawn directly as shown. The results have shown excellent correlation with echocardiographic and angiographic methods.

or through-plane (perpendicular to the valve) images (9). Using the through-plane technique the imaging plane is localized immediately distal to the valve to obtain the peak velocity at the vena contracta. For in-plane measurement the VENC must be parallel to the jet. If aortic stenosis is evaluated using the in-plane technique, the valve area can be calculated with the continuity Equation (6):

$$A_{Ao} = (A_{OT} \times V_{OT})/V_{Ao}$$

where A_{Ao}, A_{OT} are the areas and V_{Ao}, V_{OT} the peak velocities, respectively, of the ascending aorta and of the outflow tract.

Causes of underestimation of peak velocity may be in-plane averaging (limited spatial resolution of VENC), wide slice thickness (the margins of the jet may include convergent and divergent flow up- and downstream the valve), low temporal resolution, and intravoxel dephasing (turbulent flow). Only voxels with velocities greater than 50% of the peak velocity should be included in the orifice determination.

The pressure gradient can be calculated from the modified Bernoulli equation. Mean pressure gradients correspond well with cardiac catheterization and Doppler, echo, and CMR. Accuracy rates are greater than 85% with inter-observer reproducibility of 93% (10).

Flow velocity mapping measures correlated well with Doppler echocardiography ($r = 0.96$) and cardiac catherization ($r = 0.97$) (11). Better results are obtained with CMR in patients with limited acoustic window or complex flow patterns as the entire jet can be displayed.

Follow Up

CMR is able to provide fundamental information for the follow up of aortic stenosis. Progression of lesion is low: an annual CMR study is recommended for monitoring LVH and LV function. In symptomatic patients with severe aortic stenosis, valve replacement is recommended (average survival 2–3 years). Myocardial fibrosis associated with LVH may preclude functional recovery. In asymptomatic patients with severe aortic stenosis and LVH/reduced LV function valve replacement is recommended.

Aortic Insufficiency

Aortic regurgitation is due to abnormalities of the cusps, lesions of the annulus or to dilatation of the aortic root. The most frequent causes of aortic insufficiency are:

- rheumatic heart disease
- endocarditis
- congenital bicuspid aortic valve
- aortic-annular ectasia related to Marfan's syndrome or collagen diseases
- hypertensive aortic root dilatation
- aortic dissection.

Symptomatic patients, patients with reduced LVEF at rest and/or LV dilatation [End-diastolic volume endothelium dependent dilation (EDD) $\geq$ 75 mm] should undergo valve replacement. CMR accurately determines LV function and volumes.

Spin Echo

Black blood fast spin echo and fast gradient echo images provide excellent visualization of the aortic valve morphology. It is possible to demonstrate the number of leaflets and to quantify the valve area.

Spin echo images are also useful to assess the dimension of the aortic root. An aortic root dilatation may be the cause of the aortic valve insufficiency (Fig. 13). Acute regurgitation is often related to aortic dissection. The ascending aorta should undergo replacement if exceeding 50 mm.

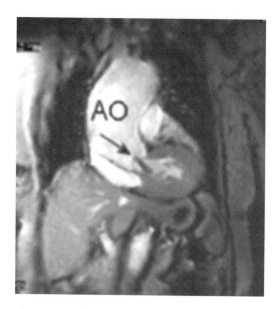

Figure 13 Coronal gradient echo sequence shows dilated aortic root and ascending aorta in Marfan's syndrome. Note the resulting aortic insufficiency (*arrow*). *Abbreviation*: AO, ascending aorta.

Gradient Echo

Turbulence jets of aortic regurgitation are diastolic and directed backward from the valve plane toward the LV outflow tract. Regurgitant jets are best visualized in the coronal oblique plane (Figs 3 and 4). Flow turbulence area and width, and the time persistence of the jet are indirect measures of regurgitant volume (6). Multiple angulated planes could be necessary to appreciate the full extent of the jet.

GRE images allow accurate assessment of ventricular volumes and function. Aortic regurgitation causes LV volume overload. In the acute regurgitation there is only a modest increase in EDD and of total systolic volume (SV). In the compensated state of chronic regurgitation, there is eccentric hypertrophy with increased EDD but normal ejection performance despite elevated afterload.

With the progression of the disease there is decompensated volume hypertrophy with reduction of the EF. An increase of the endsystolic volume or a reduction of the EF may signal the onset of LV failure and indicate the need for surgery. The comparison between left and right stroke volumes in case of a single regurgitant aortic valve allows the determination of the regurgitant volume and fraction.

(A)

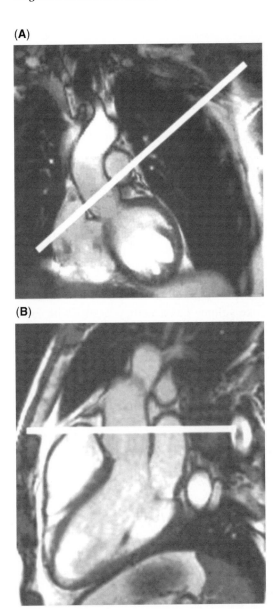

(B)

Figure 14   Coronal gradient echo (**A**) and axial oblique three-chamber (**B**) views of the aortic valve. These views can be used to acquire velocity-encoded sequences perpendicular to the flow of blood through the aortic valve (*lines*). Through-plane phase contrast imaging is an excellent method for evaluating aortic insufficiency.

Velocity Mapping

CMR can be considered the method of choice in patients with aortic regurgitation to directly quantify the regurgitant volumes (9). Velocity mapping can measure the LV stroke volume, regurgitant volume and fraction. The most accurate method is the through-plane measurement in an oblique axial plane between the aortic valve and the coronary ostia (Fig. 14). Using principles already explained in this chapter, flow can be quantified using velocity and area in forward and reverse direction. By integrating the areas under the curves, direct assessment of forward flow, reverse flow, and net forward flow can be made (Fig. 15). This has been verified against echo and angiographic methods and has excellent accuracy.

A movement of the imaging plane toward the ascending aorta leads to pitfalls due to coronary flow and aortic compliance. The reverse flow into the coronary arteries accounts for 6.3% of total flow volume (10). This can falsely reduce the regurgitant volume (measured $2\,m^3$ distal to the sinotubular region) by approximately 70% in mild and 30% in severe regurgitation.

The quantification of stroke volume has accuracy $> 90\%$ with inter-observer reproducibility of 94%. CMR has accuracy of 89% for assessment of the regurgitant fraction and 84% for regurgitant volume (10).

Significant findings in the determination of aortic regurgitation are: the slope of diastolic flow velocity, the degree of flow reversal in the descending aorta, and the comparison of stroke volume measure in the other intact valves with the regurgitant aortic valve.

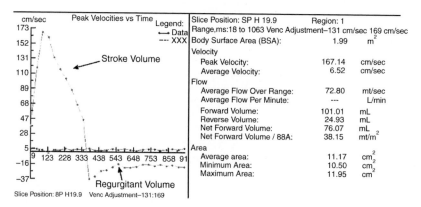

Figure 15 (*See color insert*) Flow volume curve versus time in the aorta shows the stroke volume in the initial part of the curve and regurgitant volume in diastole. Integrating the area under each curve yields numbers displayed in the right; forward volume, reverse volume, net forward volume. The regurgitant fraction can be calculated as regurgitant volume divided by stroke volume.

MITRAL VALVE DISEASE

Mitral Stenosis

Mitral stenosis (MS) occurs when mitral valve diastolic opening is restricted: if the valve orifice is narrowed by scarring or if flow through the mitral valve is obstructed by other pathology (12). Left ventricular inlet obstruction results with a diastolic pressure gradient between the left atrium and the left ventricle (13). MS is more prevalent in women. Once symptoms develop, the 10-year survival in untreated patients is 50% to 60% (14). Causes of MS are summarized below (12):

Rheumatic fever
Congenital
Parachute mitral valve
Carcinoid syndrome
Eosinophilic endocarditis
Systemic lupus
Rheumatoid arthritis
Left atrial myxoma
Secondary tumors growing into the mitral orifice (hypernephroma or lymphoma)
Thrombus

Rheumatic fever is the most frequent cause of MS (12,15). At least 60% of patients with MS have a remote history of rheumatic fever, and nearly all valve specimens have evidence of rheumatic deformities (14).

Isolated mitral valve involvement is most common, as approximately 40% of these patients present with isolated stenosis (15), followed by a combination of mitral and aortic valve disease (1). Pedunculated left atrial myxomas may prolapse into the valve orifice, obstructing flow with functional stenosis. It is often associated with the murmur of MR. Carcinoid valve disease may involve the MV but is predominantly right sided and related to hepatic metastases from a primary bowel carcinoid.

In a patient with MS, CMR can assess (15)

1. The morphology of the mitral valve apparatus
2. The hemodynamic severity of the stenosis

The valve leaflets become thickened, immobile, and encrusted by lumps of calcified fibrous tissue. The process may cause fusion of the commissures (13), and eventually involve the chordae tendinae (12,13). MS may be pure, although tethering and fibrosis of the chordae often result in varying degrees of regurgitation. The LV is not enlarged in the absence of MR (12). The left atrium is typically dilated. Enlargement of the left atrial appendage is more common than in other causes of pulmonary venous hypertension (12). Thrombus may form within the left atrial appendage.

Pulmonary venous hypertension causes interstitial and alveolar edema. Pulmonary arterial hypertension with dilatation of both main and proximal pulmonary arteries may subsequently develop. At last, the right ventricle fails and the right-sided cardiac chambers dilate (12).

Doppler echocardiography is the modality of choice in evaluating the degree of MS and is usually sufficient for therapeutic treatment planning (13). Since two-dimensional Doppler echocardiography provides the necessary information to monitor most patients with MS, there is generally no need for additional MR studies (15).

CMR may be useful in those cases in which there is a discrepancy between symptoms and Doppler echocardiography findings, where the acoustic window is limited or in presence of complex flow patterns (13). CMR study may add confirmatory data regarding the severity of the transvalvular pressure gradient, especially in MS with concomitant regurgitation (15). Atrial fibrillation develops in 30% to 40% of patients with symptomatic MS (14). This may lead to an inaccurate MR quantitative analysis, as a reliable and reproducible electrocardiographic gating cannot be obtained (13,14).

Mitral stenosis is typically graded by valve area and transvalvular pressure gradient (14). The normal adult mitral orifice area is 4 to 6 cm^2. When narrowed to 2 cm^2, there is minor elevation of left atrial pressure and a gradient across the valve during exercise. Further reduction to 1 cm^2 produces severe pressure overload leading to an increase in left atrial size, which does not correlate with the degree, severity, or duration of the disease (12).

Spin echo CMR imaging can demonstrate thickening and bulging of the leaflets and dilatation of the left atrium, whereas the left ventricle appears small (13). Cine CMR shows several signs of MS. Mitral leaflet thickening and bulging (Fig. 16), reduced diastolic opening, abnormal valve motion toward the LV outflow tract, and left atrial enlargement are all common features (13,16). In diastole, there is doming of the valve leaflets with the mitral inflow becoming funnel-like as the chordae become progressively shorter. MS is characterized by a diastolic jet of turbulence that extends from the mitral valve into the LV (Fig. 17). The degree of MS can be evaluated on the size and extent of the abnormal flow jet in the left ventricle in diastole (13). Abnormal flow jets are accurately displayed in any plane or direction with CMR (13). The optimal planes for identifying the signal void corresponding to the abnormal flow jet are the four-chamber view and the sagittal plane encompassing the left atrium and the left ventricle (17).

Velocity-encoded cine-magnetic resonance imaging (VEC-MRI) measures high-velocity jets across stenotic valves. Transmitral peak velocity in MS can be calculated in planes either perpendicular or parallel to the direction of flow. Images can be obtained in the LV short axis plane at three consecutive slices beginning proximal to the mitral coaptation point

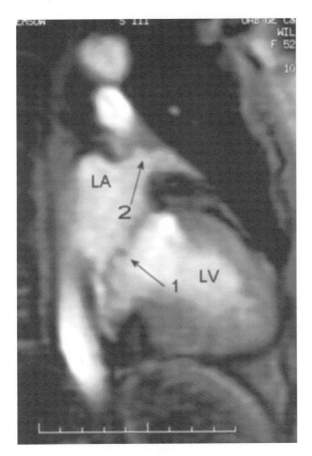

Figure 16 Sagittal two-chamber gradient echo acquisition shows the bulging of the mital valve leaflets (*arrow 1*) into the left ventricle. This plane offers an excellent view of the left atrial appendage (*arrow 2*) for assessment of a clot (not present in this figure). *Abbreviations*: LA, left atrium, LV, left ventricle.

(where the leaflets meet the annulus). Strong correlations were found for measurements of peak velocity and of mitral valve gradient between VEC-MRI and Doppler (18,19).

By using Doppler echocardiography as reference technique, an accuracy rate of 87% was found, whereas the inter-observer reproducibility rate was 96% (20). The pressure gradient across the stenotic mitral valve can be derived using the modified Bernoulli equation (13).

Mitral valve area measurements are strongly related to peak velocity. In MS intervention may be by balloon valvuloplasty or by surgery. Mitral balloon valvulotomy has immediate and longer-term results similar to those of open commissurotomy. Assessment of mitral valve suitability for

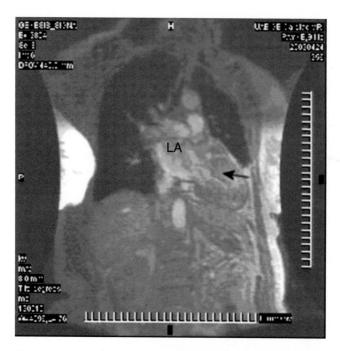

Figure 17   Sagittal two-chamber gradient echo acquisition shows the stenotic jet of mitral stenosis (*arrow*). Note the left atrium is dilated. The severity of stenosis will correlate with the extent of signal void in the left ventricle. *Abbreviation*: LA, left atrium.

percutaneous valvulotomy is of major importance in the management of MS patients, particularly in patients with mild symptoms (15).

For patients with severe MS and grade 3 or 4 mitral regurgitation, percutaneous balloon valvulotomy is contraindicated and VEC-MRI-based quantification of regurgitation may identify patients that qualify for open commissurotomy (15).

Valvuloplasty is most successful when the mitral valve leaflets are mobile and uncalcified but can also be used when the patient is unfit for surgery. Valve area may increase by 50% to 100% with a concomitant fall in pressure gradient, but results are generally less satisfactory than with valve replacement (12).

Mitral Regurgitation

Mitral regurgitation (MR) is related to inadequate closure of the mitral valve so that during systole regurgitant blood is ejected into the left atrium. Anatomic causes are numerous. Mitral regurgitation can be due to abnormalities of the mitral annulus, mitral leaflets, chordae tendinae, or papillary muscles (13,17). MR may be either functional or anatomic.

Rheumatic fever, in which the cusps are scarred and fibrotic is the most common cause worldwide (12). Mitral valve prolapse is the most common cause of regurgitation in the Western world (12). Idiopathic mitral prolapse is usually due to myxomatous degeneration with enlargement of the valve leaflets and elongation of the chordae. Regurgitant jet is usually eccentric and rarely severe (12), while in collagen disorders, such as Marfan's syndrome, a significant regurgitation is more frequent. Congenital abnormalities such as a valvular cleft, accessory or deficient leaflet tissue can cause MR (12).

In endocarditis, MR is caused by destruction or perforation of the cusps (12). Functional lesions are usually related to LV dilatation (12,13), and enlargement of the left atrium. Disturbance of papillary muscle function can be a consequence of ischemic heart disease and dyskinesia. Acute MR may follow chordae tendinae or papillary muscle rupture or valve perforation. There is severe pulmonary hypertension without enlargement of the left atrium (12).

A comprehensive assessment of patients with mitral regurgitation requires:

1. Quantification of regurgitation
2. Assessment of LV function
3. Anatomy of mitral valve and subvalvular apparatus (15)

Whereas CMR satisfies points 1 and 2, the method of choice for assessment of valve anatomy is still echocardiography (15). Spin echo sequences only assess the enlargement of the left ventricle and left atrium secondary to MR (13).

Cine GRE imaging demonstrates, during systole, the presence of a turbulent jet extending from the valve into the left atrium and corresponding to the regurgitant flow (Figs 1–3) (21,22).

In evaluating the accuracy of diagnosis of valvular regurgitation on the basis of the presence of signal loss in the recipient chamber, sensitivity was found to be 93.5% for CMR (23). The area, width, and length of the regurgitant jet or the ratio of the flow void area to the left atrial and LV area can be used to grade the severity of mitral regurgitation (Fig. 7) (13); Lederbogen et al. graded the degree of regurgitation as small if the regurgitant jet area divided by the left atrial area was less than 0.2, moderate if 0.2 to 0.4, and marked if more than 0.4 (24). Good agreement has been found with pulsed and color Doppler echocardiography (13); for regurgitant jet area, r values were 0.93 and 0.89 (24). Nishimura et al. found that the ratio of the area of signal loss to the recipient chamber had the best correlation with angiography (23). The length and area of signal void were planimetered in any view with the largest area, and its ratios to the length and area of the recipient chamber of view were calculated. Each index was significantly higher than the degree calculated by cineangiography.

The measure of the proximal flow convergence zone (PISA) may also offer an accurate method of determining regurgitant volume (25). Thus, cine CMR is a clinically useful noninvasive method in the identification and semi-quantitative assessment of regurgitation severity.

This signal void is often eccentric and should be demonstrated both on the four-chamber view and the vertical long axis view, choosing the image on which the signal void appears larger (13). Cine CMR allows to identify mitral valve prolapse detecting morphological abnormalities such as flail mitral valve leaflets (15). High-resolution images are needed to identify small, mobile vegetations, and nodules (12). Flow velocity mapping techniques allow the quantitative assessment of the mitral regurgitation. Mitral valve flow velocity mapping of forward flow through the mitral annulus has shown an accuracy rate of 90% and an inter-observer reproducibility rate of 93% (20).

Direct measurement of regurgitation is made difficult by signal loss from turbulence, complexity of the mitral apparatus geometry, the frequent occurrence of eccentric jets and the movement of the atrioventricular valves during the systole (26). Mitral motion may be corrected using different imaging planes and using the slice positioned at the annulus, or by automatic correction for through-plane motion (20), with moving slice velocity mapping technique (27). A consequence of mitral regurgitation is an increase in the total stroke volume of the left ventricle (13,17).

In patients without aortic insufficiency, the regurgitant fraction can be indirectly evaluated by measuring ventricular volumes with cine CMR sequences and Simpson's rule. Mitral regurgitant volume corresponds to the difference between the left and right ventricular stroke volume (13,20). Hundley et al. found excellent correlation between cardiac catheterization and CMR assessments of left regurgitant fraction ($r = 0.96$) (28).

In single valve disease, mitral regurgitation can also be quantified with VEC-MRI using forward flow through the mitral annulus and in the ascending aorta in a plane perpendicular to the vessel (13). Normally these values are identical. As LV inflow is increased in mitral regurgitation, the difference between the areas of the two curves gives the mitral regurgitation volume (13).

Fujita et al. found that the regurgitant fraction correlated well with the echocardiographic severity of mitral regurgitation ($r = 0.87$) (29). The best way to quantify the volume of mitral regurgitation is probably to combine ventricular volume measurements obtained with cine gradient echo CMR imaging with measurements of forward flow in the aorta obtained with VEC MRI (13). The regurgitant volume index is calculated by subtracting the forward flow volume in the proximal aorta from the LV stroke volume obtained with volume measurements.

Echocardiography easily determines mitral valve morphology and provides a grading of regurgitation severity. However, measurements of the length and area of the mitral regurgitant jet obtained with this technique are only semiquantitative (13). CMR imaging allows a quantitative assessment of the regurgitant volume (13), so that severity of mitral regurgitation is quantified/confirmed by CMR (15). Moreover, CMR is an alternative for the evaluation of patients with suboptimal echocardiographic windows. Patients with ischemic mitral regurgitation have a considerably worse prognosis than that in other causes of mitral regurgitation (15). CMR can play a major role in patient management, accurately assessing LV function, morphology and quantifying the severity of the regurgitation.

Pulmonic Stenosis

Pulmonic stenosis is usually congenital and the result of the fusion of the commissures. If severe enough, it can lead to right ventricular hypertrophy and dilatation or even right heart failure. Echocardiography has traditionally been the first test but CMR affords a far better look at the right ventricle and its outflow tract. Therefore, CMR can be used as first line in assessment of pulmonic valve disease. Spin echo sequences can show the morphology of the valve, although this information can be obtained from gradient echo cine sequences as well (30). Axial or coronal planes can be used to set up a gradient echo cine sagittal plane (Fig. 18) that provides an excellent look at the right ventricular outflow tract and the pulmonic valve. The degree of abnormal flow jet is indicative of the severity of the stenosis just as it is in the case of aortic stenosis or mitral regurgitation. This plane can be used to do PC imaging to obtain maximum velocity and calculate maximum gradient across the valve (Fig. 19) (31). This information can assist in the timing of intervention, usually percutaneous valvuloplasty.

Pulmonic Regurgitation

The ability of CMR ability to view the right ventricular outflow tract and pulmonic valve makes it the ideal method to evaluate pulmonic regurgitation. The underlying causes of pulmonic regurgitation include annular dilatation as a result of pulmonary hypertension or surgical correction of tetralogy of Fallot, pulmonic stenosis, or other malformations of the pulmonic valve or right ventricular outflow tract. Traditional methods used to study this abnormality include echocardiography and X-ray angiography but neither can provide the type of evaluation that CMR makes possible.

Cine gradient echo sequences in sagittal plane (Fig. 19) are the best to view the right ventricular outflow tract, pulmonic valve, and proximal portion of main pulmonary artery. In this view, a semi-qualitative assessment of pulmonic regurgitation can be made based on the degree of signal void in the right ventricle in diastole proximal to the pulmonic valve. Also, with this

(A)   **(C)**

(B)

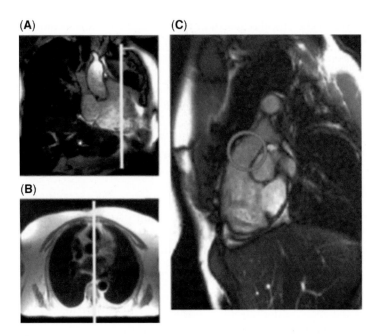

Figure 18 Coronal gradient echo (**A**) and axial spin echo (**B**) sequences can be used to get a sagittal view (**C**) of the right ventricular outflow tract and pulmonic valve (*circle*).

view along with the coronal GRE or axial four-chamber view, it is possible to assess right ventricular volumes and function.

PC imaging is an ideal tool to assess the regurgitant volume and fraction directly (31,32). Using the sagittal images of the right ventricle, PC sequence can be set up perpendicular to the direction of the flow between the pulmonic valve and pulmonary artery bifurcation (Fig. 20). Resulting magnitude and phase images are used to calculate average velocity, while the product of area and velocity gives flow in each time frame. The velocity can be integrated to give forward flow, regurgitant flow, and net forward flow for the cycle. This is a direct method of quantifying the regurgitant volume and fraction in pulmonic regurgitation.

Tricuspid Regurgitation

Tricuspid regurgitation occurs as a consequence of a number of cardiac disorders such as pulmonary hypertension, Ebstein's anomaly, right ventricular pressure overload as a result of pulmonic stenosis, carcinoid syndrome, Marfan's syndrome, rheumatic disease, and endocarditis. The best views for assessment of tricuspid regurgitation are four-chamber axial and two-chamber sagittal (Fig. 21). It is possible to overlook the signal void caused

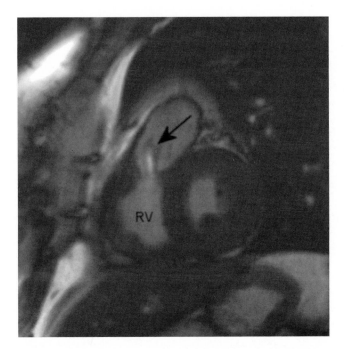

Figure 19 Sagittal cine gradient echo acquisition shows a high velocity jet (*arrow*) through the stenotic aortic valve. This is the best view to evaluate the right ventricular outflow tract and pulmonic valve and also the best plane to use for planning the PC sequence to quantify the degree of stenosis. Also, note right ventricular hypertrophy. *Abbreviation*: RV, right ventricle.

by tricuspid regurgitation in the steady-state free precession sequences because they are not as sensitive to dephasing due to their shorter TE times. Also, since the right ventricle is a lower pressure chamber and the velocities generated may not be as high as those generated by the left ventricle, the signal void generated by tricuspid regurgitation may not be as obvious as mitral or aortic regurgitation. When assessing tricuspid regurgitation, gradient echo sequences with longer TE should be used to assure detection of the regurgitant jet. VENC can be used to obtain the maximum velocity across the tricuspid valve in tricuspid regurgitation. By using the modified Bernouli's equation right atrial pressure and pulmonary artery systolic pressures can be estimated. PC imaging can also be used to get the regurgitant volumes (33).

Prosthetic Valves

Patients with prosthetic valves can be safely imaged with CMR (34). However, there is a local artifact produced by the metal in the prosthetic valve.

(A)   (B)

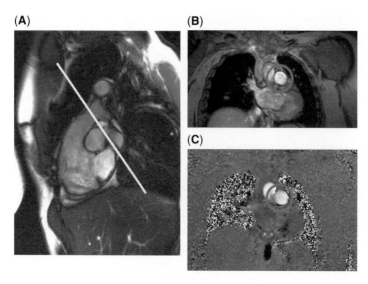

(C)

Figure 20 (A) Sagittal gradient echo through the right ventricle and pulmonic valve is the best plane to use to do velocity-encoded sequences on the pulmonic valve. Note the (B) magnitude images and (C) phase images.

Spin echo images do not show the artifact and are helpful in evaluating the area around the valve. It is also possible to see vegetations or clots around the valve with these sequences. Gradient echo sequences, however, show an obvious artifact around the valve. It is not possible to assess for vegetations

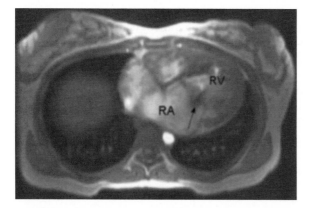

Figure 21 Axial gradient echo four-chamber acquisition shows tricuspid regurgitation (*arrow*) in corrected transposition of great arteries. Note the anatomical RV posterior and to the left. There is an Ebstein's malformation of the tricuspid valve and most of the RV is atrialized. RA is dilated. *Abbreviations*: RV, right ventricle; RA, right atrium.

or clots with these sequences. GRE sequences, however, can assess for presence of stenosis or regurgitation that may be beyond what would normally be expected with a prosthetic valve. Using PC imaging, maximum velocity across the valve can be measured and from that, the gradient calculated using Bernouli's equation (35–37). Also, regurgitant volume and fraction can be quantified using these sequences.

Endocarditis

Echocardiography remains the gold standard in assessment of vegetations or clots on the valve leaflets. Transesophageal echocardiography affords an excellent look at the structure of the valve and its supporting structures. CMR imaging does not show the valvular structure as well because of the motion of the valves. However, with the introduction of pulse sequences based on steady-state free precession, the visualization of the valvular apparatus has improved significantly (38–40). Spin echo and GRE sequences allow visualization of the paravalvular apparatus better than echocardiography because of the larger field of view and resolution. PC sequences permit the quantification of hemodynamic abnormalities associated with endocarditis.

CONCLUSIONS

While echocardiography remains the non-invasive gold-standard for direct imaging of normal and diseased valves, CMR also can provide a means to depict and quantitate valvular disease and its severity. This chapter describes the CMR findings in valvular stenosis, regurgitation, vegetations, and other valvular pathologies. CMR can accurately assess the volumes and masses of the RV and/or LV enable reliable determination of stroke volumes and reguritant volumes. Another approach to assessment of the severity of valvular regurgitation and stenosis is analogous to Doppler ultrasonography and is known as velocity mapping. CMR and echocardiography are complementary technologies for the assessment of patients with valvular heart disease, providing a comprehensive picture of the severity of disease of the valve and the impact of that disease on atrial and ventricular function.

REFERENCES

1. Natale L, Meduri A, Caltavuturo C, Palladino F, Marano P. MRI assessment of ventricular function. Rays 2001; 26:35–44.
2. Schmidt M, Crnac J, Dederichs B, Theissen P, Schicha H, Sechtem U. Magnetic resonance imaging in valvular heart disease. Int J Card Imaging 1997; 13:219–231.
3. Didier D, Ratib O, Lerch R, Friedli B. Detection and quantification of valvular heart disease with dynamic cardiac MR imaging. Radiographics 2000; 20:1279–1299.

4. Lotz J, Meier C, Leppert A, Galanski M. Cardiovascular flow measurement with PC MR imaging: basic facts and implementation. Radiographics 2002; 22: 651–671.
5. Tan RS, Mohiaddin RH. Cardiovascular applications of magnetic resonance flow measurement. Rays 2001; 26:71–91.
6. Didier D. Assessment of valve disease: qualitative and quantitative. Magn Reson Imaging Clin N Am 2003; 11:115–134.
7. John AS, Dill T, Brandt RR, et al. Magnetic resonance to assess the aortic valve area in aortic stenosis: how does it compare to current diagnostic standards? J Am Coll Cardiol 2003; 42:519–526.
8. Kupari M, Hekali P, Keto P, et al. Assessment of aortic valve area in aortic stenosis by magnetic resonance imaging. Am J Cardiol 1992; 70:952–955.
9. Schwitter J. Valvular heart disease: assessment of valve morphology and quantification using MR. Herz 2000; 25:342–355.
10. Sondergaard L, Stahlberg F, Thomsen C. Magnetic resonance imaging of valvular heart disease. J Magn Reson Imaging 1999; 10:627–638.
11. Eichenberger AC, Jenni R, von Schulthess GK. Aortic valve pressure gradients in patients with aortic valve stenosis: quantification with velocity-encoded cine MR imaging. Am J Roentgenol 1993; 160:971–977.
12. Lipton MJ, Coulden R. Valvular heart disease. Radiol Clin North Am 1999; 37:319–339.
13. Didier D, Ratib O, Lerch R, Friedli B. Detection and quantification of valvular heart disease with dynamic cardiac MR imaging. Radiographics 2000; 20:1279–1299; discussion 1299–1301.
14. Glockner JF, Johnston DL, McGee KP. Evaluation of cardiac valvular disease with MR imaging: qualitative and quantitative techniques. Radiographics 2003; 23:e9.
15. Schwitter J. Valvular heart disease: assessment of valve morphology and quantification using MR. Herz 2000; 25:342–355.
16. Casolo GC, Zampa V, Rega L, et al. Evaluation of mitral stenosis by cine magnetic resonance imaging. Am Heart J 1992; 123:1252–1260.
17. Didier D. Assessment of valve disease: qualitative and quantitative. Magn Reson Imaging Clin N Am 2003; 11:115–134, vii.
18. Heidenreich PA, Steffens J, Fujita N, et al. Evaluation of mitral stenosis with velocity-encoded cine-magnetic resonance imaging. Am J Cardiol 1995; 75:365–369.
19. Kilner PJ, Manzara CC, Mohiaddin RH, et al. Magnetic resonance jet velocity mapping in mitral and aortic valve stenosis. Circulation 1993; 87:1239–1248.
20. Sondergaard L, Stahlberg F, Thomsen C. Magnetic resonance imaging of valvular heart disease. J Magn Reson Imaging 1999; 10:627–638.
21. Kizilbash AM, Hundley WG, Willett DL, Franco F, Peshock RM, Grayburn PA. Comparison of quantitative Doppler with magnetic resonance imaging for assessment of the severity of mitral regurgitation. Am J Cardiol 1998; 81:792–795.
22. Higgins CB, Wagner S, Kondo C, Suzuki J, Caputo GR. Evaluation of valvular heart disease with cine gradient echo magnetic resonance imaging. Circulation 1991; 84(3 suppl):I198–I207.

23. Nishimura F, Yoshino Y, Mihara J, Kamiya H, Ichikawa S, Kimura M. Advantage of cine-MR imaging for the evaluation of valvular regurgitation. Jpn Circ J 1990; 54:288–291.

24. Lederbogen F, Rottbauer W, Krahe T, Schanzenbacher P, Nellessen U. Noninvasive quantification of aortic and mitral insufficiency. Comparison of dynamic magnetic resonance imaging and Doppler color echocardiography. Dtsch Med Wochenschr 1994; 119:611–617.

25. Schmidt M, Crnac J, Dederichs B, Theissen P, Schicha H, Sechtem U. Magnetic resonance imaging in valvular heart disease. Int J Card Imaging 1997; 13:219–231.

26. Tan RS, Mohiaddin RH. Cardiovascular applications of magnetic resonance flow measurement. Rays 2001; 26:71–91.

27. Kozerke S, Schwitter J, Pedersen EM, Boesiger P. Aortic and mitral regurgitation: quantification using moving slice velocity mapping. J Magn Reson Imaging 2001; 14:106–112.

28. Hundley WG, Li HF, Willard JE, et al. Magnetic resonance imaging assessment of the severity of mitral regurgitation. Comparison with invasive techniques. Circulation 1995; 92:1151–1158.

29. Fujita N, Chazouilleres AF, Hartiala JJ, et al. Quantification of mitral regurgitation by velocity-encoded cine nuclear magnetic resonance imaging. J Am Coll Cardiol 1994; 23:951–958.

30. Kivelitz DE, Dohmen PM, Lembcke A, et al. Visualization of the pulmonary valve using cine MR imaging. Acta Radiol 2003; 44:172–176.

31. Reid SA, Walker PG, Fisher J, et al. The quantification of pulmonary valve hemodynamics using MRI. Int J Cardiovasc Imaging 2002; 18:217–225.

32. Li W, Davlouros PA, Kilner PJ, et al. Doppler-echocardiographic assessment of pulmonary regurgitation in adults with repaired tetralogy of Fallot: comparison with cardiovascular magnetic resonance imaging. Am Heart J 2004; 147:165–172.

33. Kayser HV, Stoel BC, van der Wall EE, et al. MR velocity mapping of tricuspid flow: correction for through-plane motion. J Magn Reson Imaging 1997; 7:669–673.

34. Wyttenback R, Bremerich J, Saeed M, et al. Integrated MR imaging approach to valvular heart disease. Cardiol Clin 1998; 16:277–294.

35. Botnar R, Nagel E, Scheidegger MB, et al. Assessment of prosthetic aortic valve performance by magnetic resonance velocity imaging. MAGMA 2000; 10:18–26.

36. Hasenkam JM, Ringgaard S, Houlind K, Botnar RM, et al. Prosthetic heart valve evaluation by magnetic resonance imaging. Eur J Cardiothorac Surg 1999; 16:300–305.

37. Walker PG, Pederson EM, Oyre S, et al. Magnetic resonance velocity imaging: a new method for prosthetic heart valve study. J Heart Valve Dis 1995; 4:296–307.

38. Botnar R, Nagel E, Scheidegger MB, et al. Assessment of prosthetic aortic valve performance by magnetic resonance velocity imaging. MAGMA 2000; 10:18–26.

39. Hasenkam JM, Ringgaard S, Houlind K, et al. Prosthetic heart valve evaluation by magnetic resonance imaging. Eur J Cardiothorac Surg 1999; 16:300–305.

40. Walker PG, Pederson EM, Oyre S, et al. Magnetic resonance velocity imaging: a new method for prosthetic heart valve study. J Heart Valve Dis 1995; 4:296–307.

7

Magnetic Resonance Imaging of Congenital Heart Disease

Ronald M. Razmi

Cardiovascular MR/CT Center and Heart Center of Indiana, The Care Group, LLC, Indianapolis, Indiana, U.S.A.

Benigno Soto

Department of Radiology and Medicine, Cardiovascular MRI Laboratory, University of Alabama, Birmingham, Alabama, U.S.A.

INTRODUCTION

Cardiovascular magnetic resonance (CMR) examination of congenital heart disease has significant advantages over existing technologies. Due to its large field of view and superior resolution, CMR enables the clinician to study the complex relationship between various structures in great detail. Many of the patients with congenital heart disease live to adulthood nowadays and some have undergone multiple surgeries. CMR offers different methods of evaluating patency of conduits and existence of leaks in baffles. These include cine CMR, dark-blood spin echo, and phase contrast imaging. Due to its unlimited choice of imaging planes, CMR enables the clinicians to find answers critical to medical or surgical management of these patients.

Not only does CMR afford the visualization of complex anatomy and surgical results, but also it provides important hemodynamic information. Using velocity mapping, CMR can quantitate shunt fractions and obtain data on stenotic and regurgitant valves or surgically created connections.

Although the CMR examination of children with congenital heart disease is more challenging due to their inability to hold their breath, CMR still offers a wealth of anatomical information with spin echo sequences.

ATRIAL MORPHOLOGY AND ISOMERISM

The right or left atria are characterized by their atrial appendages. The right atrial appendage is a triangular structure with a broad junction with the rest of the atrium. The pectinate muscles extend from the appendage to the vestibule of the right atrioventricular (AV) junction. Crista terminalis divides the right atrium into a smooth posterior portion and a trabeculated anterior part. In contrast, the left appendage is a tubular structure with a narrow junction with the rest of the atrium. The left atrium's pectinate muscles are confined to the anterior quadrant of the vestibule. It does not have a crista terminalis (1). The right atrium receives drainage and inferior and superior vena cava. The left atrium receives from the pulmonary veins. The morphology of the normal appendages is well visualized on axial and sagittal sections of the heart and on sections which follow the long axis of each appendage (Figs. 1 and 2).

Atrial isomerism is a condition in which the right-sided and left-sided atria, normally different, instead are morphologically similar (2,3). There are two varieties of atrial isomerism: the hearts with right isomerism have the right- and left-sided atrial appendages with the morphology of a normal right atrial appendage. In left atrial isomerism, the two atrial appendages have the morphology of the normal left atrial appendages. Atrial isomerism

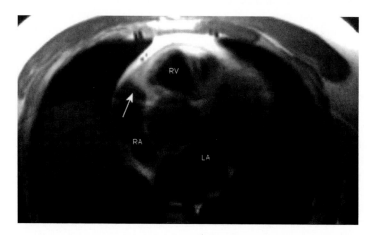

Figure 1 Axial spin echo acquisition shows the right atrial appendage (*arrow*). Note the wide orifice of the appendage. *Abbreviations*: LA, left atrium; RA, right atrium; RV, right ventricle.

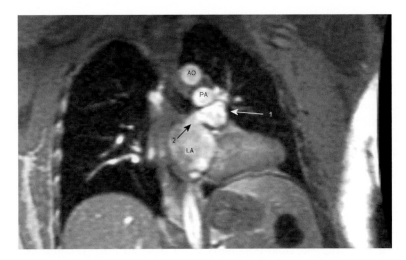

Figure 2 Right anterior oblique sagittal gradient echo acquisition shows the left atrial appendage (*arrow 1*). Note the narrow junction (*arrow 2*) with the left atrium. *Abbreviations*: PA, pulmonary artery; AO, aortic arch.

is usually associated with visceral heterotaxy. The right isomerism is associated with asplenia and left isomerism with polysplenia, however, this association is not invariable. Thoracic isomerism is usually present in patients with atrial isomerism (4).

Hearts with atrial isomerism show ambiguous AV connections. Two varieties are described: right ambiguous AV connection, in hearts with normally related ventricles; and left ambiguous AV connections, in hearts with the ventricles in an inverted relationship (2). Atrial isomerism is usually associated with a wide variety of cardiac and extracardiac malformations: anomalies in the systemic venous return are common in hearts with left atrial isomerism; such as absence of inferior cava vein with the azygos extension of the Inferior vena cava (IVC), which enters the superior caval vein. Bilateral superior vena cava occurs in 85% of patients with left atrial isomerism.

Axial and coronal sections of the heart on spin echo sequences will delineate the cardiac axis, the positions of the atrial and ventricular chambers and great arteries as well as the abdominal viscera. The morphology of the atrial appendages is well seen on planes along the longitudinal sections of these cavities (Fig. 2). The systemic and pulmonary venous connection is depicted on three-dimensional (3D) thoracic angiograms.

A complete analysis of the entire cardiovascular system is mandatory in patients with atrial isomerism, due to high incidence of the associated anomalies. The associated thoracic isomerism can be identified in coronal sections of the thorax, which will show the bronchial morphology of the isomeric lungs.

ANOMALIES OF THE AV CONNECTION

The AV connection describes the junction of the atria and ventricles. In a normal heart, the right atrium connects with the right ventricle through the tricuspid valve and the left atrium connects to the left ventricle through the mitral valve; the AV connection is concordant. Discordant AV connection occurs when each atrium is connected to a morphologically inappropriate ventricle. In hearts with atrial isomerism, the AV connection is nor concordant or discordant but ambiguous. It is then categorized by the ventricular relationship as: normally related ventricles or inverted ventricles. When the right and left atria are connected to one ventricular chamber by two AV valves, the AV connection considered a double inlet to the morphological right or left ventricle. In such arrangement, the ventricle, which does not have AV valve, is hypoplastic and usually incomplete (Fig. 3) (3). The anomaly is also defined as univentricular AV connection of right or left type. The final possibility is for both atria to be connected to a solitary or indeterminate ventricle; the condition is double inlet to indeterminate ventricle. In this context, one AV valve may be connected to both ventricular chambers; the valves are then overriding the ventricular septum. In addition, the chordae tendinae, supporting leaflets of the over-riding valve, may be straddling the ventricular septum.

A discordant AV connection describes a congenital anomaly in which the right atrium connects with the morphologically left ventricle; and the left

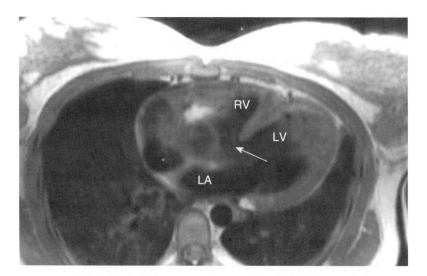

Figure 3 Axial spin echo acquisition of a heart with one functional ventricle; left ventricle. The right ventricle is hypoplastic. Notice the large ventricular septal defect (*arrow*). There is only one functional atrioventricular connection. *Abbreviations*: LV, left ventricle; RV, right ventricle; LA, left atrium.

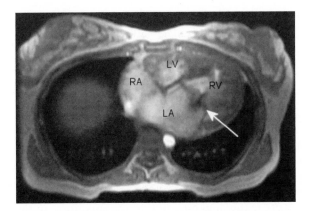

Figure 4   Gradient echo axial acquisition of a 23-year-old female with congenitally corrected transposition of great arteries. Note the morphologic right ventricle is posterior and to the left. The morphologic left ventricle is anterior and to the right. Note the Ebstein's abnormality (*arrow*) involving the left atrioventricular valve. *Abbreviations*: LV, left ventricle; RV, right ventricle; LA, left atrium; RA, right atrium.

atrium connects with the morphologically right ventricle. AV discordant connection may occur in hearts with atrial situs solitus or in hearts with situs inversus. The ventricles are themselves abnormally located: the right ventricle is in posterior and left position and the left ventricle is anterior and to the right (Fig. 4). The ventricular septum is usually straight and oriented from left to right. The cardiac axis is oriented anterior, inferior and to the left. However, dextrocardia is present in 25% of the patients. The ventriculo-arterial connection in hearts with discordant AV connections is also discordant; the association is called congenitally corrected transposition of the great arteries. Less common ventriculo-arterial connections are: double outlet right ventricle, double outlet left ventricle, and concordant ventriculo-arterial connection, also called isolated ventricular inversion.

CMR imaging of these patients involves axial multislice spin echo and cine gradient echo sequences to view the connections between the atria and ventricles, as well as the postoperative patency of conduits and baffles. From the axial slices, oblique coronal or sagittal planes can be prescribed to further delineate connections. Cine sequences are especially useful in assessment of shunts and leaks.

THE VENTRICULO-ARTERIAL CONNECTION

The majority of the hearts have two ventriculo-arterial connections, guarded by two arterial valves or by a common arterial valve. In the presence of a common arterial valve, there is a common arterial trunk. But, single outlet of the heart can also exist when the pulmonary trunk or the aorta is atretic.

In summary, the ventriculo-arterial connections are: concordant, discordant, (also called transposition), double outlet and single outlet of the heart. Transposition of the great arteries describes a cardiac malformation in which the pulmonary artery arises from the left ventricle and the aorta from the morphologically right ventricle, which results in a parallel systemic–pulmonary circulation (Fig. 5). The life in the days after birth depends on the patent foramen ovale. At the closure of the foramen ovale, the intracardiac shunt will end and life support will not be possible (5).

The anatomy of the atria is basically normal in hearts with situs solitus; although there is frequently a patent foramen ovale or an atrial septal defect (ASD). The ventricular anatomy is not quite normal; the right ventricular outflow tract is parallel to the left ventricle outlet; in such a manner that the septum is a straight structure and does not do the curvatures of the normal septum. The pulmonary valve is not wedged as deep as is the aorta in normal hearts. The result is a short AV septum in complete transposition of the arteries. The ventricular thickness is abnormal. The left ventricle is mildly thicker than the right ventricle at birth. The right ventricle rapidly becomes thicker in the first two years of life and it becomes thicker than the left (6).

The segmental chamber localization in complete transposition of the great arteries shows situs solitus of the atria, normally related ventricles, concordant AV connection and discordant ventriculo-arterial connection. The anatomy is well visualized on axial, coronal, and sagittal sections (Fig. 5). The caval veins terminate at the right atrium and the pulmonary veins into the left atrium. The ventricular chambers are in normal relationship. The outlets, however, are parallel to each other, making the entire septum visible in coronal sections. The arterial valves are also seen clearly in these sections. In hearts with cardiac axis malposition, the images are prescribed following the long axial diameter. Short axis section of the ventricles and atria is ideal to verify the morphology and calculate functional parameters. Cine CMR pulse sequences allow assessment of valvular function and chamber volumes, and phase velocity mapping provides a means to quantitate flow.

Atrial Septal Defect

Magnetic resonance offers multiple methods for assessment of interatrial shunts, such as ASDs. The true ASD can exist only within the area of the fossa ovalis. The defect is called secundum ASD (7). Although spin echo sequences in axial or short axis can reveal a structural defect in the interatrial septum, care must be taken to not diagnose an ASD based solely on this observation. This is due to the fact that normal septa can some times appear as though they have a break in their contour. The most definitive way of making this diagnosis would be to observe a jet from left to right or right to left in the area of the defect (Fig. 6). One of the best ways to

(A)   (B)

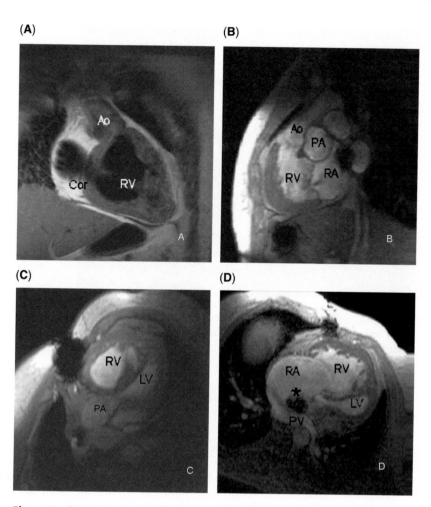

(C)   (D)

Figure 5   Complete transposition of great arteries postoperative after atrial switch. (A) Spin echo coronal. The right coronary artery can be seen. (B) Cine Gradiant Recalled Echo (GRE) along the right ventricular outflow tract. The aorta is connected to the right ventricle; mild tricuspid insufficiency. (C) Cine GRE along the left ventricular outflow tract. The pulmonary artery is connected to the left ventricle. (D) Axial GRE evidence of the previous atrial switch surgery. Pulmonary veins blood is redirected toward the right artrium. A metallic artifact (∗) is related to the atrial septum defect closure device. *Abbreviations*: Ao, aortic arch; Cor, coronary artery; RV, right ventricle; LV, left ventricle; RA, right atrium; PA, pulmonary artery.

diagnose an ASD is to inject gadolinium-DTPA and observe its passage through the right atrium (8). As the contrast brightens the signal in the right atrium, a dark jet can be observed coming through the atrial septum from the left atrium (Fig. 7). Conversely, if there is a right to left shunt, a leak

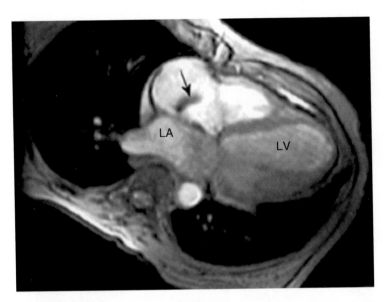

Figure 6 Axial gradient echo acquisition shows the left atrium to right atrium jet of an ostium secundum atrial septal defects (*arrow*). *Abbreviations*: LA, left atrium; LV, left ventricle.

of the contrast agent into the left side can be seen. To assure a complete evaluation of the atria, the best sequence will be short axis cine with a long echo time, using thin slices without a gap between them. The ratio of the pulmonary flow to systemic flow can be quantified by obtaining right and left stroke volumes with phase contrast imaging at the level of the aortic and pulmonic valves (9,10).

The sinus venosus defect provides the potential for interatrial shunting either because the caval veins or the right pulmonary veins are connected to both the right and left atrial chambers. Sinus venosus ASD is often associated with a partial anomalous return of the right superior pulmonary vein. Performing axial cine slices with thin sections near the top of the heart offers an excellent view of the superior vena cava and the right superior pulmonary vein and their connections to the right and left atria. In the case of a sinus venosus ASD, the right superior pulmonary vein is often visualized joining the superior vena cava and this, in turn, connects to the both atria through a high defect (Fig. 8).

Ostium premum ASD involves the AV valves and often involves other septal defects. Axial cine slices with long Echo Time (TE) often show the left to right shunting (Fig. 9). Patent foramen ovale (PFO) in the absence of atrial shunting is difficult to verify by CMR. A right to left shunt through PFO in patients with normal intracavitary pressures occurs immediately after valsalva maneuver. The diagnosis of PFO on CMR should include:

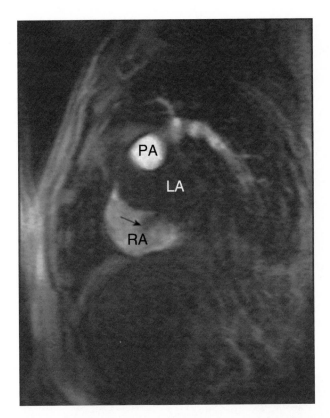

Figure 7 Short axis first-pass acquisition through the atria in atrial septal defect. Note the dark jet (*arrow*) from the dark left atrium into the bright right atrium. The contrast has arrived in the right atrium and pulmonary artery but has not yet arrived in the left atrium. *Abbreviations*: PA, pulmonary artery; LA, left artrium; RA, right artrium.

size, the degree of the septum premum defect during normal respiration and during valsalva maneuver, aneurysm of the artial septum and Chiari network. Short axis first-pass cine sequence with injection of gadolinium-DTPA at atrial level, immediately after Valsalva respiration, has been utilized recently for detecting right to left shunt. CMR angiography of the thorax with low doses of contrast is another new development that allows for images to be acquired in a shorter period of time and allows visualization of the contrast media in a similar manner to standard angiography.

Ventricular Septal Defect

Perimembranous ventricular septal defects (VSDs) are characterized by their relation to the central fibrous body; the aortic valve, septal leaflet of the

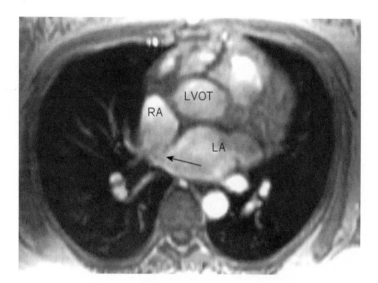

Figure 8 Axial gradient echo acquisition showing sinus venosum atrial septal defect. Note the defect in the interatrial septum (*arrow*). *Abbreviations*: LA, left atrium; RA, right atrium; LVOT, left ventricular outflow tract.

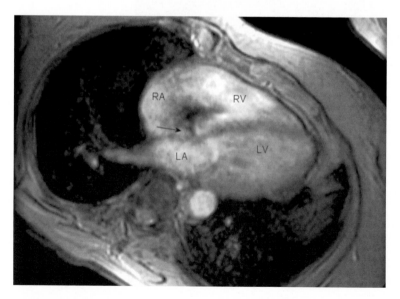

Figure 9 Axial gradient echo acquisition shows left to right jet (*arrow*) near the atrioventricular valves indicating an ostium premum atrial septal defect. There is also tricuspid insufficiency. *Abbreviations*: LA, left atrium; LV, left ventricle; RA, right atrium; RV, right ventricle.

tricuspid valve, and the AV septum (11,12). These are seen through axial four-chamber views at multiple levels. The inlet extension of the perimembranous defect is best seen on sections transverse to the aortic valve (Fig. 10), where the imaging void will show its presence upward around the crista supraventricularis. Tricuspid insufficiency involving the most medial part of the leaflet is seen in four-chamber cine sequences as a signal void in the right atrium during ventricular systole.

Juxta arterial VSDs are best demonstrated by their relation or contiguity with aortic or pulmonic valves. Multiple spin echo sections perpendicular to the outlet septum shows the borders of the defect and its extension into the muscular component (13).

Muscular defects are located in the inlet, trabecular and outlet; they are not contiguous with the arterial or AV valves (11,12). Short axis slices through the interventricular septum with no gap between the slices, and long TE should reveal a high velocity jet from left to right (Fig. 11).

The status of the aortic and pulmonic valves is important to verify in patients with VSDs in juxtaarterial positions. CMR flow studies are able to estimate the degree of left to right shunt; large defects with large left to right shunt are candidates for early repair.

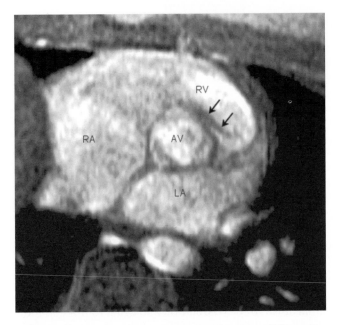

Figure 10 Gradient echo oblique sections parallel to the aortic valve show a perimembranous ventricular septal defect. Note the dark jet (*arrows*) into the right ventricle under the aortic valve. *Abbreviations*: LA, left atrium; RA, right atrium; RV, right ventricle; AV, aortic valve.

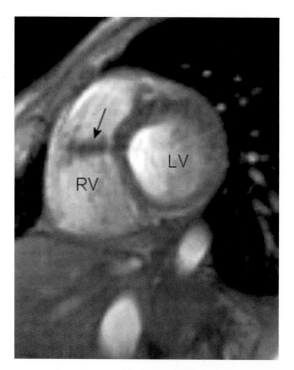

Figure 11 Short axis gradient echo acquisition shows a left to right jet (*arrow*) of muscular ventricular septal defect. *Abbreviations*: LV, left ventricle; RV, right ventricle.

Coarctation of the Aorta

Coarctation of the aorta is a congenital narrowing of the upper descending thoracic aorta adjacent to the site of attachment of the ductus arteriosus, which is sufficiently severe that there is pressure gradient across the area. Coarctation varies in severity; when it is localized, the lumen must be reduced in cross-sectional area by more than 50% before there is pressure gradient across it, but longer tubular coarctation may be hemodynamically significant with lesser narrowing. Occasionally the adult aorta may be redundant and severely kinked opposite to the ligamentum arteriosum without a significant pressure gradient, the so-called pseudocoarctation or non-obstructive coarctation.

Coarctation may be associated with anomalies of the aortic arch, VSD, bicuspid aortic valve, and sub-aortic stenosis. The collateral circulation between proximal aorta to the coarctation and distal to it is common. CMR is an extremely effective tool in assessment of these patients. Sagittal right anterior oblique slices prescribed using the axial slices can show the entire length of the ascending aorta, aortic arch, and descending aorta (Fig. 12) (14). This affords an excellent view of the stenosis and its

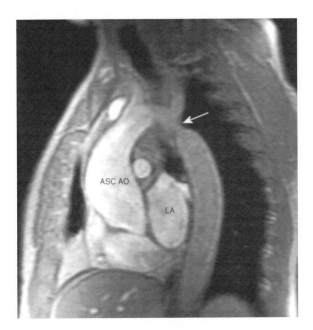

Figure 12 Gradient echo sagittal section through the thorax shows the ascending aorta, aortic arch, and descending aorta. Note the stenosis in proximal descending aorta (*arrow*). This is the best view to see the abnormality of coarctation in relation to the surrounding structures. *Abbreviation*: LA, left atrium; ASC AO, ascending aorta.

relationship with the surrounding structures. Phase contrast imaging allows quantification of the degree of stenosis. Oblique cine sequences to view the morphology of the aortic valve are mandatory since there is a high incidence of bicuspid aortic valve in patients with coarctation (Fig. 13). Short axis cine slices through the ventricles allow assessment of left ventricular function assessment and presence of VSDs and hypertrophy.

ANOMALOUS PULMONARY VENOUS CONNECTIONS

Anomalous pulmonary venous connection describes an abnormal connection of the pulmonary veins to the right atrium either directly or through venous tributaries. The anomalous connection may include the entire venous return; the total anomalous venous connection or only a portion of the venous return; the partial form.

In total anomalous venous return, the entire pulmonary venous return is connected with the right atrium either directly or through venous tributaries. There are three varieties of this connection according to the way the venous return reaches the right atrium: (i) *supracardiac*: the pulmonary venous return connects with the systemic venous channel above the right

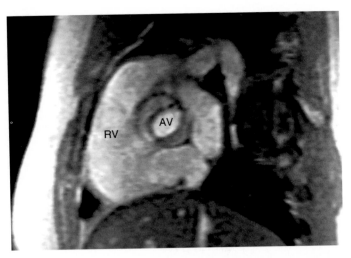

Figure 13 Oblique gradient echo acquisition in a plane parallel to the aortic valve in a 28-year-old with coarctation. This demonstrates the morphology of the aortic valve, which is bicuspid in this patient. *Abbreviations*: AV, aortic valve; RV, right ventricle.

atrium; (ii) *cardiac*: the pulmonary venous return connects directly to the right atrium or to the coronary sinus; and (iii) *infracardiac*: the venous return connects with a separate vascular structure, which, in turn, connects with the systemic veins below the diaphragm (15). In some hearts with supracardiac total anomalous venous return, the common pulmonary venous sinus, while separate from the left atrium, is in potential contact with this structure, resembling the morphology seen in certain cases of cor triatriatum (16).

Hearts with total anomalous venous return show significant changes: enlargement of the right ventricle due to volume. Stenosis in the anomalous venous channel may result in venous obstruction and pulmonary edema. The most common variety with this complication is the infra-cardiac venous return, less common is in the supracardiac variety and rare in the cardiac variety.

The abnormal connection of the common venous channel is well seen on spin echo and gradient echo cine sequences viewing the coronal, transverse, and sagittal planes. The morphology of the left atrium is characterized by the absence of its normal superior border. The draining channels are usually well seen on the standard sections. Three-dimensional angiography of the thorax with gadolinium-DTPA enhancement is able to show the entire thoracic vasculature and its abnormal connections. In the postoperative period, CMR studies may detect errors, which are fortunately rare. Residual stenosis in the pulmonary veins may result in increasing the pulmonary vascular resistance. CMR flow studies of individual pulmonary veins may detect the abnormality.

In partial anomalous pulmonary venous return, there is an anomalous connection of the individual pulmonary veins to the right atrium or its tributaries. They are as follows: (i) anomalous pulmonary venous connection to the right atrium associated with ASD of sinus venous type (Fig. 14), (ii) anomalous venous connection to the superior vena cava, not associated with ASD (Fig. 15); (iii) partial anomalous pulmonary venous connection to the left brachiocephalic vein, and (iv) anomalous venous connection to the inferior vena cava. The lungs from which the anomalous veins come from are usually hypoplastic. In half of the patients, the abnormal lung is supplied by systemic arteries originating in the thoracic aorta (17).

Axial cine sequences are the best sequences to visualize the connection of the anomalous pulmonary vein to various structures such as superior vena cava. Oblique planes are often necessary to view the connection clearly. Three-dimensional CMR angiography of the thorax will depict the entire vascular structure in great detail. The anomalous venous return results in a left to right shunt, with right heart overload and dilated pulmonary arteries. The severity of the shunt can be estimated by phase velocity mapping of flow.

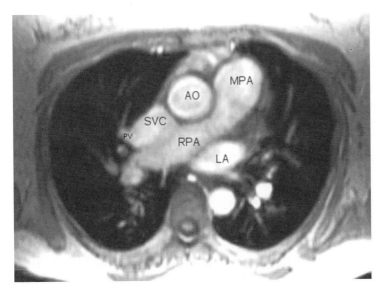

Figure 14 Axial gradient echo acquisition shows the right upper pulmonary vein join the SVC as it is about to enter the right atrium in a patient with sinus venosum defect. The SVC joins the right and left atrium at the point of their septal defect. Note the dilated pulmonary arteries. *Abbreviations*: MPA, main pulmonary artery; RPA, right pulmonary artery; AO, ascending aorta; SVC, superior vena cava. LA; left atrium.

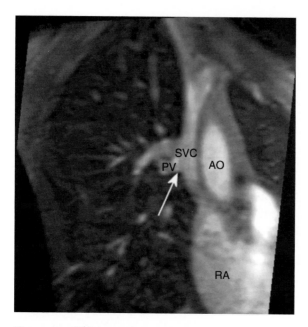

Figure 15 Oblique sagittal gradient echo section shows the anomalous right upper pulmonary vein connecting (*arrow*) with the superior vena cava before it enters the right atrium. *Abbreviations*: SVC, superior vena cava; PV, pulmonary vein; RA, right atrium; AO, ascending aorta.

COR TRIATRIATUM

Cor triatriatum describes an anomaly of the atria in which all pulmonary veins enter a common pulmonary venous chamber, located behind the heart and separated from the true left atrium by a diaphragm in which there are one or more restrictive ostia (18). The left atrium contains the atrial appendage and mitral valve. The clinical presentation of the classical cor triatriatum is that of pulmonary venous hypertension without left atrial appendage enlargement. Patients with cor triatriatum associated with an ASD present with manifestations of right-to-left shunt (19).

Multiple transverse and sagittal planes on spin echo and gradient echo cine sequences demonstrate the morphology of the atria and the pulmonary vein connections (Fig. 16). The anomalous pulmonary venous chamber is depicted better in the four-chamber section as well as in the two-chamber slices (Fig. 17), which shows the relationship between the mitral valve and the atrial membrane.

The identification of the associated anomalies is mandatory before surgical approach. Partial anomalous venous connection, coarctation of the aorta, and anomalies of the systemic venous drainage are among the most common. A comprehensive assessment of cardiac and associated vascular

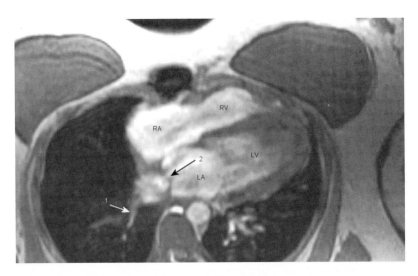

Figure 16 Axial gradient echo acquisition shows the pulmonary veins (*arrow 1*) draining into a chamber separated from the left atrium with a membrane (*arrow 2*) in a patient with cor triatriatum. *Abbreviations*: RA, right atrium; RV, right ventricle; LV, left ventricle.

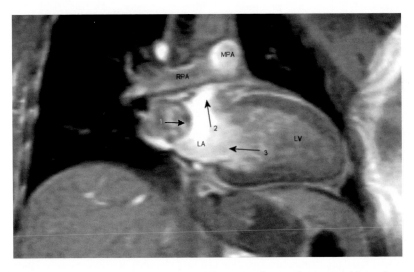

Figure 17 Sagittal right anterior oblique gradient echo acquisition shows the relationship of the posterior chamber membrane (*arrow 1*) to the left atrium, left atrial appendage (*arrow 2*) and mitral valve (*arrow 3*). *Abbreviations*: LV, left ventricle; MPA, main pulmonary artery; RPA, right pulmonary artery; LA, left atrium.

structures using multislice axial sequences is necessary to rule out associated abnormalities.

Resection of the membrane in the left atrium and reestablishing the free flow in the left atrium is the goal of the surgical treatment in cor triatriatum. In the postoperative period, it is necessary to assess residual obstruction and ventricular performance.

EBSTEIN'S MALFORMATION

Ebstein's malformation is an anomaly of the tricuspid valve characterized by apical displacement of the septal and inferior leaflets of the tricuspid valve. The tricuspid leaflets are plastered to the right ventricular endocardium. The annular attachment of the anterior leaflet of the valve is normally positioned, while the septal and inferior leaflets are attached to the right ventricle below the AV junction (20,21). The right ventricular musculature, papillary muscles, and cords are abnormally formed. The right ventricle is divided into two parts. The inlet part is covered by the tricuspid leaflet. Meanwhile, the portion of the right ventricle that is distal to the line of malattachment of the tricuspid leaflet is formed by both the trabecular and outlet segments. The right atrium and ventricle are usually dilated and the

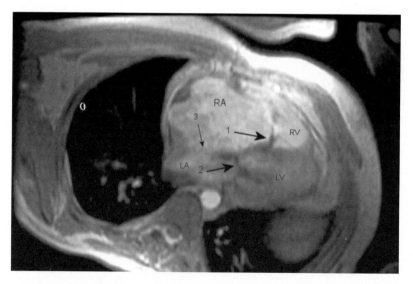

Figure 18 Axial gradient echo acquisition in a four-chamber position. Note the apical displacement of the tricuspid valve (*arrow 1*) compared with the mitral valve (*arrow 2*). The right atrium is enlarged compared with the left atrium. Right ventricle is a very small chamber distal to the tricuspid valve. Also, notice the atrial septal defect (*arrow 3*). *Abbreviations*: LV, left ventricle; LA, left atrium; RV, right ventricle.

tricuspid valve is incompetent. The fossa ovalis type of ASD is common in Ebstein's malformation. The most commonly associated lesion is pulmonary valve stenosis (20,21).

Axial cine sequences confirm the apical displacement of the tricuspid valve leaflets and show the large right atrium (Fig. 18). Many times a left-to-right shunt can be seen on these sequences but if there is high degree of suspicion for the presence of an ASD, contrast injection and first-pass visualization of the contrast through the heart needs to be undertaken (Fig. 7). Phase contrast imaging can quantify the volume of regurgitation and the degree of the shunt, if present.

CONGENITALLY CORRECTED TRANSPOSITION OF THE GREAT ARTERIES

This anomaly describes a discordant AV connection associated with a discordant ventricle–arterial connection. The right-sided left ventricle is anterior and to the right, with the right ventricle is in a posterior and left position. The ventricular septum is straight, due to the malposition of the ventricular outlets (22–24). The ventriculo-arterial connection is discordant. The left ventricular outlet is anterior and to the right and the left-sided right ventricular outlet is anterior and to the left. The ascending aorta is anterior and to the left in relation to the pulmonary artery (Fig. 19).

The right ventricle being a systemic chamber is large and hypertrophied and it supports the aorta. The left ventricle supports the pulmonary valve through an outlet, which is partially fibrous. The pulmonary and

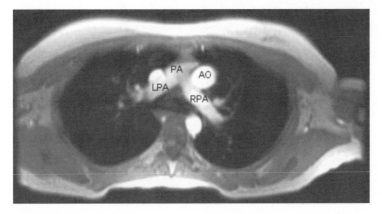

Figure 19 Axial gradient echo acquisition shows the ascending aorta to the left of the pulmonary artery in a patient with congenitally corrected transposition of great arteries. *Abbreviations*: RPA, right pulmonary artery; LPA, left pulmonary artery; PA, pulmonary artery; AO, aortic arch.

systemic circulations in a corrected transposition are in series. Associated lesions may be clinically detected such as ASD and tricuspid insufficiency (Fig. 4) (22–24). Malformation of the tricuspid valve occurs in about 25% of the patients, which results in congestive heart failure. Ebstein's malformation of the left-sided tricuspid valve is common in this condition (Fig. 4).

The anatomy of hearts with corrected transposition is depicted through spin echo and cine gradient echo sequences using transaxial, sagittal, and coronal planes. Oblique and specially designed planes are usually necessary for demonstrating specific segments of the cardiovascular system (Fig. 20) (25,26). Four chambers and short axial multiple sections are useful for localizing septal defects and the functioning of the valves. The four-chamber section of the heart with corrected transposition shows the position of the cardiac septa. The left ventricular outlet is well depicted on coronal section. The right-sided left ventricle–pulmonary artery junction is to the right of the right ventricle–aortic arch junction. The anomaly of the tricuspid valve in the corrected transposition is well demonstrated in the four-chamber section but its extension is seen better on two-chamber section of the left-sided AV connection (Fig. 20). Flow studies are necessary for estimating the magnitude of the intracardiac shunts.

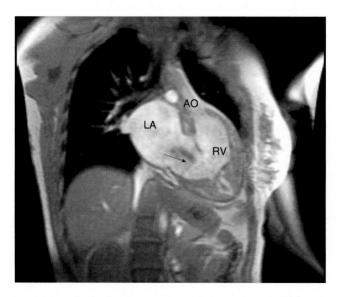

Figure 20 Sagittal right anterior oblique view of the left atrium connecting to the anatomical right ventricle. Note the Ebstein's malformation and tricuspid insufficiency (*arrow*). The anatomical right ventricle is connected to the aorta. *Abbreviations*: LA, left atrium; AO, aortic arch; RV, right ventricle.

TETRALOGY OF FALLOT

Tetralogy of Fallot is a congenital malformation of the right ventricular outflow tract; the result of an anterior leftward and cephalad displacement of
the infundibular septum. The anatomical changes result in an infundibular
VSD, stenosis of the right ventricular outlet and anterior and leftward
position of the aortic valve, which overrides the ventricular septum and originates partially from the right ventricle. Hypertrophy of the right ventricle
due to pressure and volume overload is always present. The VSD is perimembranous with outlet extension in the majority of the cases (27,28).
The defect is contiguous with the tricuspid and mitral valve in majority of the
cases. Aortic regurgitation is common and is found in over three quarters of
the adult patients with tetralogy of Fallot. Associated anatomical changes in
patients with tetralogy of Fallot include stenosis of the pulmonary valve and
stenosis of the pulmonary artery. Peripheral pulmonary artery stenosis
occurs at the central as well as in the periphery. In severe cases,
the stenosis is significant enough to result in an absence of central part
of the pulmonary artery.

CMR evaluation of patients with tetralogy of Fallot involves characterization of VSD, assessment of right ventricular outflow tract for the
degree of obstruction and pulmonary artery morphology (29). Axial sections
of the heart with high-resolution spin echo and cine gradient echo sequences
from the base to the thoracic outlet will show the basic anatomy of the heart
with tetralogy of Fallot (Fig. 21). The surgical correction may be obtained
by resection of the muscular structures of the infundibulum, insertion of a
transanular patch, or in severe stenosis, by an external conduit inserted
between the right ventricle and pulmonary artery. The outlet of the left

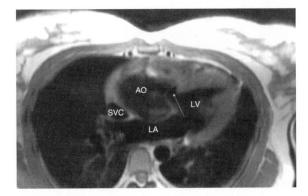

Figure 21 Sagittal gradient echo view of the right ventricular outflow tract (RVOT)
in tetralogy of Fallot. Notice the ridge causing obstruction in the RVOT (*arrow*).
There is right ventricular hypertrophy. *Abbreviations*: LV, left ventricle; AO, aortic
arch; LA, left atrium; SVC, superior vena cava.

ventricle and the aortic valve will show the aortic valve annulus and the location of the VSD. The outflow tract of the right ventricle can be best assessed on sagittal sections though the right ventricle. In order to obtain a sagittal section throughout the outflow tract, first coronal sections are used to find the best sagittal plane (Fig. 22).

The pulmonary artery anatomy is well depicted by 3D pulmonary angiography. The flow through each pulmonary artery and its branches can be assessed by phase contrast studies.

In the immediate postoperative period, CMR provides images that can confirm the patency of the right ventricular outflow tract, residual septal defects, and pulmonic valvular insufficiency. Gadolinium-enhanced pulmonary angiograms delineate the morphology and flow of the pulmonary arteries (30). In late postoperative status, CMR can assess the ventricular performance, the valvular function, particularly the pulmonary valve.

Patent Ductus Arteriosus

Ductus arterisus extends from the underside of the aortic arch just distal to the origin of the left subclavian artery to the left pulmonary artery near its

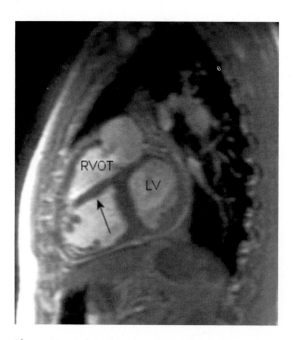

Figure 22   Axial spin echo acquisition shows the overriding aortic valve (*arrow*) in tetralogy of Fallot. Note the dilation of the aortic root and how the right ventricular outflow tract is not visible. *Abbreviations*: LV, left ventricle; RVOT, right ventricular outflow tract.

origin (Fig. 23). It is the persistent distal left sixth aortic arch. It is usually left-sided, though if there is a right-sided arch, right patent ducutus arteriosus has been reported. CMR does an excellent job of showing the connection between the aortic arch and the left pulmonary artery with sagittal right anterior oblique plane cine sequences. Since blood is bright with cine gradient echo sequences and the left-to-right shunt causes a turbulent jet, CMR may be the ideal tool to visualize this abnormality. Also, axial cine gradient echo slices will demonstrate a turbulent jet in the proximal left pulmonary artery. In most cases, the connection can be seen so well that there is no need to perform 3D angiography.

Tricuspid Atresia

Tricuspid atresia describes an absence of the AV connection of the right atrium to the right ventricle in the presence of a rudimentary right ventricle (31,32). The malformation results in an obligatory admixture of systemic and pulmonary venous return before reaching the ventricular mass. The absence of the right AV connection is the result of the hypoplasia or atresia of the inlet to the right ventricle. There is usually a large ASD. The resulting arrangement is that the parietal wall of the right atrium and the ventricle are in continuity not with each other but with the central fibrous body. A space exists between the continuous layer of the atria and ventricular myocardium,

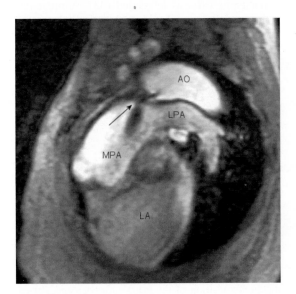

Figure 23 Sagittal gradient echo view of the patent ductus arteriosus. Note the jet (*arrow*) from the underside of the aortic arch into the proximal part of the left pulmonary artery. *Abbreviations*: MPA, main pulmonary artery; LA, left atrium; LPA, left pulmonary artery; AO, aortic arch.

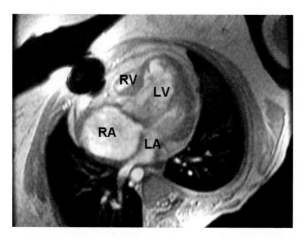

Figure 24 Axial gradient echo acquisition in a patient with tricuspid atresia. Note that the right ventricle is hypoplastic and is not connected to the right atrium. The left ventricle is dilated. *Abbreviations*: LA, left atrium; LV, left ventricle; RA, right atrium; RV, right ventricle.

which is usually occupied by AV groove tissue (Figs. 24 and 25). In hearts with situs solitus of the atria and ventricular inversion, the AV connection is discordant and the atretic tricuspid valve is left sided (33). A muscular VSD is usually present. The anomalies associated with tricuspid atresia

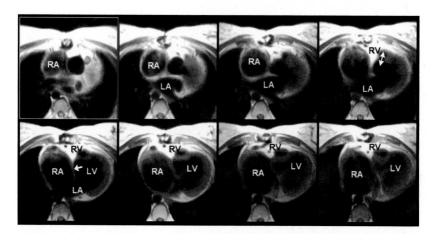

Figure 25 Multislice axial spin echo acquisition of the heart with tricuspid atresia. Note the small right ventricle and ventricular septal defect (*double arrow*). Also, note the space that separates the continuous layer of atrial and ventricular myocardium (*single arrow*). *Abbreviations*: LV, left ventricle; LA, left atrium; RA, right atrium; RV, right ventricle.

include fossa ovalis ASD, muscular trabecular VSDs, and stenosis of the right ventricular outlet.

The anatomical and functional changes in heart with classical tricuspid atresia can be seen in multislice axial spin echo and cine sequences (Fig. 25). Short axis cine sequences can show the presence of VSD (34). Ventricular morphology is well depicted in four-chamber sections (Fig. 24) and in multislice short axis cine gradient echo sequences. The ventriculo-arterial connection is well depicted on the coronal plane. Hearts with tricuspid atresia, associated with pulmonary atresia, have one arterial trunk that arises from the heart and it is the aorta.

The status of the pulmonary circulation is important for advising a surgical palliative procedure. The pulmonary artery size should be appropriate and the flow normal. The pulmonary resistance should be low. This information is provided by phase studies.

UNIVENTRICULAR AV CONNECTIONS

Univentricular AV connection describes a group of cardiac malformations in which the atria are connected to one ventricular chamber through: two AV valves, a common AV valve, or a single AV valve in the absence of its counterpart valve. The ventricular chamber, which receives the AV valves, makes three varieties of hearts with univentricular AV connection: right ventricular type, left ventricular type, and indeterminate type. The ventricular chambers are usually uneven; dominant being the chamber receiving the AV valves. The mode of AV connection describes how the junction is guarded: by one AV valve in the absence of its counterpart (Fig. 26); by two well-formed valves or by a common valve. In addition, the valve or valves may override and/or straddle the ventricular septum. The ventriculo-arterial connection is usually concordant; but the discordant ventriculo-arterial connection is not uncommon, particularly in hearts with ventricles in inverted relationship (35–37).

The hearts with double inlet left ventricle usually show one of these characteristics: situs solitus of the atria, inverted ventricles, and discordant ventriculo-arterial connection. The right and left atria are connected to the left ventricle through two well-defined valves. The ventricles are inverted in relation to the ventricular septum. The left ventricle is anterior and to the right and the right ventricle is in posterior and left position. The right ventricle is an incomplete ventricular chamber. A muscular VSD is almost always present. The ventriculo-arterial connection is discordant. The aortic valve is related to a small incomplete right ventricle and the pulmonary artery arises from the morphologically left ventricle (35–37).

The morphology of the hearts with univentricular AV connections is well depicted by CMR. The imaging planes are fundamental for proper depiction. The axial sections will show the position of the cardiac chambers

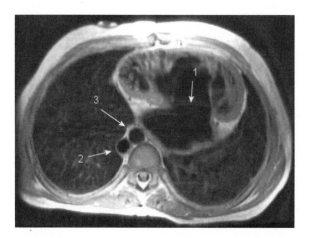

Figure 26   Axial spin echo acquisition of the univentricular heart. Note that there is only one atrioventricular valve (*arrow 1*). Also, the descending aorta is right-sided (*arrow 2*) and next to the inferior vena cava (*arrow 3*).

and septum (Fig. 26). From this set of sections, we prescribe a series of cine short axis sections, which depict the size and functioning of the ventricles. The AV valve or valves are well seen on cine four chambers and short axis sections. The ventriculo-arterial junction is easily identified on coronal sections. The semilunar valves are evaluated on sagittal sections passing through their junction. The morphology of the venous return should be assessed in each patient, in order to rule out pulmonary vein stenosis. The ratio of the pulmonary flow to systemic flow is estimated by flow CMR studies.

CONCLUSIONS

Cardiovascular magnetic resonance is useful for assessing anatomy and function of various cardiac congenital malformations. The detail and resolution exceeds all other forms of imaging, making it a key diagnostic modality, particularly in the perioperative time. Function studies and angiography provide a complete picture of the defects. Furthermore, because CMR allows image acquisition in three dimensions, virtually any view of the heart is feasible, which aids in the understanding, diagnosis, monitoring, and operative treatment of congenital heart defects. It is recommended that the reader consult the special section of the JCMR on congenital heart disease for further information (38).

REFERENCES

1. Sharma S, Devine W, Anderson RH, et al. The determination of atrial arrangement by examination of atrial appendage morphology in 1842 heart specimens. Br Heart J 1988; 60:227–231.

2. Macartney FJ, Zuberbuhler JR, Anderson RH. Morphological considerations in atrial isomerism. Br Heart J 1980; 44:657–667.
3. Anderson RH, Jo SY. Sequential segmental analysis- description and categorization for the millennium. Cardiol Young 1997; 7:98–116.
4. Soto B. Identification of the thoracic isomerism from the plain chest radiography. AJR Am J Roentgenol 1978; 13:1995–1002.
5. Anderson RH, Becker AE, Soto B. Complete transposition. Morphology of Congenital Heart Disease. Kent, U.K.: Castle House Publications Ltd, 1983: 84–100.
6. Smith A, Wilkinson JL, Arnold R, Anderson RH. Growth and development of ventricular walls in complete transposition of the great arteries with intact ventricular septum. Am J Cardiol 1982; 49:362–336.
7. Bedford DF, Sellors TH, Sommerville W, Belcher JR, et al. Atrial septal defect and its surgical treatment. Lancet 1957:1255–1261.
8. Manning WJ, Atkinson DJ, Parker JA, Edelman RR. Assessment of intracardiac shunts with gadolinium-enhanced ultrafast MR imaging. Radiology 1992; 184:357–361.
9. Arheden H, Holmqvist C, Thile U, et al. Left-to-right cardiac shunt: comparison of measurements obtained with MR velocity mapping and with radionuclide angiography. Radiology 1999; 211:453–458.
10. Hundley WG, Hong F, Li BS, Lange RE, Peshok RM. Assessment of left-to-right intracardiac shunting by velocity-encoded, phase-difference magnetic resonance imaging. Circulation 1995; 91:2955–2960.
11. Soto B, Becker AE, Moulaert AH, Anderson RH. Classification of ventricular septal defects. Br Heart J 1980; 43:332–343.
12. Kirklin JW, Barrant-Boyes BG. Ventricular Septal Defect. Cardiac Surgery. New York: John Wiley and Sons, 1986:599–664.
13. Didier D, Higgins CB. Identification and location of ventricular septal defect by gated magnetic resonance imaging. Am J Cardiol 1986; 57:1363–1368.
14. Von Shulthess GK, Higashino SM, Higgins SS, et al. Coarctation of the aorta: MR imaging. Radiology 1986; 158:469–474.
15. Brody H. Drainage of the pulmonary veins into the right side of the heart. Arch Pathol 1942; 33:221.
16. Kirklin JW, Barratt-Boyes BG. Total anomalous venous connection. In: Cardiac Surgery. New York: John Wiley and Sons:499–523.
17. Soto B, Pacifico AD. Anomalous pulmonary venous connection. Angiography of Congenital Cardiac Malformations. New York: Futura Publishing Co., 1990:121.
18. Miller G, Onley PA, Anderson RH. Cor triatriatum: hemodynamics and angiocardiographic diagnosis. Am Heart J 1964; 68:298.
19. Marin GJ, Tandon R, Edwards JE. Cor triatriatum. Study of 20 cases. Am J Cardiol 1975; 35:59–66.
20. Eagle MA, Paine TP, Bruins C. Ebstein's anomaly of the tricuspid valve. Report of three cases and analysis of the clinical syndrome. Circulation 1950; 1: 1246–1260.
21. Zuberbuhler JR, Allwork SP, Anderson RH. The spectrum of Ebstein's anomaly of the tricuspid valve. J Thorac Cardiovasc Surg 1979; 77:202–211.

22. Reddy GP, Caputo GR. Congenitally corrected transposition of the great arteries. Radiology 1999; 213:102–106.
23. Allwork SP, Bentall HH, Becker AE, Anderson RH. Congenitally corrected transposition of the great arteries: morphological study of 32 cases. Am J Cardiol 1976; 38:910–923.
24. Losekoot TG, Anderson RH, Becker AE, et al. Congenitally Corrected Transposition. New York: Churchill Livingstone, 1983.
25. Higgins CB, Caputo GR. Role of MR imaging in acquired and congenital cardiovascular disease. AJR Am J Roentgenol 1993; 161:13–22.
26. Choe HY, Kim MY, Han KV. MR imaging in the morphological diagnosis of congenital heart disease. Radiographics 1997; 17:403–422.
27. Anderson RH, Becker AE, Meier M, Soto B. Morphology of Congenital Heart Disease. Tunbridge Wells, U.K.: Castle House Publications Ltd, 1983:36–50.
28. Kirklin JW, Barratt-Boyes BG. Tetralogy of Fallot. Cardiac Surgery. New York: John Wiley and Sons, 1986:699–819.
29. Wyttenbach R, Bremerich J, Higgins CB. Cardiovascular Magnetic Resonance in Complex Congenital Heart Disease in Adult. Cardiovascular Magnetic Resonance. Churchill Livingstone, London: Manning and Pennell, 2002:311–322.
30. Geva T, Greil G, Marshall A, et al. Gadolinium-enhanced 3 dimensional Magnetic resonance angiography of pulmonary blood supply in patients with complex pulmonary stenosis or atresia. Circulation 2002; 106:473–478.
31. Anderson RH, Wilkinson JL, Gerlis LM, et al. Atresia of the right atrioventricular orifice. Br Heart J 1977; 39:414–428.
32. Dickson DF, Wilkinson JL, Smith A. et al. Atresia of the right atrioventricular orifice with atrioventricular concordance. Br Heart J 1979; 42:9–14.
33. Patterson W, Baxley WA, Karp RB, et al. Tricuspid atresia in adults. Am J Cardiol 1982; 49:141–152.
34. Fletcher BD, Jacobstein MD, Abramowsky CR, et al. Right atrioventricular valve atresia: anatomic evaluation with MR imaging. AJR Am J Roentgenol 1987; 148:671–674.
35. Anderson RH, Macartney FJ, Tynan M, et al. The univentricular atrioventricular connections: getting to the root of a thorny problem. Am J Cardiol 1984; 34:822–828.
36. Keeton BR, Macartney FJ, Hunter S, Wilkinson JL, Anderson RH. Univentricular heart of right ventricular type with double or common inlet. Circulation 1979; 59:403–411.
37. Soto B, Pacifico AD, D'Siacio G. Univentricular heart. An angiographic study. Am J Cardiol 1982; 49:787–794.
38. Fogel MA (Guest Ed.). Journal of Cardiovascular Magnetic Resonance. Focus Issue on CMR Applications in Congenital Heart Disease 2006: 8(4):569–670.

8

Ischemic Heart Disease: Stress and Vasodilator Testing

Radha J. Sarma and Gerald M. Pohost

*Department of Medicine, Division of Cardiovascular Medicine,
Keck School of Medicine, University of Southern California, Los Angeles,
California, U.S.A.*

INTRODUCTION

The advantages and disadvantages of cardiovascular magnetic resonance (CMR) stress testing have been previously described in the literature (1,2). In this chapter, CMR "stress" testing includes not only inotropic and chronotropic agents such as dobutamine and atropine, and physical stress with handgrip exercise, but also vasodilators such as adenosine and dipyridamole which do not cause actual stress but instead cause perturbation in perfusion. The techniques causing actual stress are used to induce ischemia in the myocardium which is demonstrated by perfusion defects and wall motion abnormalities. Meanwhile, the vasodilator techniques can be used to detect abnormal distribution of myocardial perfusion in healthy and diseased coronary arteries. CMR stress and vasodilator testing has been shown to have better sensitivity and specificity compared with dobutamine stress echocardiography to detect coronary artery disease (CAD) (3,4). At present stress echocardiography and radionuclide stress testing are widely available compared with CMR stress and vasodilator testing. However, CMR has evolved into a useful method with the potential to resolve important limitations of stress echocardiography and radionuclide testing. Some of these limitations in echocardiography include: (i) difficulty in finding good acoustic window to get satisfactory images, (ii) variable skill levels between sonographers in acquiring proper images, and (iii) inter-reader variability in interpreting images. It is estimated that about 10% to 15% of patients undergoing stress echocardiography have poor images. Even with the addition of echo-contrast agents, it is expected that there will be some patients who will not have adequate images of diagnostic quality. In these patients with poor echocardiography studies, fast cine CMR has been shown to be capable of detecting ischemia (5). Radionuclide testing suffers from (i) attenuation artifacts and (ii) a relatively poor resolution. On the other hand, CMR stress and vasodilator testing has very good temporal and spatial resolution of the cardiac images. In addition, cardiac structure, left ventricular function, myocardial perfusion, and infarct localization all can be performed in one single session. With new advances in CMR technology such as real-time image acquisition, CMR pharmacological testing will potentially become the non-invasive imaging test of choice for detecting CAD (1).

Indications and Contraindications for CMR Stress Testing

The indications and contraindications for CMR stress testing are generally the same as for stress echocardiography (Table 1). Few additional contraindications specific for CMR stress testing are shown in Table 2.

Careful screening of patients is very important prior to placing them in the magnetic field because treating emergencies while the patient is in the magnet is very difficult.

PROTOCOLS USED FOR CMR STRESS APPROACHES

Treadmill stress testing and upright bicycle are not feasible in the MR environment. Due to the strong magnetic field, the electrocardiogram (ECG) can only be used to monitor the heart rate and rhythm; meanwhile, evaluation of ischemia using ST segment changes is not possible. Hence the protocols use either physical exercise such as sustained isometric handgrip, handgrip using special handgrip dynamometers (Fig. 1), and supine bicycle ergometry with compatible CMR equipment (Fig. 2) or pharmacological stress testing with dobutamine and/or adenosine. Pharmacological stress has been found to be both feasible and safe in the MR environment (6,7). Among the dobutamine and adenosine protocols, dobutamine has been observed to be superior for inducing detectable wall motion abnormalities (8). Regardless of the method of stress or vasodilation, all protocols will acquire resting CMR images followed by imaging during or after the stress or vasodilation.

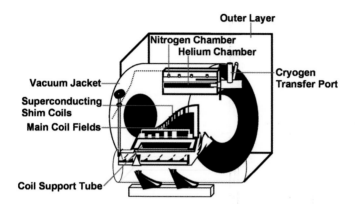

Figure 2.1 A cylindrical bore superconducting magnet showing the arrangement of main field, shim, and gradient coils within the cryostat housing. (*See p. 32*)

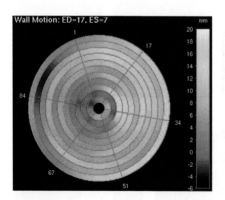

Figure 3.12 Bull's eye display of left ventricle wall motion, showing reduced function at the apex. (*See p. 65*)

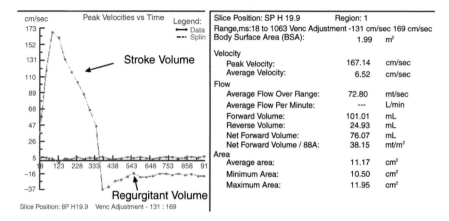

Figure 6.15 Flow volume curve versus time in the aorta shows the stroke volume in the initial part of the curve and regurgitant volume in diastole. (*See p. 128*)

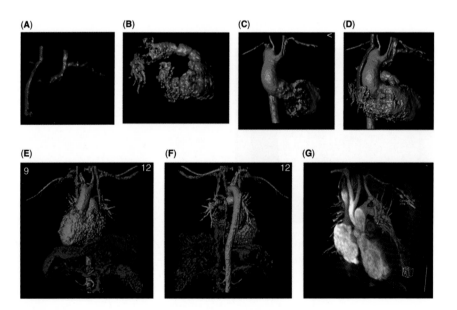

Figure 18.8 Congenital heart disease. (*See p. 409*)

Table 1 Indications and Contraindications for Cardiovascular Magnetic Resonance Stress and Vasodilator Testing

Indications
Suspected significant coronary artery disease
Preoperative risk assessment
Inability to exercise on the treadmill
Poor quality 2D echocardiogram
Contraindications
Related to dobutamine
Severe hypertension (>220 systolic, >120 diastolic)
Uncontrolled arrhythmias
Unstable angina
Severe aortic stenosis (gradient >50 mmHg, valve area <1.0 cm^2)
Hypertrophic cardiomyopathy
Myocarditis, pericardtis, or endocarditis
Related to dipyridamole or adenosine
Unstable angina or myocardial infarction <3 days
Reactive airway disease and/or asthma
Severe hypotension or hypertension
Bradycardia and heart block >2nd degree

MECHANISM OF DEVELOPING ISCHEMIA-RELATED WALL MOTION ABNORMALITIES DURING PHARMACOLOGIC STRESS TESTING

Dobutamine infusion increases both the heart rate and systolic blood pressure simulating exercise. The increased demand causes the myocardium supplied by a stenotic artery to develop wall motion abnormalities. Intermediate

Table 2 Contraindications Specific for Cardiovascular Magnetic Resonance Stress and Vasodilator Testing

Severe obesity preventing the patient from fitting in the machine
Cardiac pacemakers and pacemaker leads
Automatic implantable cardioverter defibrillators
Certain foreign bodies, tattoos, and clothes containing ferromagnetic material
[a]Other incompatible ferromagnetic metal objects such as
Metallic aneurysm clips
Cochlear implants and many inner ear wires
Periorbital metallic foreign bodies and implants
Claustrophobia (relative)

Note: Check for the manufacturer's safety information.
[a]For a complete list, please see http://www.mrisafety.com.

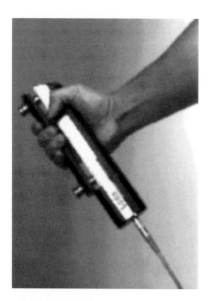

Figure 1 Handgrip dynamometer.

doses of dobutamine (i.e., 20 µg/kg/min) have been shown to have better detection of CAD compared with stress echo where higher doses (up to 50 µg/kg/min) of atropine are added to increase the heart rate (9).

Dipyridamole or adenosine cause intense vasodilatation of all normal blood vessels but diseased vessels may not show the same degree of

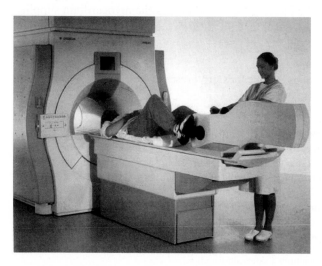

Figure 2 Magnetic resonance compatible supine bicycle ergometer.

Table 3 Protocols for Pharmacologic Stress Testing

Stress test	Test protocol
Dobutamine/ atropine	5, 10, 20, 30, 40 µg/kg body weight/min for 3 min at each dose and 0.25 mg of atropine X4, until the heart rate is at least 85% of age-predicted maximal heart rate
Dipyridamole infusion	Infusion of a fixed dose (0.56 mg/kg of body weight/min) for 4 minutes
Adenosine infusion	Infusion of adenosine at 140 µg/kg/min for 6 minutes

vasodilatation (Table 3). Known as the "coronary steal phenomenon" the healthier and more dilated arteries will "steal" blood from the diseased and less dilated arteries. With the vasodilators dipyridamole and adenosine, there is usually a 20 mmHg drop in systolic blood pressure and no significant change in the heart rate. When there is significant coronary obstruction in any of the three coronary arteries, the myocardium supplied by the diseased coronary artery is expected to be developing wall motion abnormality compared with the normal segments. However, if all three main coronary arteries are diseased, vasodilation may be limited across all three leading to "balanced ischemia," and a false-negative result.

PATIENT PREPARATION

Initial Evaluation

Prior should have a complete history and physical examination pertinent to the CMR study to evaluate the risk factors, symptoms, and any potential contraindications such as AICD for the planned study (10). Depending on the facility a proper informed consent may be obtained from all patients undergoing stress testing.

Need for Sedation

If patients are anxious or mildly claustrophobic, it may be necessary to give some mild sedation prior to the testing. Electrodes for monitoring the ECG should be properly placed on the chest. Blood pressure cuff of appropriate size and a pulse-oxymeter should be connected and baseline values are recorded. If the blood pressure, cardiac rhythm or rate is in the range for the laboratory's list of contraindications, the test may have to be rescheduled for a later time when it will be safe to conduct the test.

PATIENT MONITORING

Heart rate and rhythm, blood pressure, pulse oxymetry, and symptoms are monitored continuously for any type of stress testing. Wall motion

Table 4   Criteria for Termination of the Drug Infusion

Dobutamine	Dipyridamole/adenosine
Target heart rate achieved (85% PMHR)	Patient develops moderate/ severe angina
Systolic blood pressure drops by > 20 mmHg. Below baseline value or > 40 mmHg. From a prior recording during the infusion	Systolic blood pressure drops to < 100 mmHg
Blood pressure increase >240/120 mmHg	
Moderate angina, complex arrhythmia, new or worsening wall motion abnormality	

Abbreviation: PMHR, predicted maximal heart rate.

abnormalities are monitored at each dose increase for dobutamine with or without atropine, but only at the end of infusion (peak stress) for the dipyridamole or adenosine protocols (Table 4). ECG is only useful for monitoring the heart rate but not to detect ischemia due to baseline artifacts. As the emergency equipment is not immediately next to the patient, it is important to establish good communication with the patient during examination to evaluate the symptoms and to terminate the test if the safety is in question. A video monitor and some kind of audio monitor should be available for communicating with the patient in the MR machine. It is essential that all staff members are familiar with the emergency policies and procedures for their laboratory.

Interpretation

Resting and stress images are viewed either using a format where all images are seen at the same dose of infusion, or using the same views at different doses of the infusion. The myocardial segments are identified as proposed in the statement for healthcare professionals from the Cardiac Imaging Committee of the Council on Clinical Cardiology of the American Heart Association. Wall motion can be assessed either quantitatively or qualitatively (11). Although quantitative methods are available for research purposes (12,13), most clinical interpretation may be done by visual estimation.

Ischemia is reliably diagnosed when there are no resting wall motion abnormalities and new wall motion abnormalities develop, associated with anginal symptoms, after increasing doses of dobutamine are infused. However if there are wall motion abnormalities present at rest, new wall motion abnormalities under stress are less specific unless the magnitude of wall motion, symptoms, and the work load all are supportive of the diagnosis of ischemia (14). In patients with prior myocardial infarction, a new wall motion abnormality in a segment that was normal at rest and becomes abnormal after stress indicates ischemia, especially if there is also the presence of stress-induced anginal symptoms. Dobutamine-induced wall motion abnormalities were shown to have prognostic value in patients with suspected CAD (15).

CONCLUSIONS

CMR is the gold-standard for the assessment of ventricular function and wall motion and thickening due to its ability to image in three dimensions with excellent spatial resolution. CMR imaging with stress testing by exercise through handgrip or supine bicycle ergometry or by pharmacological methods allow for the assessment of ischemic heart disease. The pharmacological stressor, dobutamine, provides a means to define the physiological significance of CAD by inducing wall motion abnormalities in the appropriate coronary distribution(s). Phophorus-31 CMR spectroscopy is used in conjunction with handgrip dynamometry to detect myocardial ischemia which, in the absence of significant disease of the large coronary vessels, suggests microvascular disease. Use of vasodilator agents such as adenosine or dipyridamole provide a means of determining the physiological importance of coronary artery stenosis using a bolus injection of paramagnetic contrast agent generating images of myocardial perfusion. Rest and vasodilator studies are compared to identify the involved territories. In view of the high resolution of CMR it is incrementally more accurate when compared to radionuclide SPECT and PET. CMR provides a comprehensive approach to the assessment of myocardial ischemia using studies at rest, with stress and/or with vasodilators. Under these circumstances function, perfusion and metabolism can be assessed, providing the comprehensive examination that CMR has been known for.

REFERENCES

1. Pohost GM, Biederman RW. The role of cardiac MRI stress testing: "make a better mouse trap...". Circulation 1999; 100:1676–1679.
2. Zoghbi WA, Barasch E. Dobutamine MRI: a serious contender in pharmacological stress imaging? Circulation 1999; 99:730–732.
3. Nagel E, Lehmkuhl HB, Bocksch W, et al. Noninvasive diagnosis of ischemia-induced wall motion abnormalities with the use of high-dose dobutamine stress MRI: comparison with dobutamine stress echocardiography. Circulation 1999; 99:763–770.
4. Nagel E, Lorenz C, Baer F, et al. Stress cardiovascular magnetic resonance: consensus panel report. J Cardiovasc Magn Reson 2001; 3(3):267–281.
5. Hundley WG, Hamilton CA, Thomas MS, et al. Utility of fast cine magnetic resonance imaging and display for the detection of myocardial ischemia in patients not well suited for second harmonic stress echocardiography. Circulation 1999; 100:1697–1702.

 6. Kuijpers D, Janssen CH, van Dijkman PR, Oudkerk M. Dobutamine stress MRI. Part I. Safety and feasibility of dobutamine cardiovascular magnetic resonance in patients suspected of myocardial ischemia. Eur Radiol 2004; 14(10): 1823–1828.
 7. Ott R, Bathagate B, Cozum-Poetica C, Banach R, Heinz K, Volkhard F. Safety and feasibility of high-dose dobutamine stress MRI for detection of myocardial ischemia: experience in 400 consecutive in- and outpatients. J Cardiovasc Magn Reson 2005; 7(1):91.
 8. Paetsch I, Jahnke C, Wahl A, et al. Comparison of dobutamine stress magnetic resonance, adenosine stress magnetic resonance, and adenosine stress magnetic resonance perfusion. Circulation 2004; 110:835–842.
 9. Power T, Kramer CM, Shaffer AL, et al. Breathhold dobutamine magnetic resonance tissue tagging: normal left ventricular response. Am J Cardiol 1997; 80: 1203–1207.
10. Ahmed S, Shellock FG. Magnetic resonance imaging safety: implications for cardiovascular patients. J Cardiovasc Magn Reson 2001; 3(3):171–182.
11. Cerqueira MD, Weissman NJ, Dilsizian V, et al. Standardized myocardial segmentation and nomenclature for tomographic imaging of the heart: a statement for healthcare professionals from the Cardiac Imaging Committee of the Council on Clinical Cardiology of the American Heart Association. Circulation 2002; 105:539–542.
12. Kraitchman DL, Sampath S, Castillo E, et al. Quantitative ischemia detection during cardiac magnetic resonance stress testing by use of FastHARP. Circulation 2003; 107:2025–2030.
13. Van Rugge FP, van der Wall EE, Spanjersberg SJ, et al. Magnetic resonance imaging during dobutamine stress for detection and localization of coronary artery disease. Quantitative wall motion analysis using a modification of the centerline method. Circulation 1994; 90:127–138.
14. Kuijpers D, Janssen CH, van Dijkman PR, Oudkerk M. Dobutamine stress MRI. Part II. Risk Stratification with dobutamine cardiovascular magnetic resonance in patients suspected of myocardial ischemia. Eur Radiol 2004; 14(10): 2046–2052.
15. Hundley WG, Morgan TM, Neagle CM, et al. Magnetic resonance imaging determination of cardiac prognosis. Circulation 2003; 106:2328–2333.

9

Ischemic Heart Disease: Myocardial Perfusion Imaging

Krishna S. Nayak

Departments of Electrical Engineering and Medicine, Division of Cardiovascular Medicine, Viterbi School of Engineering, Keck School of Medicine, University of Southern California, Los Angeles, California, U.S.A.

Gerald M. Pohost

Department of Medicine, Division of Cardiovascular Medicine, Keck School of Medicine, University of Southern California, Los Angeles, California, U.S.A.

INTRODUCTION

Myocardial perfusion imaging is the most commonly employed approach to noninvasively detect significant coronary artery disease (CAD) (1,2). To date, radionuclide methods are widely available and easily performed. They have provided the basis for the utility of myocardial perfusion imaging. Usually, imaging is performed with radiotracers, such as thallium or technitium-based agents, injected intravenously at rest and with stress (or vasodilation). Rest and stress images are compared to identify transient defects in flow related to significant disease of the epicardial coronary arteries.

Myocardial perfusion defects do not represent metabolic ischemia. Rather, they represent the abnormal blood supply to the myocardium that provides the basis for myocardial ischemia. Accordingly, myocardial perfusion imaging is a means to evaluate the significance of the CAD that may lead to myocardial ischemia.

WHAT IS PERFUSION?

Myocardial perfusion is defined as the blood supply to the myocardium, carrying oxygen and oxidizable substrate, needed for maintenance of the high-energy phosphates (e.g., adenosine triphosphate) essential for myocardial contractile function. Myocardial perfusion imaging depicts the regional distribution of blood supply. In this way, the presence of flow-limiting CAD is determined.

Myocardial perfusion imaging defines the physiological basis for myocardial ischemia. It uniquely demonstrates the physiological effects when CAD is significant and flow-limiting. Coronary angiography detects luminal narrowing in the major coronary arteries, but does not allow for the assessment of the physiological impact of these narrowings. Angiography cannot depict disease of the microvasculature due to its limited resolution. Microvascular disease has become increasingly important in the diagnosis of chest pain syndromes in the large population (especially in women). Other methods use stress to induce regional wall-motion abnormalities which are related to inadequate perfusion and metabolism.

Clinical Indications for a Myocardial Perfusion Imaging Examination

In patients with symptoms suggesting myocardial ischemia (e.g., angina pectoris), there are several approaches for detecting the presence of CAD, with a high degree of certainty. The most commonly employed approach is exercise stress testing with ECG monitoring; however stress or vasodilator myocardial perfusion imaging and stress echocardiography provide more precise indicators of CAD. Since echocardiography at this time is largely a two-dimensional approach, and frequently uses the stress agent, dobutamine, it is not as commonly performed as myocardial perfusion imaging with radionuclides. If regional wall motion abnormalities with echo or myocardial perfusion defects on radionuclide study are detected, CAD is almost certainly present. Once the diagnosis is suggested by echo or radionuclide approaches, coronary angiography is performed and percutaneous coronary intervention or cardiothoracic surgery is used for treatment. Cardiovascular magnetic resonance (CMR) can image regional myocardial perfusion non-invasively with higher spatial resolution and without ionizing radiation, when compared with radionuclide studies, making it the most accurate and effective means for noninvasively detecting CAD.

IMAGING METHODS TO ASSESS MYOCARDIAL PERFUSION

Several imaging modalities can be used to assess myocardial perfusion. The most popular and clinically established approach is based on radionuclide imaging, and uses single photon emission computed tomography (SPECT).

Another radionuclide approach, albeit considerably more expensive than SPECT, is positron emission tomography (PET). Magnetic resonance imaging (MRI) is a newer and emerging technology. There are also approaches based on echocardiography using micro-bubbles as the contrast agent, and multi-slice computed tomography (MSCT) that should be considered as research at this time.

Radionuclide Imaging

Single photon emission computed tomography imaging of perfusion is based on myocardial uptake of the single photon emitting radionuclides thallium-201 (physical half life of $\sim$73 hours) or technetium-99m-based radiopharmaceuticals (physical half life of $\sim$6 hours) such as technetium Sestamibi (3,4). These agents are introduced intravenously. Low-energy gamma photons are emitted due to the natural decay of these radionuclides, and are detected by gamma cameras that rotate around the chest. Reconstruction is similar to X-ray computed tomography. SPECT suffers from attenuation artifacts as well as limited spatial resolution, on the order of 1 cm. Its primary advantages are wide clinical availability, moderate equipment cost, and a substantial body of published literature.

Positron emission tomography imaging of perfusion is based on myocardial uptake of positron emitting radionuclides such as rubidium-82 or nitrogen-13 ammonia (5,6). As with SPECT agents PET agents are introduced intravenously but in contrast to SPECT agents, PET agents have very short half-lives (e.g., rubidium-82 has a physical half life of 75 seconds). The decay process produces emission of positrons, which, during interaction with electrons, produce two "annihilation" photons, which are detected by positron cameras. PET suffers from instrumentation expense and somewhat limited spatial resolution (albeit considerably less limited than SPECT), on the order of 6 mm.

Echocardiography

Myocardial contrast echocardiography involves peripheral injection of transpulmonary "micro-bubbles" which are on the order of 2 to 8 μm in diameter (7,8). Bubbles are monitored using a two-dimensional focused ultrasound beam. Accordingly, regional myocardial perfusion is assessed, but suffers from low signal-to-noise ratio (SNR), and is highly dependent on operator as well as reader expertise.

Computed Tomography

Perfusion imaging using MSCT is based on the dynamic imaging of iodinated contrast agents passing through the myocardium (9,10). Measurements of myocardial perfusion can be performed, but are limited due to several factors including image artifacts, X-ray dose, and the nephrotoxicity of radiopaque contrast agents.

Cardiovascular Magnetic Resonance

Cardiovascular magnetic resonance has become a gold standard for the imaging of cardiac morphology, ventricular function and myocardial viability, and is emerging as an effective means for assessing myocardial perfusion and the native coronary arteries (11). Because CMR can produce many types of image contrast, a wide variety of perfusion imaging techniques using CMR are available. The most popular technique utilizes the first-pass of a paramagnetic contrast agent traversing the myocardial vascular bed (12). This contrast agent makes tissue appear "brighter" in conventional T1-weighted images. Imaging is performed at rest and during the infusion of a vasodilator such as adenosine or dipyridamole, or physiologic stressor such as dobutamine. CMR permits perfusion assessment with substantially higher resolution, than with radionuclide methods, and because it involves no ionizing radiation, can be used serially for tracking disease or the effectiveness of a therapy. The detection of myocardial perfusion deficits using rest and vasodilator/stress perfusion CMR has been recently evaluated clinically and demonstrated high sensitivity and specificity compared with SPECT (13,14) and invasive coronary angiography (15,16). The primary challenges are temporal resolution, volumetric coverage, and quantitation of perfusion.

CMR APPROACHES

Cardiovascular magnetic resonance has the ability to produce image contrast based on a variety of physiological and functional parameters including proton density, magnetic relaxation times T1 and T2, flow and motion, tissue structure, and blood oxygenation. For that reason, there are many possible methods for assessing perfusion in vivo using CMR. These include contrast agent "first-pass" methods (using T1 contrast), spin labeling techniques (using flow), magnetization transfer techniques (using tissue structure), and blood oxygen-level dependent techniques (using blood oxygenation). Many of these are still being investigated.

The most robust and widely used method to date utilizes the first-pass of an intravenously injected contrast agent. First-pass methods are the focus of this chapter, and are the basis of our recommended protocols.

First-Pass Perfusion Imaging

First-pass perfusion imaging requires the use of special contrast agents, pulse sequences, and post processing techniques. The contrast agents used in perfusion studies affect the local spin relaxation parameters, and are identified using appropriate CMR pulse sequences. The most common class of contrast agents is gadolinium-based chelates, which have a T1 shortening effect. In conjunction with conventional heavily T1-weighted imaging sequences, they produce brightness in areas of higher concentration. A well-designed protocol will produce image intensity that is roughly proportional to contrast agent concentration. A series of images at different times post-injection are acquired, and are qualitatively examined to determine which areas of myocardium are perfused insufficiently or not at all. Quantitation of perfusion requires accurate modeling of the relationship between signal intensity time course and contrast agent concentration time course, and the relationship between the contrast agent concentration time course in myocardium and supplying arteries with myocardial perfusion rate.

Contrast Agents

Gadolinium-based chelates are currently the most widely used contrast agents in clinical MR first-pass perfusion imaging and produce the most reliable image quality (17). These include Gd-DTPA (Magnevist(R), Berlax Imaging, Inc., Seattle, WA), Gd-BOPTA (Multihance(R), Bracco Diagnostics, Inc., Princeton, NJ), Gd-DTPA-BMA (Omniscan(R), GE Healthcare, Waukesha, WI), Gd-DOTA (Dotarem(R), Guerbet Group, France), and Gd-HP-D03A (ProHance(R), Bracco Diagnostics, Inc., Princeton, NJ), among others.

The main considerations for a contrast agent are: (i) that it should have high relaxivity (defined as the rate at which $R1 = 1/T1$ increases as a function of concentration) (Fig. 1) and (ii) that it should be safe in humans at the required concentrations. At 1.5 T, these agents listed above have relaxivity on the order of 5 to 10 s^{-1} mM^{-1}.

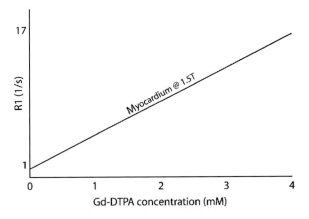

Figure 1 Plot of myocardium R1 ($R1 = 1/T1$) as a function of Gd-DTPA concentration at 1.5 T. R1 is approximately a linear function of contrast agent concentration. The slope is termed the "relaxivity" of the contrast agent ($\sim5/s/mm$ for Gd-DTPA at 1.5 T). Higher relaxivity means that the agent produces more T1 shortening for the same contrast agent concentration.

Pulse Sequences

Pulse sequences are of critical importance as they determine the image contrast, spatial resolution, and coverage. The main requirements of a first-pass perfusion imaging sequence are: (i) to provide strong T1 contrast to differentiate contrast-enhanced from non-contrast enhanced myocardium, (ii) to provide volumetric coverage with high temporal resolution (to gather first-pass information from the whole heart from a single bolus injection), and (iii) to provide adequate spatial resolution (to be able to resolve small regional defects or sub-endocardial defects).

Figure 2 contains a generalized picture of a typical first-pass imaging sequence which has all the elements described above. Strong T1 contrast is generated using inversion recovery (IR) or saturation recovery (SR) preparation. IR provides the strongest T1 contrast, and can be used when only one or two slices are of interest and the heart rate is stable. SR is the current "standard," and is compatible with higher numbers of slices (such as six to eight), and provides stable image contrast regardless of heart rate variation.

Rapid volumetric coverage is accomplished through interleaved acquisition of multiple slices. Figure 2 illustrates the acquisition of six slices every two heartbeats. The number and position of slices should be chosen to appropriately cover the entire left ventricle. The temporal resolution will be roughly 2 seconds (for a 60-beat/minute heart rate) which is adequate for capturing the first-pass which takes roughly 15 to 25 seconds in normal myocardium. Note that the slices have different cardiac phase, but do so

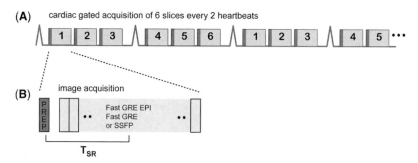

Figure 2 Cardiovascular magnetic resonance first-pass perfusion pulse sequence. (A) Acquisitions are cardiac-gated using Vector-ECG, ECG, or plethysmograph. Multiple slices are acquired consecutively (as shown: six slices in two R–R intervals). This is repeated continuously during the first-pass and washout of contrast agent, which takes roughly 40 to 60 seconds. (B) T1 contrast is generated using saturation or inversion recovery preparation (dark gray). Fast "snapshot" imaging of each slice is performed using fast gradient echo or fast steady–state free precession acquisitions (light gray). Image contrast is primarily determined by the type of preparation and the recovery time T_{SR}.

consistently. In other words, all images of slice no. 1 are from systole, while all images of slice no. 3 are from late diastole (Fig. 2).

In order to achieve this level of imaging speed, contrast preparation and full image acquisition of each slice can take at most 200 to 250 msec. This requires an ultrafast acquisition scheme, typically fast gradient echo (FGRE) or steady–state free precession (SSFP, also known by the trade names: True-FISP, FIESTA, and Balanced-FFE). FGRE can be used in combination with echo–planar (EPI) or spiral readouts for further speedups. SSFP has higher SNR compared with FGRE, but can suffer from off-resonance artifacts which limit the repetition time (TR) to less than 4 ms at 1.5 T. Multi-slice saturation recovery FGRE and SSFP are the basis of today's most robust protocols.

Processing and Analysis

As breathing motion predominantly causes bulk motion (translation and rotation) in short-axis images, first-pass images should be registered in order to improve the tracking of individual segments. At this time, qualitative evaluation of first-pass myocardial perfusion imaging is most commonly practiced, because of image artifacts (discussed later in this chapter) and difficulty with quantitation. After contrast agent injection, poorly perfused myocardial segments will enhance or brighten slowly compared with better-perfused segments, and therefore will appear dark relative to nearby better-perfused myocardium.

Quantitation is an active area of research, and is typically performed by plotting regional signal intensity as a function of time during the first-pass. Time–intensity curves are normalized, and the signal intensity slope is computed. The slopes for each segment are compared to establish perfusion differences. A simple quantitation method uses the signal intensity upslope. More accurate measures can be performed using time–intensity curve deconvolution using a measured arterial input function (usually in the ascending aorta) (18,19). Signal saturation and sensitivity to the accuracy of the input function has led to the "double-bolus" method (20,21), which involves measurement of the input function using a separate low-dose injection and fast imaging in the ascending aorta, prior to the full-dose injection used for the measurement of myocardial enhancement.

RECOMMENDED PROTOCOLS

Cardiovascular magnetic resonance myocardial perfusion imaging is optimally performed in a single examination, with scans performed at rest and with the administration of vasodilators (e.g., adenosine or dipyridamole) or pharmacologic stress-inducing agents (e.g., dobutamine). This requires two separate contrast agent injections during two sequential "first-pass" scans, one at rest and one during vasodilation/stress.

Cardiovascular magnetic resonance-delayed enhancement (Chapter 12) has become a clinically trusted approach for the assessment of myocardial viability. The approach requires imaging at 5 to 15 minutes after the injection of contrast. If a myocardial viability examination is ordered, resting myocardial perfusion can also be assessed during the "first-pass" at no additional cost in contrast agent and minor additional cost in examination time. Our recommended protocols for resting-only and rest plus vasodilator/stress are outlined in Tables 1 and 2.

Tips for patient preparation: (i) warn the patient that they may experience certain sensations during the injection of vasodilator or physiological stressor (e.g., transient lightheadedness for adenosine and palpitations for dobutamine), and (ii) instruct the patient on approaches for breath-holding at the start of the injection of contrast agent, and on breathing shallowly thereafter.

Table 1 Cardiovascular Magnetic Resonance Perfusion Imaging—Resting Protocol

Localization	Perform real-time interactive localization of four-chamber and two-chamber long-axis views. Verify patient comfort, reliable gating, and appropriate coil positioning	5 min
Perfusion prescription	Saturation-recovery fast gradient echo: two R–R interval temporal resolution, six short-axis slices spanning apex to base (use more slices if heart rate is slower than 75 beats/min)	3 min
Precontrast calibration	With saturation pulse turned OFF, scan once to verify appropriate slice positioning (e.g., if patient has moved, coach them to stay still, and start from beginning)	5 min
	With saturation pulse turned ON, scan once to verify maximal suppression of normal myocardium (if suppression is inadequate, adjust the saturation pulse area, or the saturation recovery time; methods for performing these adjustments are vendor-specific)	
	Prepare the sequence to scan with saturation pulse ON for at least 50 sec (the minimum duration for first-pass studies)	
First-pass scan	Coach the volunteer to perform a breath-hold (if possible) for the initial 20 sec, and shallow breathing thereafter	3 min
	Request breath-hold, begin the scan, and after 2 sec, start the contrast agent injection	

Note: A majority of the time is spent preparing and calibrating the sequence to ensure satisfactory image quality during the first-pass scan. The total scan time is less than 20 minutes.
Abbreviation: CMR, cardiovascular magnetic resonance.

Table 2 Cardiovascular Magnetic Resonance Perfusion Reserve Protocol—Rest and Vasodilator/Stress

Localization	Perform real-time interactive localization of four-chamber and two-chamber long-axis views. Verify patient comfort, reliable gating, and appropriate coil positioning	5 min
Perfusion prescription	Saturation-recovery fast gradient echo: two R–R interval temporal resolution, six short-axis slices spanning apex to base (use more slices if heart rate is slower than 75 beats/min)	3 min
Pre-contrast calibration	With saturation pulse turned OFF, scan once to verify appropriate slice positioning (e.g., if patient has moved, coach them to stay still, and start from beginning)	5 min
	With saturation pulse turned ON, scan once to verify maximal suppression of normal myocardium (if suppression is inadequate, adjust the saturation pulse area, or the saturation recovery time; methods for performing these adjustments are vendor-specific)	
	Prepare the sequence to scan with saturation pulse ON for at least 50 sec (the minimum duration for first-pass studies)	
Adenosine/ dipyridamole	*Note*: While adenosine is more commonly used, dipyridamole has been used historically and is still an alternative to adenosine	5 min
Vasodilator first-pass scan	Begin adenosine infusion	
	Coach the volunteer to perform a breath-hold (if possible) for the initial 20 sec, and shallow breathing thereafter	
	Shortly after the start of adenosine infusion, request a breath-hold, begin the scan, and after 2 sec, start the contrast agent injection. Follow with a saline flush	
	Immediately after the end of scanning, stop the adenosine infusion, flush with saline	
Wait	Wait for the washout of contrast agent Left ventricular function and delayed enhancement scanning may be performed during this time	15–25 min

(*Continued*)

Table 2 Cardiovascular Magnetic Resonance Perfusion Reserve Protocol—Rest and Vasodilator/Stress (*Continued*)

Resting First-pass scan	Coach the volunteer to perform a breath-hold (if possible) for the initial 20 sec, and shallow breathing thereafter Request breath-hold, begin the scan, and after 2 sec, start the contrast agent injection	3 min

Note: While this protocol specifies adenosine, the preparation and timing will differ for alternative vasodilator or stress agents (such as dipyridamole). Total examination time should be approximately 45 to 60 minutes (including function and delayed enhancement).

CLINICAL ASPECTS

The results of myocardial perfusion imaging with CMR are similar to those of myocardial perfusion imaging with radionuclides. Briefly, when there is myocardial scar, there are persistent defects in the distribution of gadolinium at both rest and vasodilator/stress. When there is obstructive CAD in the absence of scar, there are transient defects in the distribution of gadolinium during vasodilator/stress that are not present at rest.

Persistent Defects

With radionuclide thallium studies, perfusion is evaluated with vasodilation/stress. In regions of scar, thallium activity is persistently reduced, while in viable regions, thallium activity fills in over time.

When using CMR with a paramagnetic contrast agent (generally a gadolinium chelate), the presence of a perfusion defect both at rest and during vasodilation/stress is an indication of non-viable myocardium. CMR also detects non-viable myocardium using the approach of delayed contrast enhancement (Chapter 12). The delayed enhancement approach is the more sensitive means for detecting non-viable myocardium, as it depicts the non-viable territory with higher spatial resolution and higher contrast compared with perfusion-based approaches.

Several other pathologies can lead to persistent defects. These include myocardial sarcoidosis and myocardial tumors (primary or metastatic).

Transient Defects

Large-vessel CAD demonstrable by coronary angiography generally produces perfusion defects in the distribution of the obstructed coronary artery or arteries (Figs. 3 and 4). Images during the passage of contrast agent in the presence of vasodilator infusion will delineate territories supplied by coronary arteries with flow-limiting disease. Territories with transient defects do not exhibit delayed enhancement. Recent studies by Bernhardt et al. (15)

(A)

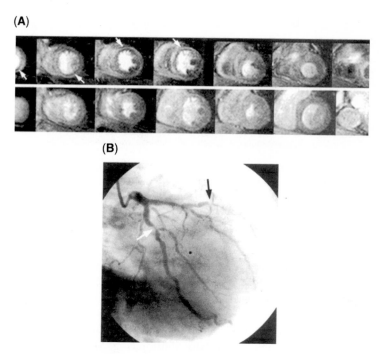

(B)

Figure 3 Correspondence between (**A**) cardiovascular magnetic resonance detected perfusion defects and (**B**) angiographically significant disease. *Source*: Figure 1 from Ref. 16.

and Wolff et al. (21) have shown that the sensitivity and specificity of first-pass CMR perfusion imaging for detecting CAD are 93% to 96% and 75% to 87%, respectively.

Diffusely Distributed Defects

A unique aspect of CMR perfusion imaging is that it allows imaging of perfusion abnormalities associated with microvascular disease. Microvascular

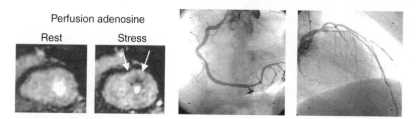

Figure 4 Transient defect detected by cardiovascular magnetic resonance perfusion at rest and during the infusion of adenosine in a patient with angiographically significant coronary artery disease. *Source*: Figure 2 from Ref. 22.

(A)   (B)   (C)

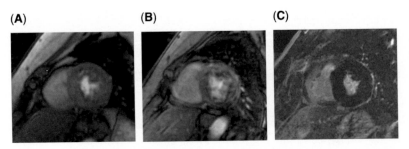

Figure 5   CMR first-pass perfusion and delayed enhancement images from a 63-year-old woman with chest pain and no significant angiographic coronary artery disease (CAD). Resting perfusion imaging (**A**) shows homogeneous distribution of contrast (the normal pattern). Adenosine perfusion imaging (**B**) demonstrates patchy distribution of perfusion defects not suggestive of any specific coronary arterial distribution. High-resolution delayed enhancement imaging (**C**) shows no evidence of myocardial scar. The pattern of patchy perfusion is consistent with microvascular disease (dysfunction) that is commonly observed in women without angiographically significant CAD. *Source*: Courtesy of Gerald M. Pohost, MD, Division of Cardiovascular Medicine, University of Southern California, Los Angeles, California, U.S.A.

disease cannot be seen by conventional coronary angiography and produces perfusion defects in a widespread patchy distribution (Fig. 5), or a subendocardial distribution (Fig. 6) (23). This is possible because of the high spatial resolution and good contrast of CMR perfusion imaging. Microvascular

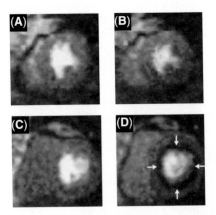

Figure 6   Images of myocardium at peak contrast enhancement during the first-pass of gadolinium at rest (**A, C**) and during adenosine infusion (**B, D**), in a control subject showing normal uniform myocardial signal enhancement and a patient with Cardiac Syndrome X showing a ring of reduced signal around the left ventricular cavity. The authors interpreted this pattern as sub-endocardial ischemia. *Source*: Figures 2 and 3 from Ref. 23.

disease has recently been demonstrated by CMR perfusion in a large percentage of women with chest pain and no angiographically significant CAD (24).

ARTIFACTS

There are many types of artifact that are observed with CMR. Many can be easily avoided at the pre-contrast calibration step (Tables 1 and 2). These include:

1. Aliasing—if aliasing occurs in the precontrast images, increase the field-of-view.
2. Inadequate saturation—if myocardium is not saturated before contrast administration, rerun prescan, and if that does not improve saturation, adjust the tip angle of the saturation pulse.
3. "Ghosting" artifacts—if using an EPI-based acquisition, timing errors and eddy currents may cause ghosting artifacts. When this happens, repeat the EPI reference scan and retry. If artifacts do not improve, switch to a simple gradient echo acquisition.
4. "Banding" artifacts—if using an SSFP-based acquisition, off-resonance may cause banding artifacts over the heart (dark bands). When this happens, reduce the TR and perform localized shimming. If both fail, switch to an FGRE acquisition.

An artifact of critical importance in dynamic contrast-enhanced studies is the "dark rim" artifact, which has been under investigation for some time (25). In first-pass perfusion studies, this could cause an erroneous diagnosis of a sub-endocardial perfusion defect, since the dark rim appears at the boundary between myocardium and blood pool (Fig. 7). Potential causes of this artifact include susceptibility, motion, and T1 recovery during a segmented acquisition.

A recent analysis by Di Bella et al. (26) identified inadequate spatial resolution as a definite and important contributor, where limitations in the extent of acquired k-space causes Gibbs ringing (27) in the image. This can be addressed by increasing spatial resolution and windowing the acquired k-space data (consult with your vendor to implement these solutions).

CONCLUSIONS

Myocardial perfusion imaging using CMR generates accurate, high-resolution, high-contrast images. Generally, imaging relies on the use of T1-shortening contrast agents and pulse sequences that produce image intensity proportional to contrast agent concentration. Persistent defects and transient defects are easily observed. Quantitation can be performed using a double-bolus approach, which is a slight modification to the standard acquisition protocol. In the near future, we expect improvements in

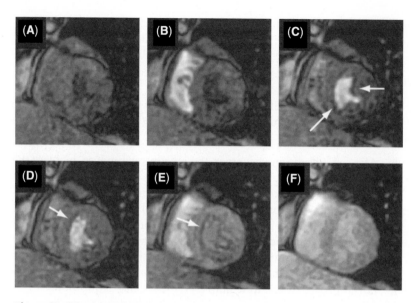

Figure 7 "Dark rim" artifacts. Images from a healthy volunteer which show artifacts mimicking subendocardial perfusion defect (*white arrows*). The artifact is seen at many stages during the first-pass of contrast. These images were acquired using a saturation recovery FGRE pulse sequence on a clinical 3 Tesla scanner. *Source:* Courtesy of Scott B. Reeder, MD, PhD, Departments of Radiology and Medical Physics, University of Wisconsin, Madison, Wisconsin, U.S.A.

contrast, volumetric coverage, and spatial resolution as a result of higher field strengths, improved contrast preparation schemes, and novel pulse sequences. We also anticipate improved approaches for quantitation.

The difference between perfusion imaging with CMR and radio-nuclides is the lack of ionizing radiation, higher resolution, and improved SNR. Myocardial perfusion imaging is improved when CMR studies are performed at higher magnetic field strengths, such as 3 T compared with the more widely available 1.5 T (28). Myocardial perfusion imaging using radio-nuclides has become a standard approach for the noninvasive detection of CAD. With present CMR technology, and anticipated future improvements, CMR should become the standard approach for myocardial perfusion imaging.

One of the most important and unique contributions of CMR perfusion imaging is the ability to identify patterns indicative of microvascular disease. There are no other noninvasive technologies at the present time that can demonstrate perfusion changes related to microvascular disease. We can anticipate improved microvascular disease detection using high-field systems, which achieve higher spatial resolution and contrast.

REFERENCES

1. Pohost GM, Zir LM, Moore RH, McKusick KA, Guiney TE, Beller GA. Differentiation of transiently ischemic from infarcted myocardium by serial imaging after a single dose of Thallium-201. Circulation 1977; 55(2):294–302.
2. Hachamovitch R, Berman DS, Kiat H, Cohen I, Friedman JD, Shaw LJ. Value of stress myocardial perfusion single photon emission computed tomography in patients with normal resting electrocardiograms: an evaluation of incremental prognostic value and cost-effectiveness. Circulation 2002; 105(7):823–829.
3. Hor G. Myocardial scintigraphy—25 years after start. Eur J Nucl Med 1988; 13:619–636.
4. Keijer JT, Bax JJ, van Rossum AC, Visser FC, Visser CA. Myocardial perfusion imaging: clinical experience and recent progress in radionuclide scintigraphy and magnetic resonance imaging. Int J Card Imaging 1997; 13:415–431.
5. Muzik O, Duvernoy C, Beanlands RS, et al. Assessment of diagnostic performance of quantitative flow measurements in normal subjects and patients with angiographically documented coronary artery disease by means of nitrogen-13 ammonia and positron emission tomography. J Am Coll Cardiol 1998; 31: 534–540.
6. Schwaiger M, Muzik O. Assessment of myocardial perfusion by positron emission tomography. Am J Cardiol 1991; 67:35D–43D.
7. Mulvagh SL. Myocardial perfusion by contrast echocardiography: diagnosis of coronary artery disease using contrast-enhanced stress echocardiography and assessment of coronary anatomy and flow reserve. Coron Artery Dis 2000; 11: 243–251.
8. Senior R, Kaul S, Soman P, Lahiri A. Power Doppler harmonic imaging: a feasibility study of a new technique for the assessment of myocardial perfusion. Am Heart J 2000; 139:245–251.
9. Schmermund A, Bell MR, Lerman LO, Ritman EL, Rumberger JA. Quantitative evaluation of regional myocardial perfusion using fast X-ray computed tomography. Herz 1997; 22:29–39.
10. Georgiou D, Wolfkiel C, Brundage BH. Ultrafast computed tomography for the physiological evaluation of myocardial perfusion. Am J Card Imaging 1994; 8:151–158.
11. Higgins CB, Sakuma H. Heart disease: functional evaluation with MR imaging. Radiology 1996; 199:307–315.
12. Atkinson DJ, Burstein D, Edelman RR. First-pass cardiac perfusion: evaluation with ultrafast MR imaging. Radiology 1990; 174:757–762.
13. Sakuma H, Suzawa N, Ichikawa Y, et al. Diagnostic accuracy of stress first-pass contrast-enhanced myocardial perfusion MRI compared with stress myocardial perfusion scintigraphy. Am J Roentgenol 2004; 185:95–102.
14. Fenchel M, Helber U, Kramer U, et al. Detection of regional myocardial perfusion deficit using rest and stress perfusion MRI: a feasibility study. Am J Roentgenol 2005; 185:627–635.
15. Bernhardt P, Engels T, Levenson B, et al. Prediction of necessity for coronary artery revascularization by adenosine contrast-enhanced magnetic resonance imaging. Int J Card. In press.

16. Wolff SD, Schwitter J, Coulden R, et al. Myocardial first-pass perfusion magnetic resonance imaging a multicenter dose-ranging study. Circulation 2004; 110: 732–737.

17. Weiskoff RM, Caravan P. MR contrast agent basics. In: Lardo A, Chronos NA, Fayad ZA, Fuster V, eds. Cardiovascular Magnetic Resonance: Established and Emerging Applications. Chapter 2. Taylor & Francis, Spain, 2004; 17–38.

18. Jerosch-Herold M, Wilke N, Stillman AE. Magnetic resonance quantification of the myocardial perfusion reserve with a Fermi function model for constrained deconvolution. Med Phys 1998; 25(1):73–84.

19. Jerosch-Herold M, Swingen C, Seethamraju RT. Myocardial blood flow quantification with MRI by model-independent deconvolution. Med Phys 2002; 29(5): 886–897.

20. Christian TF, Rettmann DW, Aletras A, et al. Absolute myocardial perfusion in canines measured by using dual-bolus first-pass MR imaging. Radiology 2004; 232(3):677–684.

21. Hsu LY, Rhoads KL, Holly JE, Kellman P, Aletras AH, Arai AE. Quantitative myocardial perfusion analysis with a dual-bolus contrast-enhanced first-pass MRI technique in humans. J Magn Reson Imaging 2006; 23(3):315–322.

22. Paetsch I, Jahnke C, Wahl A, et al. Circulation 2004; 110:835–842.

23. Panting JR, Gatehouse PD, Yang GZ, et al. Abnormal subendocardial perfusion in cardiac syndrome X detected by cardiovascular magnetic resonance imaging. N Engl J Med 2002; 346(25):1948–1953.

24. Special Issue: "Coronary Artery Disease in Women." J Am Coll Cardiol Suppl, February 7, 2006.

25. Faranesh AZ, Oznur I, Kraitchman DL, Reeder SB, Bluemke DA, McVeigh ER. Hypoenhancing artifacts in contrast enhanced cardiac perfusion imaging: implications for false positive diagnosis. In: Proceedings of RSNA, 84th Scientific Meeting, Chicago, IL, 1998.

26. Di Bella EV, Parker DL, Sinusas AJ. On the dark rim artifact in dynamic contrast-enhanced MRI myocardial perfusion studies. Magn Reson Med 2005; 54(5):1295–1299.

27. Gibbs JW. Fourier series. Nature 1899; 59:200–606.

28. Strach KA, Meyer C, Naehle CP, et al. High resolution myocardial perfusion imaging at 3.0 T: comparison to standard 1.5T perfusion studies and diagnostic accuracy in patients with suspected CAD. In: Proceedings of Society for Cardiovascular Magnetic Resonance, Miami, FL, 2006:7–8.

10

Ischemic Heart Disease: Myocardial Metabolism

Steven M. Stevens, Hee-Won Kim, and Gerald M. Pohost
*Department of Medicine, Division of Cardiovascular Medicine,
Keck School of Medicine, University of Southern California,
Los Angeles, California, U.S.A.*

INTRODUCTION

The principle of nuclear magnetic resonance was first described in 1946 (1,2). A radiofrequency (RF) applied to a sensitive nucleus in the setting of a magnetic field can induce resonance ultimately resulting in a signal at a frequency that is related to the chemical and structural properties of the molecules that contain the sensitive nuclei. Different molecules and different environments of these molecules can change the frequencies of the signals emitted, allowing differentiation between nuclear species and their environments. The mathematical operation of Fourier transformation provides a means of changing the distribution of frequencies (in k-space) into spectra. A spectrum is a two-dimensional representation of the frequencies of the signals depicting the various molecular components containing the sensitive nucleus under scrutiny (Fig. 1). The magnitude of the spectral peaks (the area under the peak at each frequency) represents the concentration of the molecule being sampled in the myocardium (for example).

Cardiovascular magnetic resonance spectroscopy (CMRS) has similarities to CMR imaging but is specifically applied to evaluate the composition

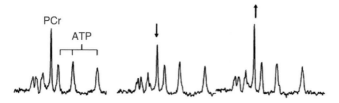

Figure 1 Phosphorus-31 spectra from the anterior myocardium of abnormal responder during rest (*left*), handgrip stress (*middle*), and recovery (*right*) at 3T. PCr drop and recovery was observed during 30% maximum handgrip stress for 6 minutes. *Abbreviations*: PCr, phosphocreatine; ATP, adenosine triphosphate.

and metabolism of cardiovascular tissue. Using an isolated perfused rat heart model, in 1977, Jacobus et al. (3) and Garlick et al. (4) were the first two groups to generate phosphorus-31 (^{31}P) spectra of heart muscle using CMRS. These spectra demonstrated phosphocreatine (PCr), adenosine triphosphate (ATP), inorganic intracellular phosphate, and other blood borne phosphates such as 2,3-diphophoglycerate (2,3-DPG). In addition to ^{31}P, other nuclear species can be studied and the concentrations of their molecular components estimated. Nuclei that have been studied in biologic systems include proton (^{1}H), carbon-13 (^{13}C), fluorine-19 (^{19}F), sodium-23 (^{23}Na), and ^{31}P. Of these nuclei, ^{31}P spectroscopy is the most well established for CMR in the clinical setting, largely due to its applicability to observe the main components in high-energy phosphate metabolism, ATP, PCr, and inorganic phosphate. The 2,3-DPG in the red blood cells is seen as two separate phosphate peaks near the intracellular inorganic phosphate peak (Pi) (Fig. 1). The ability to noninvasively monitor in vivo myocardial high-energy phosphate metabolism has tremendous potential to allow the evaluation of intracellular myocardial metabolism to determine the impact of heart disease on myocardial energetics. Clinical and basic science uses of ^{31}P-CMRS include the observation of changes in high-energy phosphate metabolism and intracellular pH related to ischemia, myocardial viability, and microvascular disease and/or endothelial dysfunction. The unique role of CMRS to monitor intracellular metabolism is especially important in microvascular disease/dysfunction, as no other imaging technique can reliably detect such abnormalities at the intracellular level. Accordingly, CMRS techniques have the great potential to study pathological conditions that have an important microvascular component such as cardiomyopathies, allograft rejection, the effects of revascularization, Cardiac Syndrome X, heart disease in women, and cardiovascular disease in diabetes. As a result, CMRS is in its developmental infancy and will continue to generate new clinically relevant applications related to cardiovascular diagnosis, prognostication, and the impact of treatment for a wide variety of cardiovascular disease states.

VOLUME LOCATION TECHNIQUES FOR IN VIVO SPECTROSCOPY

The region of the myocardium to be studied must be localized so that the signal from the volume of interest (VOI) is acquired, while signal contamination from surrounding tissue is minimized. Scout MR imaging is used to localize the VOI, which is usually on the anterior wall of the left ventricle (Fig. 2A, B). The patient is typically lying in the prone position to minimize the distance from the ^{31}P coil and the myocardium. Because skeletal muscle surrounding the myocardium contains considerable molecular phosphates, spatial localization is required to generate spectra from only myocardium. An RF pulse is applied to excite the VOI and generate free induction decay RF signals that are received by the surface coil. This time domain RF signal is converted to the MR spectrum in the frequency domain through the mathematical operation known as Fourier transformation.

The use of a surface coil has been adopted in ^{31}P-CMRS because of its sensitivity and inherent localized B_1 field close to the coil. The volume of myocardium, interrogated and the sensitivity depend on the distance between the coil and the myocardium evaluated. Several techniques combined with surface coil application such as surface-spoiling methods (6), use of depth-pulses (7), and rotating-frame methods (8) help to delineate the localized myocardial volume. In most CMRS studies techniques combine the use of the RF field (B_1) of the surface coil and the static magnetic field (B_0).

Single-Voxel MRS

Single-voxel MRS includes depth-resolved surface-coil spectroscopy (DRESS), image-selected in vivo spectroscopy (ISIS), point-resolved spectroscopy

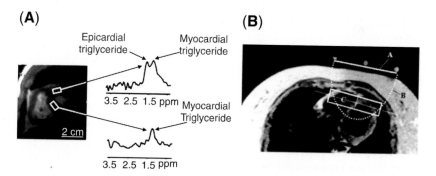

(A)

Epicardial triglyceride   Myocardial triglyceride

3.5 2.5 1.5 ppm Myocardial Triglyceride

2 cm

3.5 2.5 1.5 ppm

(B)

Figure 2 (A) Selection of volume of interest in the ventricular septum and in the left ventricular (LV) wall with corresponding spectra. Spectrum from septum displays single resonance from myocardial triglyceride. Spectrum from LV wall contains additional resonance from epicardial fat. **(B)** Scout image for single-volume localization. A: surface coil, B: effective B_1 RF field, C: volume of interest for modified oblique DRESS technique. *Abbreviations*: LV, left ventricle; DRESS, depth-resolved surface-coil spectroscopy. *Source*: From Ref. 5.

(PRESS) and stimulated-echo acquisition mode (STEAM) (9), and utilizes the slice-selective B_0 gradient and provides spectra from a single volume (voxel) (Table 1).

Using a surface coil, the DRESS sequence determines a slice by using a frequency-selective 90° pulse followed by a gradient-refocusing pulse. Since the lateral extent of the DRESS slice is defined by the sensitive volume of the surface coil, contamination from the surrounding tissue such as chest muscle or the liver is always a potential problem. In ISIS, selective inversion pulses are applied along three orthogonal axes to localize a single volume of myocardium within the sensitive region of the surface coil. The ISIS approach is less affected by the signal loss due to T_2 relaxation as this sequence does not use a refocusing pulse or an echo. On the other hand, the ISIS approach is more sensitive to motion artifacts because a series of acquisitions is necessary for defining the ISIS voxel. The STEAM approach uses three consecutive 90° slice-selective pulses applied to three orthogonal axes to generate a stimulated echo from the volume. A disadvantage of STEAM is that the stimulated echo by the sequence produces only half of the possible signal from the VOI. The PRESS sequence consists of 90°–180°–180° pulses to the three axes and retains full signal intensity. The PRESS approach cannot reduce the echo time as short as STEAM.

Table 1 Single-Volume Spectroscopic Localization Techniques

Depth-resolved surface-coil spectroscopy
Signal from the contiguous cylindrical slices
Simple and good signal-to-noise ratio
Poor lateral definition of VOI
Used extensively to study cardiac metabolism in various pathologies, including transplant rejection, myocardial ischemia and infarction, and dilated cardiomyopathy
Image-selected in vivo spectroscopy
Selective inversion pulses applied along three orthogonal axes
Excellent definition of VOI
Effective for short T_2 metabolite (^{31}P)
Sensitive to motion artifacts (localization relies on a difference scheme)
Point-resolved spectroscopy
Retaining full signal from the voxel
Good inversion pulse required
Longer echo time (mainly for not-too-short T_2 metabolite, ^1H)
Double signal-to-noise ratio over STEAM
STEAM
Stimulated echoes used
Short echo time available (for short T_2 metabolites, ^1H)
Yielding only half of signal from the voxel

Abbreviations: VOI, volume of interest; STEAM, stimulated echo acquisition mode.

Spectroscopic Imaging

Unlike single-voxel CMRS, the spatial information based on CMR spectra can be obtained using the spectroscopic imaging (MRSI) technique (Table 2). This is also known as chemical shift imaging (CSI) where the RF signals are phase-encoded by switching gradients into one- to three-dimensions, as used in CMR imaging. The raw data are processed to provide a spectral map consisting of each voxel or slice that represents the NMR spectrum at a certain position. The spatial resolution of MRSI is far less than CMR imaging because the concentrations of metabolites are three orders less than that of water in human tissue. Meanwhile proton MRSI for brain has been widely used in the clinical examination, cardiac application of SI technique has been demonstrated only by a limited number of groups (11–13).

The MRSI approach is advantageous to the efficiency of data collection as the MR signals from the whole volume are collected during acquisition. The MRSI, however, has the major drawback in which the signal from the single voxel is distributed over other voxels by the spatial response function originated from the truncation of k-dimension. In this Fourier method, the contamination arises by aliasing and also by signal bleeding when the voxel size is larger than the scale of the biological heterogeneities. This phenomenon can be alleviated by several techniques including acquisition weighting (14,15).

Table 2 Magnetic Resonance Spectroscopic Imaging and Others

MRSI
Spatial and spectral information are obtained simultaneously
Slice (1D) or voxels (2D/3D) defined by phase encoding steps
Each voxel is less well delineated than single-voxel spectroscopy
Contamination by signal bleeding as Fourier method is used
Usually requires long acquisition time (2D/3D ever worse)
Spatial localization with optimal pointspread function
Signals can be acquired from voxels of arbitrary shaped compartments
Improved SLIM method (using optimized pointspread function)
A priori knowledge used regarding anatomic structures
Absolute quantitation available
Contamination from outside the volumes of interest
Hybrid techniques
Outer volume suppressed ISIS (10)
DRESS/SI
PRESS/SI
STEAM/SI

Abbreviations: MRSI, magnetic resonance spectroscopic imaging; DRESS, depth-resolved surface-coil spectroscopy; PRESS, point-resolved spectroscopy; STEAM, stimulated echo acquisition mode; ISIS, image-selected in vivo spectroscopy.

Other Techniques

The second RF channel enables proton-decoupled ^{31}P-MRS that increases spectral resolution and increase signal-to-noise ratio by nuclear Overhauser enhancement (16). On the other hand, the very elegant method, spectral localization by imaging (SLIM), was introduced in the late 1980s by which spectral information is obtained from well-defined compartments (17). The SLIM has great potential by which MR spectra can be obtained from arbitrary-shaped compartment, but dreadful contamination is introduced by the pointspread function unless each compartment is very homogeneous. Another technique, spectral localization with optimal pointspread (SLOOP) function improves SLIM by optimizing the pointspread function using prior knowledge and iteration (18,19). This spectroscopy technique has great potential for absolute quantitation of high-energy phosphate by incorporating target volume, coil sensitivity, and pointspread effects (20).

ISCHEMIC HEART DISEASE AND MYOCARDIAL VIABILITY

The application of monitoring high-energy phosphate metabolism is exquisitely suited for ischemia detection. The most labile high-energy phosphate is PCr which serves to replete ATP when there is increased myocardial work. As ATP is hydrolyzed for energy release, the accumulation of adenosine diphosphate will favor the hydrolysis of PCr to creatine, regenerating ATP. There is a chemical equilibrium between PCr and ATP, and their ratio remains stable in the resting state. However, a change in the ratio between PCr and ATP may indicate an increase in myocardial work beyond the level that can be sustained by blood supply. For example, when the myocardium is stressed and the blood supply is inadequate, ischemia results. Under these circumstances PCr reserve is decreased and PCr/ATP decreases. This decrease in PCr/ATP with myocardial ischemia has been observed in both animal and clinical experiments. Absolute quantitation of high-energy phosphates is technically more difficult, requiring an accurate phosphate reference standard. To date only limited studies have attempted quantify these concentrations, although such quantitation has substantial advantages (e.g., to evaluated myocardial viability) over use of the ratio.

In 1990, Weiss et al. studied patients with left anterior descending (LAD) coronary artery disease (CAD) using ^{31}P spectroscopy of the spatially localized left ventricular anterior wall myocardium. The spectra were gathered before, during, and after isometric handgrip exercise. In the control group of 11 patients, no change was observed in the myocardium secondary to handgrip exercise, with mean PCr to ATP ratios of 1.72 ± 0.15. In a second group of nine patients with non-ischemic cardiomyopathy, again no change was observed; the mean ratio was 1.59 ± 0.31. However, in 16 patients with LAD CAD, the ratio decreased dramatically with hand-grip exercise, starting at a baseline of 1.45 ± 0.3; decreasing to 0.91 ± 0.24 during exercise stress; and recovering to 1.27 ± 0.38. Perhaps the most remarkable observation was in five of those patients who later underwent revascularization; their PCr to ATP ratio not only increased at baseline from 1.51 ± 0.19 to 1.60 ± 0.2, but also demonstrated no significant change during exercise, 1.62 ± 0.18. Note that the prerevascularization stress measurement was 1.02 ± 0.19 (21). Clearly, this noteworthy study showed that PCr to ATP ratio reliably monitored changes in high-energy phosphate metabolism that were representative of myocardial ischemia.

We now recognize that when myocardium becomes ischemic, its PCr to ATP ratio decreases, while normal myocardium demonstrates no such decrease. However, myocardial scar, which is by definition substantially less metabolically active, should not demonstrate a significant change in PCr/ATP. Yabe et al. demonstrated this phenomenon in 1994 by comparing 27 patients with LAD coronary artery stenosis greater than or equal to 75% and 11 normal controls (22). The DRESS single-volume localization technique was employed to isolate the VOI of the anterior wall of the left ventricle. The study patients with LAD stenosis were divided into two groups based on exercise stress testing with radionuclide imaging using thallium-201 (^{201}Tl). As expected, those with a transient defect between stress and rest images were found to have a change in PCr to ATP ratio with handgrip exercise: 1.60 ± 0.19 at rest to 0.96 ± 0.28 with stress. Meanwhile, in both the group with a fixed defect (most likely related to myocardial scar) and in the normal group, no change in the PCr to ATP ratio was observed. Therefore, ^{31}P-CMRS is useful for detecting ischemia in viable myocardium based on changes in PCr/ATP, while such metabolic changes are not observed in normal or scarred myocardium with stress.

Assessing myocardial viability is essential to clinical decisions regarding revascularization. Three methods to date have been used to assess this vital information: preserved coronary flow reserve, wall motion, and metabolism. CMR imaging can assess the first two, while for metabolism CMRS is ideal. Quantitation of ATP and PCr is useful to differentiate viable from non-viable myocardium. Ratios are only useful when there is a relative decrease in PCr. Whereas, if both ATP and PCr decrease proportionally, no change in the ratio is observed. Yabe et al. studied 41 patients with LAD stenosis greater than or equal to 50% who also underwent exercise ^{201}Tl imaging (23). Subjects were divided into three groups based on the results of exercise ^{201}Tl imaging: normal controls (C), those with a reversible defect (RD[+]), and those with a fixed defect (RD[–]). One-dimensional CSI localization techniques were employed to select anterior and apical slices of the left ventricle. ^{31}P-CMRS revealed significant differences in quantitation of PCr and ATP among the three groups, with the PCr and ATP concentrations greatest in the normal group, less in the RD[+], and least in the RD[–] group.

Metabolism in patients with non-Q-wave infarctions (NQWI) was studied by Moka et al. (24) Data was acquired from ^{31}P-CMRS detection of high-energy phosphate metabolism, left ventricular functional parameters, and technetium-99m methoxyisobutylisonitrile ([99 m]Tc-MIBI). Two groups were compared: group A consisting of 15 patients with NQWI and group B made up of 10 controls without CAD. All patients of group A displayed anterior wall hypokinesia in the infarcted area on both ventriculography and MRI. There were significant differences between groups A and B in all measurements compared: myocardial accumulation of ^{99m}Tc-MIBI ($66.3 \pm 11.8\%$ vs. $95.6 \pm 2.2\%$ in group B), mean wall thickness during the complete cardiac cycle (9.5 ± 1.8 mm vs. 13.1 ± 1.1 mm in group B, $p<0.001$), systolic wall thickening (2.6 ± 1.4 mm vs. 5.8 ± 1.5 mm in group B, $p<0.01$) and PCr/ATP (1.12 ± 0.22 vs. 1.74 ± 0.23 in group B, $p<0.01$). These results suggest that along with decreased perfusion and functional impairment following NQWI, there also exists a significant decrease in PCr/ATP, demonstrating altered myocardial high-energy phosphate metabolism.

DILATED CARDIOMYOPATHY AND HEART FAILURE

There is ample evidence that heart failure and cardiomyopathy is accompanied by metabolic changes (25). Studies using ^{31}P-CMRS have had mixed results demonstrating such changes. Several early studies looking at dilated cardiomyopathy showed no reduction in PCR/ATP (26–28). Hardy et al. were the first to demonstrate a significant reduction in PCr/ATP. They looked at patients with severe dilated cardiomyopathy and found the PCr/ATP ratio to be significantly decreased (1.46 ± 0.07) from normal patients (1.80 ± 0.06, $p<0.001$) (29). The idea that severity of failure in dilated cardiomyopathy may relate to PCr/ATP was explored in a study by Neubauer et al. in 1992 (30). ISIS was used to localize left ventricular myocardium for ^{31}P-CMRS and PCr/ATP ratios were calculated. The PCr/ATP ratios were correlated with the New York Heart Association (NYHA) class of heart failure ($r = 0.60$, $p<0.005$). Six of those patients were studied 12 ± 6 weeks after pharmacological treatment who showed improvement of the NYHA status by 0.8 ± 0.3 classes. Along with improvement of NYHA status, PCr/ATP increased from 1.51 ± 0.32 to 2.15 ± 0.27 ($p < 0.01$). A second study by Neubauer et al. in 1995 was able to correlate PCr/ATP ratio with NYHA status and function assessment, ejection fraction (EF) and end-diastolic wall thickening (31). Hansch et al. were able to correlate PCr/ATP with EF as well in more recent study using two dimensional chemical shift imaging (2D-CSI) localization (32). A third study by Neubauer et al. in 1997 used the PCR/ATP ratio to prognosticate mortality in dilated cardiomyopathy in patients classified as either NYHA I, II, or III, all with an EF $<50\%$ (33). Patients were divided into two groups,

PCr/ATP >1.60 and PCr/ATP <1.60. Patients were followed for 2.5 years. The cardiovascular mortality rate was significantly greater ($p = 0.016$) in the group with PCr/ATP <1.60 (40% or 8/20) compared to the group with PCr/ATP >1.60 (5% or 1/19). In fact, PCr/ATP predicted survival with greater accuracy than NYHA and EF in this study.

Left ventricular hypertrophy has been extensively studied using PCr/ATP. A proposed mechanism is that as the myocardium hypertrophies, the blood supply becomes inadequate causing ischemia. Aortic stenosis causes severe left ventricular hypertrophy and its relation to decreases in left ventricular ATP/PCr was first studied by Conway et al. in 1991 (8). Since then, multiple studies have found that PCr/ATP inversely correlates with left ventricular hypertrophy in aortic stenosis (34–37). Likewise, the hypertrophied septum in hypertrophic cardiomyopathy has been shown to have decreased PCr/ATP, perhaps by similar mechanism as in left ventricular hypertrophy (38–40). Left ventricular remodeling with mitral regurgitation also is accompanied by a decrease in PCr/ATP, though mitral regurgitation is often accompanied by eccentric hypertrophy of the myocardium rather than concentric hypertrophy as in aortic stenosis (41).

Remodeling in various forms of heart failure is clearly accompanied my metabolic changes which have been detected with ^{31}P-CMRS. The clinical application for this technology may be to monitor severity of disease, treatment outcome, prognostics or simply to reveal further understanding of the pathophysiology of heart failure.

CARDIAC TRANSPLANTATION

Heart transplantation has become a routine tool for the treatment of end-stage heart failure. With the improvement of surgical techniques and immunosuppressive therapy, two areas in need of improvement are predicting early graft dysfunction prior to transplantation and accurate detection of rejection to ensure optimal medical management posttransplantation. Allograft ^{31}P-CMRS may be ideal for both applications.

Donor-derived heart grafts often sustain severe physiological stress prior to explantation and transplantation. The mechanisms for this stress include the effects of: catecholamine release with brain death, cold storage, the effects of the pressors required to sustain graft viability, and the impact of graft transportation. Therefore, pretransplant assessment of the donor heart is necessary to avoid early graft rejection. Van Dobbenburgh et al. studied the energy metabolism of 25 excised human donor hearts arrested with cardioplegic solution using ^{31}P-CMRS prior to transplantation (42). Spectroscopy is performed in approximately 30 minutes, within an acceptable timeframe between harvest and implantation. PCr/ATP was directly correlated to cardiac index 1 week posttransplantation ($r = 0.49$, $p = 0.01$), while pH measured by the chemical shift of inorganic phosphate showed no relationship ($r = 0.31$, $p = 0.13$). Caus et al. showed that parameters assessed by ^{31}P-CMRS correlated with criteria used by the United Network for Organ Sharing method of determining whether hearts are fit for transplant based on echocardiographic-derived EF, amount of inotrope administration to the donor, and global visual condition of the graft determined by the surgeon. Substantial evidence for the utility of ^{31}P-CMRS pretransplant has been described by Caus et al. (43). The "CMRS score" was calculated based on metabolic criteria including pH and PCr/pH ratios, as well the more established PCr/ATP. Significant differences in all metabolic markers exist between hearts with early rejection, those not suitable for transplantation, and those transplanted without complication. The CMRS score was 100% sensitive and 86% specific for predicting early graft failure. Therefore, ^{31}P-CMR is proving to be useful for assessing heart transplant grafts pretransplantation to predict early rejection and dysfunction.

Phosphorus-31 CMRS may also be useful after cardiac transplantation for monitoring graft rejection. There have been numerous animal model studies which demonstrate that spectroscopy is useful for detecting changes in high-energy phosphate metabolism during cardiac allograft rejection (44–49). Canby et al. (44), for example, studied subcutaneously transplanted hearts from one strain of rat (Brown Norway) into another strain of rat (Lewis) and found that allograft rejection was characterized by a significant decrease in PCr/ATP. This work was the first to suggest the utility of ^{31}P-CMRS for detection of myocardial rejection. Bottomley et al. were the first to study human cardiac transplantation with ^{31}P-CMRS. They found ignificant reductions in myocardial PCr/ATP in allografts with endomyocardial biopsy proven mild rejection (1.57 ± 0.50) compared with healthy controls (1.93 ± 0.2, $p < 0.01$) (50). Unfortunately, there were no significant differences in PCr/ATP between allografts with mild and moderate rejection. To make this approach most useful, it should differentiate between mild and moderate rejection, since the mild classification is not an indication for change in immunosuppressive treatment. More patients need to be studied to explore this potentially useful tool for monitoring cardiac allograft rejection.

MICROVASCULAR DISEASE

Endothelial dysfunction and microvascular disease play a role in virtually all heart disease.^{31}P-CMRS is an approach which might be useful for detecting ischemia in patients with CAD (large or small vessel). We discussed the changes in phosphoenergetics (PCr, ATP, and pH) in large vessel CAD above, in this section we will discuss the studies that show change in the phosphoenergetics in microvascular disease or even dysfunction in the absence of microvascular disease. Other imaging modalities (e.g., myocardial perfusion imaging and coronary angiography) can detect epicardial CAD whereas changes in high-energy phosphate metabolism provide insights into the effects of disease at the intracellular level. Two situations in which the microvasculature is important are chest pain syndromes in the absence of large vessel CAD (especially in women) and diabetes mellitus.

In the Coronary Artery Surgery Study database with 12,462 men and 2366 women, 50% of women with chest pain were found to have normal coronary angiograms compared with 17% of men (51). Accordingly, Buchthal et al. used ^{31}P-CMRS to determine if women with chest pain and without evidence of significant large vessel disease by coronary angiography had changes in high-energy phosphate metabolism indicative of ischemia (52). Of the 35 women with chest pain studied, seven (20%) had a significant decrease in PCr/ATP with handgrip exercise under the 2 SD threshold determined from an 11 women control group. Therefore, microvascular disease without significant epicardial CAD may contribute to chest pain in women.

There have been several studies exploring ^{31}P-CMRS in diabetes mellitus. Type 1 diabetes was evaluated by ^{31}P-CMRS to correlate PCr/ATP with hemoglobin A1c (HbA1c) and diastolic dysfunction on echocardiography (53). There was a significant reduction in PCr/ATP in patients with type I diabetes compared with normal controls (1.90 ± 0.4 vs. 2.15 ± 0.3, $p<0.05$). Furthermore, the PCr/ATP ratio correlated inversely with HbA1c ($r = -0.41$) and diastolic function (E/A ratio) ($r = -0.42$). Similarly, in a study in patients with type 2 diabetes, myocardial PCr/ATP was significantly lower than in controls (1.47 vs. 1.88, $p = 0.01$) and inverse associations were found between myocardial PCr/ATP and E peak acceleration, E peak deceleration, and E peak filling rate (in all, $p<0.05$) (54). Additionally, significant decreases in PCr/ATP with handgrip exercise have been found in type 2 diabetes mellitus, but this study did not exclude the possibility of epicardial CAD. Most recently in a study by Varadarjan et al. (unpublished data), young patients (18–40 years) with type 1 diabetes and low risk factor profiles for CAD underwent ^{31}P-CMRS. PCr/ATP ratios with handgrip exercise were compared to markers of microvascular disease in other organs: microalbuminuria and diabetic retinopathy. Furthermore, a 3T platform was used for this study which yielded better signal-to-noise, increasing sensitivity, precision, and enabling a more accurate estimate of intracellular pH. The preliminary results showed that 50% (8/16) of patients had significant decreases in PCr/ATP ratios with handgrip stress.

NUCLEAR SPECIES OTHER THAN ^{31}P USED IN CMRS

In addition to ^{31}P, spectroscopy can be used to detect resonance signals from other nuclear species. Some that have been studied include ^{1}H, ^{13}C, oxygen-17 (^{17}O), ^{19}F, and ^{23}Na. With the exception of proton, however, the clinical application of these nuclear species is unlikely in the near future.

Table 3 Clinical Applications of ^{31}P-CMRS Now and in the Future

---

Ischemic heart disease
Normal myocardium has normal PCr/ATP that does not decrease with stress
Viable myocardium with ischemic stress has normal PCr/ATP
    that decreases with handgrip exercise
Myocardial scar had decreased PCr/ATP ratio, but no change during rest
A CMRS handgrip stress test can potentially be used as a screening test for CAD
Post-revascularization ischemia related to microvascular disease can be
    monitored by detecting PCr/ATP
Heart failure
Dilated cardiomyopathy is accompanied by decreased PCr/ATP
PCr/ATP ratio is useful to prognosticate mortality in dilated
    cardiomyopathy
Left ventricular hypertrophy, mitral regurgitation, and hypertrophic
    cardiomyopathy are all associated with decreased PCr/ATP
Heart Transplant
Exvivo donor graft can be evaluated for a decreased
    PCr/ATP pre-transplant to determine risk for early rejection
Mild rejection is associated with decreased PCr/ATP
Transplant patients can be monitored with CMRS periodically
    for signs of rejection and immunosuppressive therapy
    modified accordingly
Chest pain in women and Syndrome X
Chest pain without evidence of epicardial coronary artery disease is associated
    with decreased PCr/ATP with handgrip stress suggesting microvascular
    disease
Future applications may be useful for detecting microvascular
    ischemia in women without large vessel coronary artery disease
Diabetes
Diabetes type 1 and 2 associated with decreased PCr/ATP both at rest
    and with stress
Diastolic dysfunction in diabetes is associated with PCr/ATP
Diabetic cardiomyopathy may be a microvascular phenomenon as suggested
    decreased PCr/ATP
Nuclear species other than ^{31}P
^{1}H can be used to detect non-phosphorylated creatine kinase,
    hence depicting complete metabolic cycle between PCr/ATP/Pi
^{1}H can track intracellular fatty acid metabolism myoglobin concentration as
    markers of aerobic metabolism
^{17}O can track oxygen consumption during aerobic respiration
^{13}C can provide new insight into TCA and glycolysis cycles

---

Abbreviations: CMRS, cardiovascular magnetic resonance spectroscopy; PCr, phosphocreatine; ATP, adenosine triphosphate; CAD, coronary artery disease; TCA, tricarboxylic acid; Pi, inorganic phosphate; ^{1}H, proton; ^{13}C, carbon-13; ^{19}F, fluorine-19; ^{23}Na, sodium-23; ^{31}P, hosphorus-31.

Proton spectroscopy had been used to quantify myocardial lipids which can be used as a marker for reduced aerobic metabolism and accordingly ischemia (55). Bench research methods have been able to assess the oxygenation of myocardial myoglobin to gage ischemic severity (56,57). Recently, Bottomley et al. were able to quantify unphosphorylated creatine kinase concentration in infracted myocardium using ^{1}H spectroscopy (58). Combined with ^{31}P-CMRS, the entire cycle in high-energy phosphate metabolism can be depicted if both phosphorylated and unphosphorylated creatine kinase, ATP, and inorganic phosphate concentrations are measured.

Carbon-13 NMR is currently under investigation in the animal model, as it may provide insight into glycolysis and the tricarboxylic acid (TCA) cycle. The clinical application of ^{13}C will depend on increased signal-to-noise and sensitivity, pulse sequence methodology which include cross-polarization, heteronuclear multiple-quantum coherence, and heteronuclear chemical shift correlation.

THE FUTURE OF CMRS

Presently, CMRS can reliably monitor high-energy phosphate metabolism in a variety of cardiovascular diseases. Studies of microvascular disease and dysfunction are perhaps the most suitable application for CMRS because of its ability to evaluate intracellular metabolism. Future applications will require techniques that will allow generation of metabolite map depicting the distribution of one or more molecular species (e.g., ATP or PCr) and increase diagnostic yield to the entire left ventricle rather than its current limitation to the anterior wall. Increasing magnetic field strengths will lead to improvement in signal-to-noise and allow more precise identification of spectral peaks such as inorganic phosphate which can be used to estimate intracellular pH. As CMR scanners become more readily available, there will be an increasing need to train more spectroscopists able to harvest the immense potential of CMRS. With the resultant widespread use of CMRS, larger studies will be needed to substantiate its use in clinical practice. Applications are vast, with the most important areas are those affecting the microvasculature such as diabetes, chest pain syndromes in the absence of large vessel CAD, cardiomyopathy, rejection after heart transplantation, viability, the effects of anti-ischemic pharmaceutical agents and revascularization assessment (Table 3). Meanwhile new techniques in the application of other nuclear species may provide further understanding of myocardial metabolism. Accordingly, CMRS is able to provide new insight into intracellular mechanisms, while potentially providing novel and useful diagnostic techniques, making this an exciting and promising area of cardiovascular research.

REFERENCES

1. Bloch R, Hensen WW, Packard ME. Nuclear induction. Phys Rev 1946; 69:127.
2. Purcell EM, Torrey HC, Pound RV. Resonance absorption by nuclear magnetic moments in a solid. Phys Rev 1946; 69:37–38.
3. Jacobus WE, Taylor GJ IV, Hollis DP, et al. Phosphorus nuclear magnetic resonance of perfused working rat hearts. Nature 1977; 265:765–758.
4. Garlick PB, Radda GK, Seeley PJ. Phosphorus CMR studies on perfused heart. Biophys Res Commun 1977; 74:1256–1262.
5. Szczepaniak LS, Dobbins RL, Metzger GJ, et al. Myocardial triglycerides and systolic function in humans: in vivo evaluation by localized proton spectroscopy and cardiac imaging. Magn Reson Med 2003; 49:417–423.
6. Chen W, Ackerman JJH. Surface-coil spin-echo localization in vivo via inhomogeneous surface-spoiling magnetic gradient. J Magn Reson 1989; 82:655–658.
7. Bendall MR, Pegg DT. Theoretical description of depth pulse sequences on and off resonance. Magn Reson Med 1985; 2:91–113.
8. Conway MA, Allis J, Ouwerkerk R, Niioka T, Rajagopalan B, Radda GK. Detection of low phosphocreatine to ATP ratio in failing hypertrophied human myocardium by ^{31}P magnetic resonance spectroscopy. Lancet 1991; 338:973–976.
9. Frahm J, Merboldt KD, Hanicke W. Localized proton spectroscopy using stimulated echoes. J Magn Reson 1987; 72:502–508.
10. Connelly A, Counsell C, Lohman JAB, Ordidge RJ. Outer volume suppressed image related in vivo spectroscopy (OSIRIS), a high-sensitivity localization technique. J Magn Reson 1988; 78:519–525.
11. Schaefer S, Bober JR, Schwartz GS, Twieg DB, Weiner MW, Massie B. High-energy phosphate metabolism in patients with global myocardial disease. In vivo phosphorus-31 spectroscopic imaging. Am J Cardiol 1990.
12. Bottomley PA, Hardy CJ, Roemer PB. Phosphate metabolite imaging and concentration measurements in human heart by nuclear magnetic resonance. Magn Reson Med 1990; 14:425–434.
13. Jung WI, Widmaier S, Seeger U, et al. Phosphorus J coupling constants of ATP in human myocardium and calf muscle. J Magn Reson B 1996; 110:39–46.
14. Mareci TH, Brooker HR. Essential considerations for spectral localization using indirect gradient encoding of spatial information. J Magn Reson 1991; 92:229–246.
15. Pohmann R, von Kienlin M. Accurate phosphorus metabolite images of the human heart by 3D acquisition-weighted CSI. Magn Reson Med 2001; 45:817–826.
16. Jung WI, Sieverding L, Breuer J, et al. Detection of phosphomonoester signals in proton-decoupled 31P NMR spectra of the myocardium of patients with myocardial hypertrophy. J Magn Reson 1998; 133:232–235.
17. Hu X, Levin DN, Lauterbur PC, Spraggins T. SLIM: spectral localization by imaging. Magn Reson Med 1988; 8:314–322.
18. Von Kienlin M, Mejia R. Spectral localization with optimal pointspread function. J Magn Reson 1991; 94:268–287.
19. Loeffler R, Sauter R, Kolem H, Gaase A, von Kienlin M. Localized spectroscopy from anatomically matched compartments: improved sensitivity and localization for cardiac 31P MRS in humans. J Magn Reson 1998; 134:287–299.

20. Meininger M, Landschuetz W, Beer M, et al. Concentrations of human cardiac phosphorus metabolites determined by SLOOP 31P NMR spectroscopy. Magn Reson Med 1999; 41:657–663.
21. Weiss RG, Bottomeley PA, Hardy CJ, et al. Regional myocardial metabolism of high-energy phosphates during isometric exercise in patients with coronary artery disease. N Engl J Med 1990; 323:1593–1600.
22. Yabe T, Mitsumnami K, Okada M, et al. Detection of myocardial ischemia by 31P magnetic resonance spectroscopy during handgrip exercise. Circulation 1994; 89:1709–1716.
23. Yabe T, Mitsunami K, Inunbushi T, et al. Quantitative measurements of cardiac phosphorous metabolites in coronary artery disease by 31P magnetic resonance spectroscopy. Circulation 1995; 92:15–23.
24. Moka D, Baer FM, Theissen P, Schneider CA, Dietlein M, Erdmann E, Schicha H. Non-Q-wave myocardial infarction: impaired myocardial energy metabolism in regions with reduced 99mTc-MIBI accumulation. Eur J Nucl Med 2001; 28(5):602–607.
25. Ingwall JS. On the hypothesis: cardiac failure is due to decreased energy reserve. Circulation 1993; 87(suppl VII):VII-58–VII-62.
26. Schaefer S, Gober JR, Schwartz GG, Twieg DB, Weiner MW, Massie B. In vivo phosphorus-31 spectroscopic imaging in patients with global myocardial disease. Am J Cardiol 1990; 65:1154–1161.
27. Auffermann W, Chew WM, Wolfe CL, et al. Normal and diffusely abnormal myocardium in humans: functional and metabolic characterization with P-31 MR spectroscopy and cine MR imaging. Radiology 1991; 179:253–259.
28. Masuda Y, Tateno Y, Ikehira H, et al. High-energy phosphate metabolism of the myocardium in normal subjects and patients with various cardiomyopathies— the study using ECG gated MR spectroscopy with a localization technique. Jpn Circ J 1992; 56:620–626.
29. Hardy CJ, Weiss RG, Bottomley PA, Gerstenblith G. Altered myocardial high-energy phosphate metabolites in patients with dilated cardiomyopathy. Am Heart J 1991; 122:795–801.
30. Neubauer S, Krahe T, Schindler R, et al. 31P magnetic resonance spectros-copy in dilated cardiomyopathy and coronary artery disease. Altered cardiac high-energy phosphate metabolism in heart failure. Circulation 1992; 86:1810–1818.
31. Neubauer S, Horn M, Pabst T, et al. Contributions of ^{31}P magnetic resonance spectroscopy to the understanding of dilated heart muscle disease. Eur Heart J 1995; 16:115–118.
32. Hansch A, Rzanny R, Heyne JP, Leder U, Reichenbach JR, Kaiser WA. Non-invasive measurements of cardiac high-energy phosphate metabolites in dilated cardiomyopathy by using ^{31}P spectroscopic chemical shift imaging. Eur Radiol 2005; 15:319–323.
33. Neubauer S, Horn M, Cramer M, et al. Myocardial phosphocreatine-to-ATP ratio is a predictor of mortality in patients with dilated cardiomyopathy. Circu-lation 1997; 96:2190–2196.
34. Bottomley PA. Noninvasive study of high-energy phosphate metabolism in human heart by depth-resolved ^{31}P NMR spectroscopy. Science 1985; 229:769–772.

35. Blackledge MJ, Rajagopalan B, Oberhaensli R, Bolas NM, Styles P, Radda GK. Quantitative studies of human metabolism by ^{31}P rotating frame NMR. Proc Natl Acad Sci USA 1987; 84:4283–4287.
36. Radda GK, Rajagopalan B, Taylor D. Biochemistry in vivo: an appraisal of clinical magnetic resonance spectroscopy. Magn Reson Q 1989; 5:122–151.
37. Radda GK. The use of NMR spectroscopy for the understanding of disease. Science 1986; 233:640–645.
38. deRoos A, Doornbos J, Luten PR, et al. Cardiac metabolism in patients with dilated and hypertrophic cardiomyopathy: assessment with proton decoupled 31P MR spectroscopy. J Magn Reson Imaging 1992; 2:711–719.
39. Sakuma H, Takeda K, Tagami T, et al. 31P MR spectroscopy in hypertrophic cardiomyopathy: comparison with Tl-101 myocardial perfusion imaging. Am Heart J 1993; 125:1323–1328.
40. Jung W, Sieverding L, Breur J, et al. 31P NMR spectroscopy detects metabolic abnormalities in asymptomatic patients with hypertrophic cardiomyopathy. Circulation 1998; 97:2536–2542.
41. Conway MA, Bottomley PA, Ouwerkerk R, Radda GK, Rajagopalan B. Mitral regurgitation: impaired systolic function, eccentric hypertrophy, and increased severity are linked to lower phosphocreatine/ATP ratios in humans. Circulation 1998; 97(17):1716–1723.
42. Van Dobbenburgh JO, Lahpor JR, Wooley SR, et al. Functional recovery after human heart transplantation is related to the metabolic condition of the hypothermic donor heart. Circulation 1996; 94:2831–2836.
43. Caus T, Kober F, Mouly-Bandini A, et al. ^{31}P CMRS of heart grafts provides metabolic markers of early dysfunction. Eur J Cardiothorac Surg 2005; 28(4):576–580.
44. Canby RC, Evanochko WT, Barrett LV, et al. Monitoring the bioenergetics of cardiac allograft rejection using in vivo P-31 nuclear magnetic resonance spectroscopy. J Am Coll Cardiol 1987; 9:1067–1074.
45. Haug CE, Shapiro JI, Chan L, Weil R. III. P-31 nuclear magnetic resonance spectroscopic evaluation of heterotopic cardiac allograft rejection in the rat. Transplantation 1987; 44:175–178.
46. Fraser CD Jr., Chacko VP, Jacobus WE, et al. Metabolic changes preceding function and morphologic indices of rejection in heterotopic cardiac allografts. Transplantation 1988; 46:346–351.
47. Fraser CD Jr., Chacko VP, Jacobus WE, et al. Early phosphorus 31 nuclear magnetic resonance bioenergetic changes potentially predict rejection in heterotopic cardiac allografts. J Heart Transplant 1990; 9:197–204.
48. Walpoth BH, Galdikas J, Tschopp A, et al. Differentiation of cardiac ischemia and rejection by nuclear magnetic spectroscopy. Thorac Cardiovasc Surg 1991; 39:217–220.
49. Suzuki K, Hamano K, Ito H, Fujimura Y, Esato K. The detection of chronic heart graft rejection by ^{31}P CMR spectroscopy. Surg Today 1999; 29(2):143–148.
50. Bottomley PA, Weiss RG, Hardy CJ, et al. Myocardial high-energy phosphate metabolism and allograft rejection in patients with heart transplants. Radiology 1991; 191:67–75.

51. Davis KB, Chaitman B, Ryan T, Bittner V, Kennedy JW. Comparison of 15-year survival for men and women after initial medical or surgical treatment for coronary artery disease: a CASS Registry study. J Am Coll Cardiol 1995; 25:1000–1009.

52. Buchthal SD, den Hollander JA, Merz CN, et al. Abnormal myocardial phosphorus-31 nuclear magnetic resonance spectroscopy in women with chest pain but normal coronary angiograms N Engl J Med 2000; 342(12):829–835.

53. Metzler B, Schocke MF, Steinboeck P, et al. Decreased high-energy phosphate ratios in the myocardium of men with diabetes mellitus type I. J Cardiovasc Magn Reson 2002; 4(4):493–502.

54. Diamant M, Lamb HJ, Groeneveld Y, et al. Diastolic dysfunction is associated with altered myocardial metabolism in asymptomatic normotensive patients with well-controlled type 2 diabetes mellitus. J Am Coll Cardiol 2003; 42(2):328–335.

55. den Hollander JA, Evanochko WT, Pohost GM. Observation of cardiac lipids in humans by localized ^{1}H magnetic resonance spectroscopic imaging. Magn Reson Med 1994; 32:175–180.

56. Kreutzer U, Mekhamer Y, Chung Y, Jue T. Oxygen supply and oxidative phosphorylation limitation in rat myocardium in situ. Am J Physiol Heart Circ Physiol 2001; 280:H2030–H2037.

57. Chung Y, Jue T. Regulation of respiration in myocardium in the transient and steady state. Am J Physiol 1999; 277:H1410–H1417.

58. Bottomley PA, Weiss RG. Noninvasive localized MR quantification of creatine kinase metabolites in normal and infarcted canine myocardium. Radiology 2001; 219:411–418.

11

Coronary Artery Imaging

Robert W. W. Biederman and Mark Doyle

Division of Cardiology, Cardiovascular MRI Laboratory, Allegheny General Hospital, Pittsburgh, Pennsylvania, U.S.A.

CORONARY ARTERY IMAGING APPROACHES

Since its inception, cardiovascular magnetic resonance (CMR) has held the promise that the coronary arteries could be noninvasively imaged. Very early in the history of CMR, clinical images were produced with sufficient resolution and contrast to visualize vessels with the dimensions of the coronary arteries. However, it is universally acknowledged that heart motion, due to the cardiac cycle and to respiration has hindered attempts to image the coronary arteries. Thus, early on, motion compensation strategies were devised to accommodate both sources of motion. Cardiac synchronization of the acquisition can routinely achieve adequate compensation for cardiac motion, which can be sustained over multiple cycles. Further, accommodation of respiratory motion has fallen into two distinct approaches: (i) breath-holding and (ii) respiratory compensation. There are several features that are common to all approaches, and these will be addressed first.

COMMON FEATURES OF CORONARY ARTERY IMAGING APPROACHES

Maximal Flow

The coronary arteries should be imaged during the portion of the cardiac cycle when blood flow through them is maximal. This occurs during diastole when the myocardium is relaxed and there are no compression forces to clamp down on the arterioles such as those present during systole. Imaging during the period of maximal coronary flow ensures that the arteries are seen at their largest dimensions, allowing the best resolution and opportunity to detect a stenosis. Further, as is common practice in the catheterization laboratory, some degree of vasodilatation may be induced, possibly by administration of a sublingual dose of nitroglycerine. By inducing vasodilatation, the presence of a stenosis may be accentuated by comparison with the normally responding coronary artery segments in proximity to a localized stenosis. For the right coronary circuit, flow is present even during systole, and generally visualization of the right coronary artery (RCA) and possibly the posterior descending artery (in right dominant individuals) can be seen more reliably than any other segment. This in part is due to the sustained flow through the RCA branch and due to its relatively straight path. Flow through the left circuit, including the left main, the left anterior descending artery and the circumflex artery is generally maximal during diastole, and peaks at 50% into the cycle, then tapers off, though still present at some level for most of diastole.

Limited Acquisition Duration Within Cycle

Synchronization of the magnetic resonance imaging (MRI) acquisition to the cardiac cycle is required for most imaging approaches that require more than one cardiac cycle to build up a sufficiently large data set. Synchronization ensures that cardiac motion due to the cardiac cycle is effectively frozen. However, all CMR sequences are applied for a finite amount of time within the cycle, and this can lead to motion blur, effectively placing a limit on the resolution that can be achieved. A general principle is that the motion that takes place during sampling time limits the resolution. Because the rate of cardiac motion is lower during diastole, the coronary arteries are usually imaged during diastole. This allows data to be acquired for segments typically ranging from 50 to 100 milliseconds. During this interval, as much data as possible is acquired, which generally requires that data are acquired with rapidly repeated sequences.

Blood Contrast

In addition to resolution, it is imperative that contrast be generated between the coronary artery lumen and surrounding tissue. It is natural to look for contrast mechanisms based on blood flow. Imaging sequences that allow a high degree of flow refreshment can generate contrast (1). However, the requirement to acquire data rapidly does not lend it self to long refreshment times, and there are limits to this mechanism. Alternatively, blood signal can be enhanced by introduction of a TI relaxation contrast agent. Contrast agents that leak in to the interstitium increase blood signal, but do not necessarily produce blood contrast, due to enhancement of surrounding myocardium. Generally, this class of agent requires infusion over the duration of the imaging sequence, which may last upwards of 20 minutes. Agents that are restricted to the blood pool, do not require continuous infusion, and can also generate blood/myocardium contrast. Another mechanism that helps isolate the signal from the coronary arteries is based on the observation that in general, the coronary arteries are embed in fat-filled groves on the epicardial surface. A sequence that incorporates fat suppression can thus help produce additional contrast in the vicinity of the coronary arteries, i.e., local contrast (2). However, sequences that suppress the fat signal based on a spectrally selective pulse, may inadvertently suppress blood signal, as blood enters the heart from a remote region that experiences the suppression pulse due to field inhomogeneities (3). Another blood signal contrast mechanisms is based on its inherent T2 characteristic. In the absence of flow effects, the T2 of blood is relatively long compared to myocardium and thus a long TE sequence could potentially produce blood contrast (4). However, mechanisms that rely on T2 properties may be compromised by signal loss resulting from blood passing through stenotic regions and suffering turbulent disruption. Another mechanism is based on the proton density of blood, which is generally the highest of all tissues in the vicinity of the heart. Techniques that rely on this mechanism can produce good contrast without the use of contrast agents but generally require long repetition times.

Resolution

As alluded to above, motion limits the resolution with which the coronary arteries can be visualized. To ameliorate this problem, most coronary artery imaging approaches rely on rapidly acquiring data, limiting the opportunity for motion to take place. It is possible to acquire data very rapidly with the echo–planar imaging (EPI) approach, but this approach has had only limited success in imaging the coronary arteries. One reason for this is that its effective T2 is very long, and this produces excessive T2 blurring. The related approach of spiral imaging has proven to permit rapid coverage of k-space, while not suffering excessive T2 blurring. Spiral scans have an effectively short TE, which has good T2 and flow characteristics and signal read-out times are not excessively long, being on the order of less that 20 milliseconds. However, both EPI and spiral scans produce artifacts in the presence of inhomogeneities and fat signals (i.e., all off resonance signals) and high performance systems are required for optimal imaging. Inherent to all two-dimensional (2D) imaging sequences is the requirement to acquire data from one slice. In 2D sequences the slice dimension is generally the largest, ultimately placing a limit on the resolution achievable (5). The penalties for generating thinner slices are:

- An increase in the minimum echo time
- A decrease in the signal to noise ratio
- Reduction of the spatial coverage permissible for a given number of slices

An alternative to 2D imaging is three-dimensional (3D) imaging. In 3D imaging, a slab is selected and the "slice" dimension is spatially encoded as opposed to being selected (6). Due to the width of the slab selection, intrinsic flow refreshment is generally not a major source of contrast and many 3D approaches are supplemented with administration of a contrast agent (7). Because the slice dimension of a 3D approach is encoded, the sequence is generally longer than 2D approaches, where each 2D slice can be imaged separately, whereas they are all imaged "simultaneously" in 3D approaches. The advantages of 3D approach compared to a comparable 2D sequence are:

- Low echo times are possible
- The signal to noise ratio is higher
- Thin, contiguous slices are produced

In general, approaches that generate 3D data sets seem to have a natural advantage over 2D approaches when considering the resolution requirements for coronary artery imaging.

Signal to Noise

Considering that voxel dimensions of the order of 0.5-mm cubed are required, it is immediately apparent that excellent signal reception is required (8). This is conventionally provided by positioning cardiac-specific phased array coils around the thorax. Currently, a new generation of phased array coils are being developed to take advantage of the advanced hardware available, including higher numbers of independent receiver channels available for use by receiver coils. Phased array coils and specialized software can also be used to reduce the scan time typically by factors of two to four, but at the expense of decreasing the signal to noise ratio. These "parallel" imaging approaches such as SMASH and SENSE, effectively split up the data acquisition process and distribute them between each element of the phased array coil.

Breath-Holding

It has been demonstrated that the heart moves primarily in the cardiocranial direction with normal respiratory motion, with an excursion on the order of 2-cm. Breath-holding approaches seek to suspend this motion, and thus effectively provide a continuous period of 15–30 seconds when coronary imaging can be applied (9). Longer periods of breath holding can be achieved if the patient is in some way conditioned, either by providing oxygen during the procedure or by hyperventilating them prior to breath holding. In general, it is easier for the patient to hold their breath at close to end expiration and in our institution we employ breath holding in this manner. These approaches can be used to extend the basic breath-hold time and reproducibility. It is generally acknowledged that there is too much variation in breath-holding position between multiple breath holds for data to be effectively combined (10). Thus, due to the relatively short breath-hold period and its lack of reproducibility, breath-hold approaches are generally employed with 2D imaging. Due to their limited region of view, 2D approaches generally require expert guidance to position slices in a manner to successfully image each coronary artery segment. As gradient strengths of scanners have increased with each successive model, so has the popularity of 2D approaches, because adequate resolution and contrast are increasingly available.

Respiratory Gating

Respiratory gating is the approach whereby, under free breathing, respiratory motion is monitored and data only acquired when this motion is within predefined limits, principally centered around end expiration (11). Respiratory compensation approaches are generally about 25% to 40% efficient, i.e., data are effectively acquired for this percentage of the actual scan time. Despite this low efficiency, respiratory gating approaches are patient-friendly in that little to no patient training or special cooperation is required (12). Due to the extended time allowed by respiratory gating approaches, 3D imaging sequences are generally used, typically requiring administration of a contrast agent.

Limiting Factors of Coronary Artery imaging

In this summary of coronary artery imaging sequence considerations, it is apparent that the success of any imaging approach is dependent of several interrelated phenomenon:

- Compensation of cardiac and respiratory motion
- Generation of sufficient blood contrast
- Generation of sufficient resolution
- Acquisition of data in a limited scan time

If any one consideration is not adequately addressed then the approach is not viable. Hence, the focus of each clinical protocol that employs an imaging sequence is focused on ensuring that each element is addressed.

CLINICAL CORONARY ARTERY IMAGING

The "Holy Grail" for any noninvasive imaging modality is the ability to successfully image the coronary arteries. Historically, the "gold standard" has been the cardiac catheterization as originally described by Werner von Forssmann in 1929 and refined by Mason Sones in the mid-1950's. Nearing

1.5 million cases performed per year and a mortality that has remained essentially unchanged at one per thousand and, when combined with a normalcy rate of 40% to 50%, the risk–benefit ratio may no longer support this cavalier use (13,14). Interestingly, in an era of dramatic advances in cardiovascular medicine touching nearly every aspect of cardiology and cardiothoracic surgery, there have been only incremental gains in the catheterization lab. Certainly, image acquisition has improved, X-ray contrast has become safer, catheters have been engineered to be manipulated more easily by even more skilled cardiologists and while angioplasty/stenting advances have nearly eradicated a generation of cardiothoracic surgeons, little impact has been made towards reducing the general invasiveness, morbidity, and mortality that has remained unchanged in the last two decades (14).

General improvements have been realized in magnetic resonance angiography (MRA) not limited to the areas of respiratory compensatory, free breathing navigator-based techniques, applications either with or without gadolinium and in image resolution. Currently, CMR fidelity and reproducibility are approaching, and in limited cases, achieving, that seen with standard X-ray angiography. Such advances are contributing to the increased use of CMR-based approaches in assessing anomalous arteries, detection of coronary stenoses, coronary flow applications, coronary bypass graft imaging, and coronary fistula evaluation. More recently, vessel wall imaging has been demonstrated with and without plaque characterization. It is clearly foreseeable that an algorithm employing coronary imaging followed by perfusion sequences and viability followed with a functional assessment will be the test of choice within the next five years.

Historical uses of coronary imaging has been well reviewed elsewhere (13), and the discussion here is largely limited to pertinent studies that have been described in the last five years in the areas of imaging anomalous, native, diseased, bypassed, and ectatic coronary vessels with a discussion of CMR insights into atherosclerotic plaque imaging.

Anomalous Coronary Artery Imaging

Numerous descriptions of the ability for CMR to detect and identify anomalous coronary arteries abound in the literature. Nearly every study performed to date (and historically) has served to establish MRI/MRA as the "gold standard" for the evaluation of such pathology. The chief explanation resides, not in CMR's ability to resolve the coronary anomaly better then X-ray angiography, but with its ability to depict the coronary tree relative to the adjacent anatomy. This provides a roadmap of the coronary bed in context of its anatomic relations (Fig. 1). This capacity, counterintuitively, is not easily realized in the cardiac catheterization suite due to the obligate requirement for contrast to highlight each vasculature territory, which does not permit simultaneous delineation of neighboring structures.

(A)   (B)

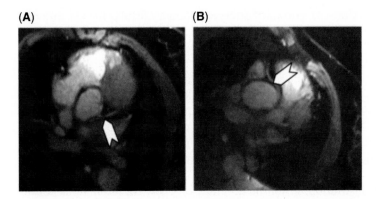

Figure 1   A 45-year-old female who presented with chest pain, underwent a nuclear stress test and was demonstrated to have inferior hypoperfusion at peak stress. A cardiac catheterization ensued with a normal left system but an right coronary artery (RCA) that arose adjacent to the left main and which traveled anteriorly but with an unknown (unclear) trajectory. (**A**) Cardiac magnetic resonance imaging with a spectral spatial pulse applied with a gradient echo, noncontrast acquisition demonstrated the left main and a hint of the adjacent takeoff of the RCA. (**B**) The anterior trajectory of the RCA between the aorta and the right ventricular outflow tract is seen. This anatomy is associated with dynamic compression and sudden death. The patient underwent coronary artery bypass grafting.

While numerous techniques for identifying anomalous coronary arteries have been described including placement of a Swan-Ganz catheter or an integrated approach with the "dot" or "i" sign, in clinical practice, most find such approaches to be time and logistically prohibitive. As such, many suspected anomalous coronary cases are referred for identification/confirmation in the using CMR. This approach has recently been borne out by Razmi et al. (15) demonstrating the ability to detect 16/16 coronary artery anomalies as compared to 16/16 by X-ray angiography or transesophageal echocardiography. Coronary anomalies diagnosed by magnetic resonance coronary angiography (MRCA) in this study included right-sided origin of left coronary artery (LCA) ($n = 7$), right-sided origin of left circumflex (LCX) ($n = 2$), slightly anterior or posterior displacement of LCA ($n = 2$), left-sided origin of RCA ($n = 3$), anterior displacement of RCA ($n = 1$), common ostium of LCA and RCA ($n = 1$). A 2D breath-hold imaging with contrast administration was employed, relying chiefly on double inversion recovery sequences and confirmation by gradient–recalled echo sequences.

In an analogous manner, Taylor et al. (16), identified abnormal coronary artery anatomy by consensus for 16 noncoronary congenital heart disease subjects in which 18 were suspected via their likely association with congenial heart disease, rather than by prior equivocal X-ray angiogram coronary anomalies. In this study, the following anomalies were seen: single coronary artery ($n = 4$), coronary artery/pulmonary fistulas ($n = 3$), anterior LCA with posterior RCA (in subjects with transposition) ($n = 3$), circumflex from the RCA ($n = 2$), abnormal RCA origin alone ($n = 3$), abnormal left anterior descending (LAD) coronary artery origin alone ($n = 2$), and LAD from RCA ($n = 1$). The magnetic resonance angiography (MRA) was compared to X-ray angiography, correctly identifying abnormal coronary anatomy in 14 of 16 subjects (sensitivity 88%, specificity 100%, and accuracy 92%). The CMR was performed predominantly with a 3D-segmented fast low-angle shot (FLASH) imaging sequence in combination with the phase-reordering algorithm hybrid ordered phase encoding imaging in mid to late diastole.

At our institution, given the accuracy of CMR for anomalous coronary arteries, a young patient presenting with typical chest pain undergoes noninvasive imaging by MRI under the presumption that the risk of an invasive approach is not warranted, ideal, or accurate enough to justify the risks (Figure 2).

Native Coronary Imaging

Traditionally, standard spin echo pulse sequences were used to image native coronary arteries, but with the introduction of rapid breath-hold 2D-segmented k-space gradient-echo approaches, a new appreciation of the utility of MRA has emerged for coronary artery imaging applications, that is defining the burgeoning CMR field that we know today.

(A)   **(B)**

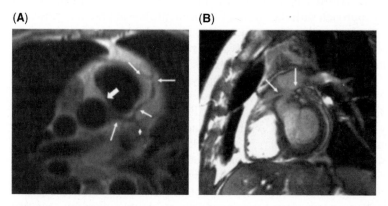

Figure 2 (A) A 55-year-old male undergoing a routine cardiac catheterization with normal left anterior descending (LAD) (*multiple small arrows*), coronary artery, left circumflex and LAD arteries. Note absent right coronory artery (RCA) ostium. (B) A sagittal oblique view of the RCA arising off the posterior and leftward Sinus of Valsalva. In (A), a subtle hint of an anterior directed vessel is seen (*large arrow*), which is diagnostic in (B) of an anomalous RCA arising off the left coronary sinus of Valsalva, but which was nondiagnostic at catheterization.

Clinical applications of existing coronary MRA techniques include:

- determining the patency and direction of flow in native coronary arteries
- evaluating the patency of coronary artery bypass grafts
- evaluating the patency of native vessels following coronary stent placement
- evaluating congenital and acquired coronary variants
- following the progress of known proximal lesions before or after treatment with angioplasty
- identifying anomalous coronary arteries and their anatomic course
- screen and evaluate patients with ischemic heart disease
- routinely portray the proximal and middle portion of major coronary arteries and some coronary artery branches in most patients.

The current limitations of coronary MRA include the inability to visualize the more distal portion of the coronary arteries and coronary artery branches (see Table 1). At its current stage of development, coronary MRA may be most helpful in excluding clinically important stenoses in patients referred for diagnostic contrast angiography. As techniques continue to improve they may become an integral part of the evaluation of patients with ischemic heart disease (Figs. 3–5).

Clinical Strategies

Both 2D and 3D MRI techniques are employed currently for coronary imaging by CMR. Recent improvements including spectrally spatially selective radio frequency RF pulses to suppress epicardial fat, phased array surface coils to increase signal-to-noise ratio (SNR). Two-dimensional techniques have been implemented using spiral scanning with interleaved spiral trajectories through k-space that provide high temporal and spatial resolution with relative insensitivity to flow and motion artifacts.

However, limitations exist to the 2D approach. Vessel tortuosity often impairs the selection of 2D imaging planes. Therefore, anatomic approaches comparable to those used with conventional angiography and echocardiography has been incorporated. Steady-state free precession (SSFP) imaging is used to provide better visualization and resolution of the coronary arteries, incorporating overlapping slice acquisitions to capture tortuous anatomy. Multiple oblique as well as fixed transverse planes are used to image the arteries (Fig. 6). Occasionally, infusion of gadolinium-Diethylenetriaminepentaacetic acid (Gd-DTPA) during the acquisition improves contrast to noise ratio of the vessel relative to adjacent tissue, especially phase sensitive techniques (Figure 4).

More recently, non–breath-hold 3D MRA techniques have been employed using navigator echo-based respiratory gating approaches to

Table 1 Comparison of Conventional and Magnetic Resonance Coronary Angiography

Conventional coronary angiography		Magnetic resonance coronary angiography	
Advantages	Disadvantages	Advantages	Disadvantages
Direct visualization of coronary anatomy	Invasive nature	Noninvasive	Need for ≥1.5T imaging unit
Usually close proximity to angioplasty team if necessary	Necessary injection of intracoronary contrast into an artery via an arterial catheter	No absolute need for intracoronary contrast, commonly done without an intravenous	Direct imaging time typically 2–3 times lengthier than conventional angiography
"Gold standard" for the last 40 yrs	Potential for marked patient discomfort	Minimal patient discomfort (except for potential claustrophobia)	Transfer required to angioplasty suite is needed
Can visualize proximal, mid, and distal vessels	Longer total time: 6–7 hrs (including recovery)	Total time: 45–60 min	Metallic foreign bodies may be contraindicated
No concern for pacemaker patients	Need for NPO status preceding 6 hrs	No post-procedure monitoring	Best at visualizing the proximal and mid vessels
Cardiac catheterization facilities common	Requires ionizing radiation	No NPO status needed	Pacemakers are a relative contraindication

		Cardiovascular Magnetic Resonance Imaging Centers less ubiquitous
Little more than vascular and organ shadows for reference	3D; theoretically any plane can be accommodated	
Risk of death 1:1000	No need for ionizing radiation	
Absolute risk of morbidity 1:1	Both anatomic and functional data are possible noninvasively when phase velocity mapping used	
4–6-hrs acute post-catheterization convalescence, subacute convalescence variable	3D relation to other structures easily visualized (ideal for anomalous vessels)	
Only anatomic data	No risk of death from intervention	
Single or biplane angiography	No risk of pericatheterization complications	
Not ideal for ostial or anomalous origins	Can be sent home immediately	
Expense: $1000–$2500	Expense: $450–$1000	

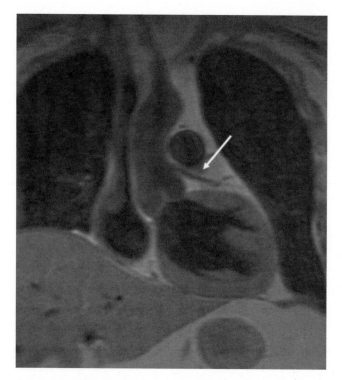

Figure 3 Breath hold spin echo image of a patient, demonstrating patent left main and proximal left anterior descending.

accommodate respiratory motion, primarily occurring in the superior–inferior direction due to diaphragmatic motion. Several thin, contiguous slices are acquired with less partial volume effects and more accurate vessel size estimation than 2D techniques. These techniques offer several advantages over 2D techniques, including higher spatial resolution, increased SNR, continuous coverage of the coronaries, a capacity for multiplanar reconstruction postprocessing, and preferential suitability for those patients who cannot cope with breath-holding requirements.

CLINICAL STUDIES: IDENTIFICATION OF NORMAL AND DISEASED VESSELS

The establishment of equivalence between MRA and X-ray angiography is nearly complete for the delineation in those with normal coronary arteries. By definition, this entails *a priori* knowledge of who possesses normal coronaries, a feat not clinically possible in a prospective study. Thus, retrospectively,

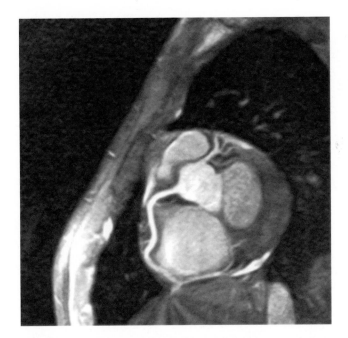

Figure 4 A 3D, segmented k-space gradient echo acquisition using a 6-element cardiac phased array coil (512 matrix, 20 slices at 1.5 mm per slice), obtained on a Philips Intera 3T under free breathing and utilizing navigator respiratory compensation with contrast. *Source*: From Ref. 17.

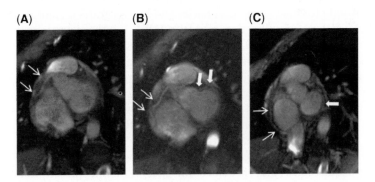

Figure 5 Three successive planes covering the right coronary artery (RCA) demonstrating in a gradient echo sequence the RCA arising off the correct, anterior-most right coronary sinus of Valsalva, the patency of the ostia, proximal (**A**), mid (**B**), and early distal (**C**) vessel. In this projection prescribed off a short axis image, no left anterior descending is visible and a hint of the left circumflex is viewed (*solid arrows*).

(A)   **(B)**

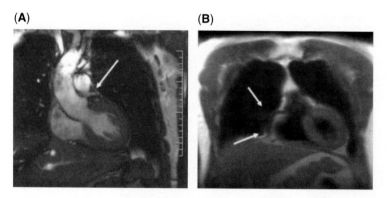

Figure 6 The left main (**A**) is seen using a 2D steady-state free precession and the right coronary artery (**B**) is seen using a 2D spin echo acquisition. Both images are acquired using a coronal plane, an acquisition not generally possible by echocardiography and a plane somewhat removed from the left anterior oblique in X-ray angiography. Important, but incomplete information concerning the vessels is acquired, demonstrating that a few key views may provide details about the presence or absence of life-threatening stenoses in a binary fashion.

if one is assigned the diagnosis of "normal" it is almost a certainty that this represents a true negative. Numerous studies completed in the early 80's through the mid-80's affirm this position. In 10 studies in which all four coronaries were visualized, correct identification of normal coronary arteries was achieved. These historical studies are summarized here, with the number of studies (out of the 10) that had 100% visualization indicated in square brackets: successful visualization ranged for the LAD [85–100% (6)], RCA [92–100% (6)], LAD [86–100% (7)], and the most difficult LCX [76–100% (3)] (18).

While the data for anomalous coronaries and bypass grafts is clinically accepted, the evidence for utilization of MRI/MRA for the detection of coronary stenosis is evolving (19,20). The evolution, however, is gaining speed (21) as evidenced by the growing sentiment, backed by compelling studies, to support the notion that such clinical utility may have already arrived in certain limited indications. The most striking description of coronary artery imaging was presented by Manning and coworkers (22). Seeking to demonstrate the utility for coronary imaging by CMR in a generic setting, they choose centers that had demonstrated prowess at cardiac, but not necessarily coronary imaging. Recognizing that there were many "recipes" for coronary acquisitions, they provided all sites with one prescription and used a vendor specific sequence and platform (Philips). Using state of the art 3D MRI technology, the multicenter, international study enrolled 109 patients who underwent MRI prior to undergoing conventional X-ray coronary angiography. Eighty-four percent of the major coronary arteries were visualized by MRI (vs. 100% by X-ray angiography). Eighty-three percent of clinically significant coronary artery abnormalities, later identified on X-ray coronary angiography, were also detected by the MRI scanner. This translated into an overall accuracy of 72% for the MRI scanner, versus 100% accuracy for the standard X-ray angiographic technique. When analyzing the accuracy of MRI in detecting patients at greatest risk of a life-threatening heart attack (i.e., patients with a diseased left main coronary artery or three-vessel coronary artery disease), the overall accuracy of MRI increased to 100%. It should be pointed out that in 16% of study patients, MRI was unable to successfully image the coronary arteries.

This important trial demonstrates a number of important concepts that will pave the way for future understanding and applications clinically. Firstly, if the coronaries are successfully imaged, life-threatening disease can be detected. Secondly, as the normalcy rate of X-ray angiography cases approaches 50% (across the United States), application of MRA technology as a screening tool in patients with a low to intermediate pretest probability is indicated. In this scenario, significant coronary disease could be detected, negating an invasive risky approach in a substantial number of patients for whom the pretest probability is not high. Thirdly, in patients who possess a cardiomyopathy, the interrogation typically proceeds to coronary artery catheterization, because, for an ischemic, cardiomyopathy is always indicated by the presence of high-grade proximal lesions which should be MRI visible. Finally, it is our belief that the incorporation of MRI/MRA into the armamentarium of clinicians creates the milieu for a more sophisticated, mature, and scientific approach. Consider that currently, if the extent of disease found in a patient is unequivocal, that patient will typically undergo either angioplasty or bypass therapy. However, for many patients following cardiac catheterization the true significance of disease remains equivocal requiring further testing to proceed to the *correct* therapeutic intervention (Fig. 7). For example, if a patient with chest pain has a 50% to 75% lesion, the physiologic consequence to that patient may range from life-threatening to no obstructive coronary flow upon provocation. One option for further evaluation is the nuclear examination, requiring a separate study, exposure to radionuclides and substantially prolonging the diagnostic assessment. Supplemental intravascular ultrasound (IVUS) could be considered, but requires further coronary intervention and usually provocation, all prolonging time that a foreign body is resident within the coronary bed. In our laboratory, if a patient presents with chest pain, they can undergo a CMR coronary examination, and if disease is seen, they can undergo a rest and stress perfusion exam (using either adenosine, dipyridamole or dobutamine) to delineate the physiologic importance of the anatomic finding. Moreover, incorporating delayed hyperenhancement while the contrast has already been administered is a unique ability of MRI to obtain essentially for free, additive clinical and prognostic information yielding the extent of scar and viable myocardium. When combined with the unparalleled accuracy

(A)   **(B)**

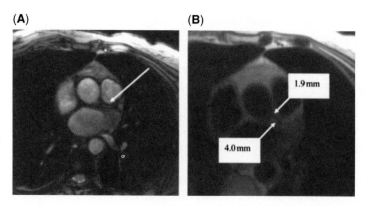

Figure 7 A 40-year-old male presented with chest discomfort prompting an X-ray angiogram. While the lumenogram suggested a 20% to 30% narrowing, the catheter damped, supporting an important stenosis, providing equivocal data for this critical clinical question. In this gradient echo axial slice, the mid-left main is narrowed, shown using a breath-hold gradient echo sequence. In this sequence (**A**) and the next (**B**), quantification using a series of 2D acquisitions demonstrated a 47% stenosis confirming the hemodynamic data acquired during the diagnostic catheterization, refuting the luminal data. This observation is not uncommon and forms the basis of nonluminal imaging such as intravascular ultrasound or, as shown here, a non-invasive evaluation in ambiguous situations; another emerging role for magnetic resonance imaging coronary angiography. These finding were confirmed at surgery for bypass grafting.

and "gold standard" of an left ventricle structure and function examination, the CMR center now becomes, not the proverbial "one-stop shop" but the "one-stop shopping mall." Such an approach is a paradigm change for both the patient and clinical setting (Fig. 8).

The successful application of MRI to the coronary arteries is an exciting development, and holds great potential for noninvasively screening high-risk patients for coronary artery disease. In the Manning study approximately one-half of the patients could have avoided the use of X-ray coronary angiography based upon the CMR findings (22). It is important to note a current limitation of CMR when compared to conventional angiography: a patient found to have clinically significant narrowing of the coronary arteries still requires X-ray angiography in order to dilate and stent the site(s) of narrowing. Based upon this study, CMR appears to be capable of accurately diagnosing significant coronary artery disease in the majority of cases, but it cannot support any of the interventions necessary to treat this disease at the present time, (considerable efforts currently in progress addresses that shortcoming). It is our impression that within five years, a patient will not arbitrarily enter the cardiac catheterization suite prior to undergoing a CMR examination for structure, function, coronary

(A)   (B)

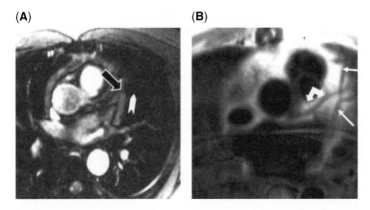

Figure 8 (A) The left main-, proximal-, and mid-sections of the left anterior descending (LAD) are seen (*arrow*). A small portion of the diagonal vessel (chevron) is also appreciated in a patient with an angiographically normal LAD (steady-state free precession 2D). (B) Is a spin echo image of another patient showing similar anatomy. Also seen is the Great Cardinal Vein (*single arrow*), often confused on magnetic resonance imaging as the LAD or it's diagonal (*double arrow heads*).

imaging, perfusion and viability. Such an approach would dramatically reduce the morbidity and mortality and provide for tangible and intangible socioeconomic benefit.

Taking this concept further, Voudris et al. (23) evaluated 48 patients undergoing CMR and X-ray diagnostic coronary angiography for angina or silent ischemia. They evaluated the angiographic and coronary flow velocity parameters that best correlated with the results of stress myocardial perfusion imaging at rest and during hyperemia for the poststenotic segment and an adjacent but, angiographically normal, branch of the LCA. They calculated the relative coronary flow velocity reserve (RCFVR) as the ratio of the coronary flow velocity reserve (CFVR) of the poststenotic vessel to the normal reference vessel. The best cutoff points for reversible perfusion defects were calculated using an Receiver Operating Characteristic (ROC) analysis. Poststenotic CFVR showed reasonable correlations to minimal lumen diameter and stenosis percentage ($r = 0.57$ and $r = 0.55$, respectively; $p < 0.001$). However, RCFVR showed stronger correlations with angiographic indexes of stenosis severity ($r = 0.66$ and $r = 0.68$, respectively; $p < 0.0001$). Based on ROC cutoff values (1.67 for poststenotic CFVR and 0.64 for RCFVR), RCFVR had better agreement with myocardial perfusion imaging results, compared to poststenotic CFVR (agreement 92% vs. 75%, respectively). As expected, the more physiologic and patient-specific the interrogation, the better the results, the authors concluded. Here, RCFVR is a better descriptor than poststenotic CFVR for functional significance of observed coronary artery stenoses.

Analogous to the physiologic understanding of an anatomic stenoses mentioned above, incorporation of CMR phase velocity mapping (PVM) to measure blood velocity adds an important feature to determining the significance of an observed lesion. This finding helps to adjudicate those lesions seen on CMR that occasionally are present but may be an artifact from a vessel traveling oblique to the image plane or a bend in the vessel, either of which is a pitfall for the clinician. Applying PVM to such a lesion slightly downstream (less than 1 cm) and, upon the finding of normal velocities) 0.8 to 1.2 milliseconds assures the physician that the vessel is patent. Provocation with dobutamine or adenosine has also been shown to correctly identify those patients with abnormal flow reserve. Two studies performed by Hundley and associates recently demonstrated the efficacy of physiologic testing by CMR. In the first study, 30 patients underwent coronary flow reserve testing using CMR to identify left main or LAD coronary artery disease (24). Utilizing a coronary flow reserve of less than 1.7 identified stenoses greater than 70% with a sensitivity of 100% and a specificity of 83%. Their second study showed that a coronary flow reserve of less than 2.0 was predictive of more than 70% restenosis following angioplasty with the same sensitivity and specificity (25).

Coronary Artery Bypass Graft

Relative to the more torturous anatomy of native arteries, the evaluation of bypass grafts is considerably less cumbersome. Not only are the vessels larger, their course more predictable, but there are an absence of side branches and the influence of cardiac motion is less severe (Fig. 9). Using PVM, velocities can be quantified or a simple binary determination can be made to determine patency. Using the former, it is now clear that bypass graft flow is typically biphasic with velocities slightly exceeding 1.0 milliseconds. Because blood flow within the bypass typically only has one exit, there is no complication due to multiple run-off vessels provided by side braches in native coronaries, and thus there is no requirement to verify the exact patency within the entire course of the graft. If biphasic flow at 1.0 milliseconds is seen, the graft is patent. However, there may be narrowing or luminal stenoses present, but necessary flow is present (during ambient testing conditions, typically resting). It should be noted, that for the RCA, flow is typically biphasic throughout the cardiac cycle, while for the left system, biphasic *systolic* flow is the norm. Thus, temporal resolution of flow is required for such determinations to be made. The ability to achieve adequate temporal resolution is limited by the number of views acquired per segment in any k-space segmenting approach. Ideally, lower segmentation factors allow increased temporal resolution, but this is achieved at the expense of increasing the scan time. Sparse dynamic sampling techniques such as BRISK offer the ability to achieve rapid scanning, while maintaining adequate temporal resolution (26).

(A) (B)

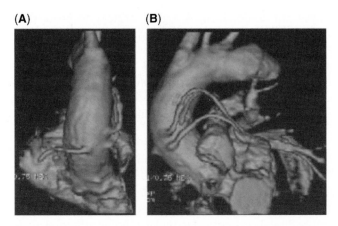

Figure 9 Surface rendering of a 22 second magnetic resonance angiogram (MRA) performed on a 56-year-old male with known arch repair following an aortic dissection. The patient returned for follow-up magnetic resonance imaging with complaints of chest pain six weeks later. While the aortic dissection had not progressed (not shown), MRA was performed specifically to interrogate the three emergently placed saphenous vein bypass grafts (SVG). Shown are two views of the 3D reconstruction of the source images demonstrating two patent SVG's on the left and the third SVG to right coronary artery on the right. The patient underwent X-ray cardiac catheterization later that day confirming the finding of patent grafts.

Langerak et al. recently evaluated 173 consecutive patients, who after receiving coronary artery bypass grafting (CABG), and subsequently presented with chest pain (27). A total of 69 eligible patients with 166 grafts (81 single vein, 44 sequential vein, and 41 arterial grafts) underwent CMR with baseline and stress flow mapping. Both scans were successful in 80% of grafts. The grafts were divided into two groups: (i) stenosis 50% ($n = 72$); (ii) greater than or equal to 70% ($n = 48$) either in the graft or recipient vessels. Multiple MRI variables were incorporated into a marginal logistic regression and used to predict the probability for the presence of stenosis for each graft type. ROC analysis was performed to assess the diagnostic value of CMR. The sensitivity and specificity with 95% confidence intervals (CI) for detecting single vein grafts with greater than or equal to 50% stenosis were 94% (86–100) and 63% (48–79), respectively; while for greater than or equal to 70% stenosis they were 96% (87–100) and 92% (84–100), respectively. The authors, using PVM demonstrated that CMR is useful for identifying grafts and recipient vessels with flow-limiting stenoses. While acceptable PVM scans could only be obtained in 80% of the grafts, once a high quality scan was obtained, the clinical accuracy was extraordinary, suggesting that CMR can be used interchangeably with X-ray angiography in situations where images can be obtained. A logical strategy to proceed in such cases may include (i) a post-CABG patient who presents with signs and symptoms consistent with a stenosed graft would enter the MRI suite and (ii) only if the images were suboptimal would the patient be required to undergo X-ray angiography. Even those in which the image strategy was less than ideal, some idea of which grafts were compromised could be transmitted to the angiographer, potentially limiting X-ray exposure and contrast.

Atherosclerotic Plaque Imaging

X-ray angiographic modalities indirectly detect the incidence of atherosclerotic plaque-based luminal perturbation. Techniques that are capable of imaging the plaque more directly are critical to understanding atherosclerosis pathophysiology. This may lead to the detection and treatment of "vulnerable plaques," which is one of the main goals of CMR. The ability to image plaques noninvasively is a major property of CMR that has only recently been capitalized on (28). CMR visualization of atherosclerotic plaque is based on the principle that different components of the plaque (lipid core, fibrous cap, hemorrhage, and calcium) produce unique and distinctive signal characteristics, permitting identification and separation of each. This is usually accomplished either by application of multiple distinct sequences, each designed to aid in separation of the anatomic details via their dissimilar relaxation or spin density properties. Using such an approach, a slice through the plaque is repeatedly imaged, each instance using a different pulse sequence. To identify individual tissue characteristics, sequences are used that weight images to enhance distinct features based on T1, T2, time-of-flight (TOF) and proton density weighting (PDW), applied with or without gadolinium contrast media. Using such an approach, Yuan et al. have provided stellar examples of the ability to distinguish the specific features of the atherosclerotic plaque (29,30). Calculation of plaque volume can be achieved by subtracting luminal volume from the total vessel wall volume. Atherosclerotic plaque characterization has been performed in ex vivo and in vivo situation in both animal models as well as in humans (30–33). The use of multispectral CMR to classify atherosclerotic plaques, based on the American Heart Association classification system has also been validated (34). Contrast-enhanced CMR can be used to detect neovasculature in carotid plaques and to identify the fibrous cap in aortic and carotid plaques (35). CMR can also be used to monitor the effects of lipid-lowering therapies on atherosclerotic plaques (36). In a case-controlled study using eight subjects from the FATS trial, it was been shown that prolonged and aggressive lipid-lowering therapy is associated with decreased lipid content and increase in fibrous tissue in carotid arterial plaques (37). In a prospective CMR study of carotid plaques, simvastatin therapy was associated with increased luminal area, decreased vessel wall area, and decreased maximal wall thickness at two years' follow up, indicating reverse arterial remodeling (38).

Kawasaki's Disease

Limiting invasive coronary imaging in young patients is an ideal goal, and one that recently became a possibility with the release of two studies in patients with coronary aneurysms (Fig. 10) demonstrating that serial

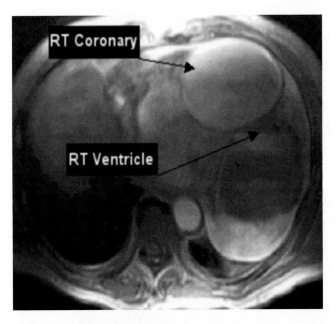

Figure 10 A 74-year-old man with a 10-week history of increasing shortness of breath and chest pressure sought evaluation at an outside hospital. Coronary angiography and a chest computed tomography were performed with the findings of a large bilobed anterior mediastinal mass. He was transferred for further evaluation whereupon he underwent further evaluation with a repeat X-ray angiogram and transesophageal echocardiogram, which only clouded the differential diagnosis [right coronary artery (RCA) was found to be "occluded"]. An atypical thymoma, consistent with the anterior mass was the chief consideration. The following day he underwent cardiovascular magnetic resonance imaging at our institution. Using a Fast Cine pulse sequence, the "mass" was demonstrated to be a $7 \times 9 \times 9$ cm aneurysm of the RCA. The aneurysm partially compressed the right ventricle confirmed by phase velocity mapping having a 35-mmHg gradient between the right ventricle (RV)/right atrium (RA). The patient was taken to the operating room the following day undergoing uneventful aneurysm resection and saphenous vein bypass graft to the proximal descending artery. Note the marked posterior displacement of the cardia, the compression of the RV, and one of two bilobed aneurysms, as large as the entire heart. The second aneurysm (not shown) is almost as large but more inferior positioned.

catheterizations could be negated. In the first study, six subjects (age 10–25 years) with known coronary artery aneurysms from Kawasaki disease underwent coronary MRA using a free-breathing T2-prepared 3D bright blood segmented k-space gradient-echo sequence with navigator gating and tracking, followed by X-ray coronary angiography within a median

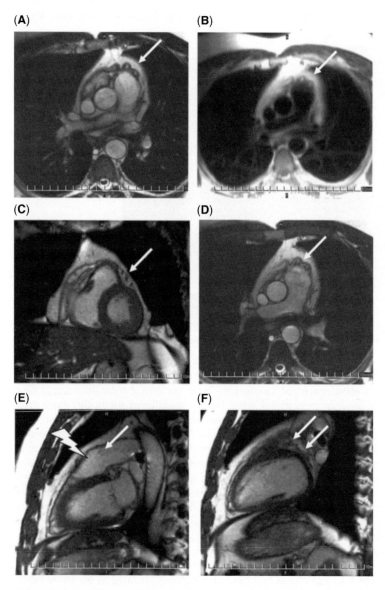

(A)   **(B)**
(C)   **(D)**
(E)   **(F)**

Figure 11   (*Caption on facing page*)

of 75 days (39). There was complete agreement between MRA and X-ray angiography in the detection of aneurysms ($n = 11$), coronary artery stenoses ($n = 2$), and coronary occlusions ($n = 2$). In the second study, 13 patients (12 male), age three to eight years, were studied using CMR and compared to X-ray angiography within one week (40). All scans were carried out with the patient free breathing using a 2D real-time navigator beam. In six patients, aneurysms of the coronary arteries were identified, while coronary ectasia alone was present in the remaining seven patients. Again CMR and X-ray angiography diagnosis of coronary artery aneurysms were in complete agreement. The maximal aneurysm diameter and length and ectasia diameter by MRA and XCA were similar and no stenotic lesion was identified by either technique. It seems clear that MRI/MRA may provide a noninvasive alternative, reducing the need for serial X-ray coronary angiography in this young patient population.

Coronary Fistula

The main predicament in examining coronary fistula, in which flow from a coronary artery is directed to one or more chambers within or adjacent to the heart, is the ability to delineate their course. The difficulty for X-ray coronary angiography is not related to the inability to detect the fine aberrant vessels, but from the failure to detect where the efflux of that vessel empties. This problem arises due to the requirement inherent to X-ray angiography for the contrast media to clearly opacify the vessel and, simultaneously, its dumping chamber, a feature not shared by CMR. Several cases have been reported highlighting the ability of CMR to delineate and demarcate the correct course of fistula, otherwise not visualized by X-ray angiography (41,42). Our experience has been similar, where we have observed cases where X-ray angiography has led to equivocal results that have been resolved by CMR with "reasonable" ease (Figs. 11 and 12). Further, we additionally calculate

Figure 11 (*Figure on facing page*) A 42-year-old presents with peculiar symptoms of dyspnea and a slightly enlarged right ventricle by echocardiography, prompting an X-ray angiogram. The catheterization demonstrates an unusual anteriorly directed vessel arising from the left anterior descending (LAD). Using a series of Steady-state free precession images (all except **B**), this vessel is seen to arise from the LAD traveling superiorly and anteriorly around the RVOT (**A, B** and **D**) to empty (arrows at two tiny dark dots **E**) into the supra-valvar pulmonary artery (lightening bolt, **E**). Another confluence of the abnormal vasculature is seen in **C**. Especially in **A, B**, and **D**, the serpentine nature of this coronary to pulmonary artery fistula is demonstrated. By phase velocity mapping the QP:QS was shown to be 1.3:1, which not significant, and the RV was shown by 3D quantification to be at the top of the normal range. Prophylactic coiling interruption was considered (as was an anterior thoracotomy approach), all of which the patient elected to forgo, pending progression.

(A)   (B)

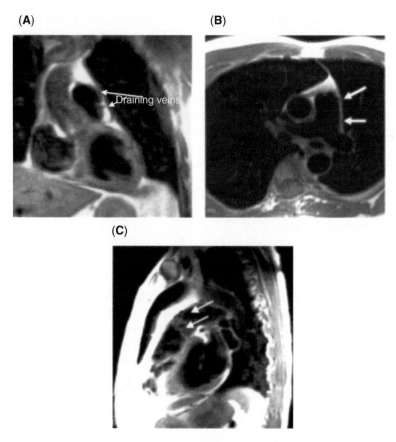

(C)

Figure 12 A 35-year-old male presented with dyspnea. (**A**) Anterior vessel arising from the left anterior descending (LAD) traveling superior and leftward was unable to be identified to its final destination prompting a cardiovascular magnetic resonance imaging. Serial multiple oblique spin echo images demonstrate several draining vessels traveling superiorly and anteriorly (**A**), traveling lateral to the main pulmonary artery (**B**), (*arrows*) entering the suprapulmonic valvular artery, diagnostic of an LAD to pulmonary artery fistula (**C**), (*arrows*).

QP:QS to quantify the shunt ratio, adding physiologic significance the observed aberrant flow.

FUTURE DEVELOPMENTS

Perfusion

Myocardial perfusion imaging can be performed using CMR either as a stand-alone study or in conjunction with coronary artery imaging. Using perfusion data acquired at rest and stress, the myocardial flow reserve (MFR) can be calculated and used as an indicator of functional capacity of the coronary vasculature. Doyle et al., as part of the NHLBI-sponsored the Women's Ischemia Symptoms Evaluation (WISE) Trial, recently reported on 184 women (the largest CMR perfusion study to date) presenting with chest pain and who underwent near simultaneous evaluation using nuclear gated-SPECT, X-ray coronary artery angiography and CMR myocardial perfusion studies. Baseline and vasodilation (dipyridamole) perfusion CMR data was used to generate a flow reserve (MFR) index (43). Following a Pilot phase, in which an understanding of CMR characteristics was gained for determination of the MFR index and of ischemic conditions. Patients were evaluated as being either (i) adequate (AMFRI) or (ii) inadequate (IMFRI) with regard to the flow reserve/(MFR) index and as being normal or positive with regard to ischemic regions. Prospectively, 138 patients were evaluated using CMR and conventional SPECT. When compared with each other, CMR and gated-SPECT demonstrated no difference in accuracy of detection of severe coronary artery stenoses (greater than or equal to 70%) when using angiography as the "gold standard." However, both CMR and SPECT demonstrated higher accuracy in the AMFRI group compared to the IMFRI group: for CMR (86% vs. 70%, $p < 0.05$) and gated-SPECT (89% vs. 67%, $p < 0.01$). The IMFRI group ($n = 55$, 30% of study population) had a higher resting double product compared with the AMFRI group ($10,599 \pm 2871$ vs. 9378 ± 2447, $p < 0.01$), consistent with augmented resting myocardial blood flow. This demonstrated the importance of being able to assess MFR when evaluating myocardial perfusion. However, this information was only available to CMR, and thus SPECT did not have intrinsic markers indicating whether adequate or inadequate MFR was achieved. Thus, when using myocardial perfusion approaches to select those that may require an intervention, CMR with its ability to assess MFR and the presence of ischemia, may become an important test.

Intravascular Agents

Intravascular contrast agents exhibit several advantages over traditional extracellular agents, including a much greater T1 relaxivity, maintenance of a higher concentration within the blood pool, and lower extravasation into the myocardium. All these features provide the potential for improved contrast to noise ratio. Recently Yucel and colleagues studied the performance of intravascular contrast agents applied to 3D coronary MRA, cine MRI, and myocardial perfusion (44). They concluded that maintaining a blood pool agent that did not leach into the myocardium improved the CNR. Additionally, the persistence of contrast within the vascular pool permitted the convenience of longer imaging times, allowing incorporation of less time-sensitive 3D acquisitions with less reliance on rapid imaging sequences.

Targeted Contrast Agents

Targeted contrast agents are under development to improve the capability of CMR as a diagnostic tool for a variety of diseases including inflammation and microthrombus within fissures of unstable atherosclerotic plaques, potentially allowing sensitive, early detection of vascular microthrombi which is the precursor to stroke and MI (45–47).

Corrective Models

The 3D respiratory influence superimposed upon an already complex cardiac motion can be isolated, leading to improved fidelity of image quality. Shechter et al. reconstructed the motion of the heart and developed a method to separate the cardiac and respiratory motion fields. Theoretically, this can lead to optimized cardiac imaging above and beyond that achievable by respiratory gating approaches (48).

CONCLUSIONS

When discussions surrounding CMR coronary artery imaging arise in conjunction with comparison to X-ray angiography, typically such considerations are limited to the pros and cons of each, assuming that as a default, the latter is the "gold standard." However, recent findings may serve to tarnish this view of X-ray angiography. Uretsy et al. evaluated 171 patients as part of the assessment of treatment with lisinopril and survival ATLAS Trial, investigating the etiology of cardiomyopathies (49). There were 92 clinical diagnoses of isolated ischemic cardiomyopathy (ICM, 54% of the study group), 17% idiopathic, 13% ICM, and hypertension, 5% with no cause listed, 4% hypertension, 2% each for valvular heart disease), ICM, and other clinical combinations, and 0.6% for each of ICM plus idiopathic and ICM plus hypertension plus idiopathic. Of those diagnosed clinically as having isolated ICM ($n = 92$) or in combination with another diagnosis ($n = 28$), at autopsy, 83% were found to have significant CAD. Of the 51 patients diagnosed clinically as having a nonischemic cause or with no diagnosis listed, at autopsy, 31% were found to have significant CAD. Unstated in the report, but mathematically derivable, of patients diagnosed with a nonischemic cardiomyopathy, nearly one-third *have* significant CAD. Even more troublesome, for patients diagnosed clinically by catheterization as having an ischemic cardiomyopathy, at autopsy 17% were show to posses *no* significant CAD. While there are many potential reasons for these findings, in aggregate, the preponderance of the discordant findings is indicative of there being substantial sources of error in the evaluation of X-ray angiograms.

Thus, there are a number of reasons to reevaluate the current standing of conventional X-ray angiography including, the morbidity and mortality levels, the approximately three- to five-fold higher tangible costs relative to CMR, as well as intangible costs relating to diagnostic accuracy and patient comfort. Analogous to the circumstances of anomalous coronary arteries, where CMR is now regarded as the "gold standard" for detection, it nevertheless took a decade of work by MRI specialists to convince the medical community of this fact. Today, it is common knowledge. However, evaluation of coronary arteries using CMR is currently on a more advanced footing, so the journey to general acceptance is not anticipated to be as long.

Today, there is no question as to the utility of CMR for application to image the coronary arteries. With improvements in hardware (e.g., 3-Tesla field strength) and acquisition techniques (parallel imaging, spiral acquisition, contrast enhancement etc.), CMR is an important noninvasive tool in the diagnosis of coronary artery stenosis. When combined with it's noninvasiveness, patient comfort, reduction in risk, and exponential improvements in speed, ease and accuracy, as well as the recent documentation of robustness in a landmark clinical trial, the next five years will see CMR become the preferred imaging modality for an increasing number of indications including cardiomyopathy, anomalous coronary arteries, and as a screening test for those with low and intermediate risk, or those not wishing to encounter the risk of invasive angiography.

REFERENCES

1. Pennell DJ, Bogren HG, Keegan J, Firmin DN, Underwood SR. Assessment of coronary artery stenosis by magnetic resonance imaging. Heart 1996; 75(2):127–133.
2. Muller MF, Fleisch M, Kroeker R, Chatterjee T, Meier B, Vock P. Proximal coronary artery stenosis: three-dimensional MRI with fat saturation and navigator echo. J Magn Reson Imaging 1997; 7(4):644–651.
3. Bornert P, Stuber M, Botnar RM, Kissinger KV, Manning WJ. Comparison of fat suppression strategies in 3D spiral coronary magnetic resonance angiography. J Magn Reson Imaging 2002; 15(4):462–466.
4. Spuentrup E, Bornert P, Botnar RM, Groen JP, Manning WJ, Stuber M. Navigator-gated free-breathing three-dimensional balanced fast field echo (TrueFISP) coronary magnetic resonance angiography. Invest Radiol 2002; 37(11):637–642.
5. Duerinckx AJ, Urman MK. Two-dimensional coronary MR angiography: analysis of initial clinical results. Radiology 1994; 193(3):731–738.
6. Lethimonnier F, Furber A, Morel O, et al. Three-dimensional coronary artery MR imaging using prospective real-time respiratory navigator and linear phase shift processing: comparison with conventional coronary angiography. Magn Reson Imaging 1999; 17(8):1111–1120.
7. Regenfus M, Ropers D, Achenbach S, et al. Noninvasive detection of coronary artery stenosis using contrast-enhanced three-dimensional breath-hold magnetic resonance coronary angiography. J Am Coll Cardiol 2000; 36(1):44–50.
8. Oshinski JN, Hofland L, Dixon WT, Pettigrew RI. Magnetic resonance coronary angiography using navigator echo gated real-time slice following. Int J Card Imaging. 1998; 14(3):191–199.

9. White CS, Laskey WK, Stafford JL, NessAiver M. Coronary MRA: use in assessing anomalies of coronary artery origin. J Comput Assist Tomogr. 1999; 23(2):203–207.

10. McConnell MV, Khasgiwala VC, Savord BJ, et al. Comparison of respiratory suppression methods and navigator locations for MR coronary angiography. Am J Roentgenol 1997; 168(5):1369–1375.

11. Stuber M, Botnar RM, Danias PG, et al. Double-oblique free-breathing high resolution three-dimensional coronary magnetic resonance angiography. J Am Coll Cardiol 1999; 34(2):524–531.

12. Achenbach S, Kessler W, Moshage WE, et al. Visualization of the coronary arteries in three-dimensional reconstructions using respiratory gated magnetic resonance imaging. Coron Artery Dis 1997; 8(7):441–448.

13. Biederman RW, Fuisz AR, Pohost GM. Magnetic resonance angiography. Curr Opin Cardiol 1998; 13(6):430–437.

14. Baim DS, Grossman W. Complications of cardiac catheterization. In: Bain DS, Grosman DW, eds. Cardiac Catheterization Angiography and Interventions. 5th ed. Baltimore: Williams and Wilkens, 1996:17–38.

15. Razmi RM, Meduri A, Chun W, et al. Coronary magnetic resonance angiography (CMRA): the gold-standard for determining the proximal course of anomalous coronary arteries. J Am Coll Cardiol 2001; 37:380.

16. Taylor AM, Thorne SA, Rubens MB, et al. Coronary artery imaging in grown up congenital heart disease: complementary role of magnetic resonance and X-ray coronary angiography. Circulation 2000; 101:1670–1675.

17. Stuber et al. Magn Reson Med 2002; 48(3).

18. Danias PG, Stuber M, Manning WJ. Coronary Magnetic Resonance Angiography-Clinical Results. In: Manning WJ, Pennell D, eds. Cardiovascular Magnetic Resonance. Livingstone Churchill, 2002:215–215.

19. Paetsch I, Gebker R, Fleck E, Nagel E. Cardiac magnetic resonance (CMR) imaging: a noninvasive tool for functional and morphological assessment of coronary artery disease: current clinical applications and potential future concepts. J Interv Cardiol 2003; 16(6):457–463.

20. Salm LP, Bax JJ, Lamb HJ, et al. Evaluation of rerouting surgery of a coronary artery anomaly by magnetic resonance angiography. Ann Thorac Surg 2003; 76(5):1748.

21. Plein S, Ridgway JP, Jones TR, Bloomer TN, Sivananthan MU. The impact of myocardial flow reserve on the detection of coronary artery disease by perfusion imaging methods: an NHLBI WISE study. Radiology 2002; 225(1):300–307.

22. Kim WY, Danias PG, Stuber M, et al. Coronary magnetic resonance angiography for the detection of coronary stenoses. N Engl J Med 2001; 27;345(26): 1863–1869.

23. Voudris V, Avramides D, Koutelou M, et al. Relative coronary flow velocity reserve improves correlation with stress myocardial perfusion imaging in assessment of coronary artery stenoses. Chest 2003; 124(4):1266–1274.

24. Hundley WG, Hamilton CA, Clarke GD, et al. Visualization and functional assessment of proximal and middle left anterior descending coronary stenoses in humans with magnetic resonance imaging. Circulation 1999; 29; 99(25): 3248–3254.

25. Hundley WG, Hillis LD, Hamilton CA, et al. Assessment of coronary arterial restenosis with phase-contrast magnetic resonance imaging measurements of coronary flow reserve. Circulation 2000; 23;101(20):2375–2381.
26. Doyle M, Walsh EG, Foster RE, Pohost GM. Rapid cardiac imaging with turbo BRISK. Magn Reson Med 1997; 37(3):410–417.
27. Langerak SE, Vliegen HW, Jukema JW, et al. Value of magnetic resonance imaging for the noninvasive detection of stenosis in coronary artery bypass grafts and recipient coronary arteries. Circulation 2003; 25;107(11):1502–1508.
28. Fayad ZA, Fuster V, Fallon JT, et al. Noninvasive in vivo human coronary artery lumen and wall imaging using black-blood magnetic resonance imaging. Circulation 2000, 102: (5) 506–510.
29. Yuan C, Beach KW, Smith LH, et al. Measurement of atherosclerotic carotid plaque size in vivo using high resolution magnetic resonance imaging. Circulation 1998; 98:2666–2671.
30. Yuan C, Mitsumori LM, Ferguson MS, et al. In vivo accuracy of multispectral magnetic resonance imaging for identifying lipid-rich necrotic cores and intraplaque hemorrhage in advanced human carotid plaques. Circulation 2001; 104:2051–2056.
31. Shinnar M, Wehrli S, Levin M, et al. The diagnostic accuracy of ex vivo MRI for human atherosclerotic plaque characterization. Arterioscler Thromb Vasc Biol 1999; 19:2756–2761.
32. Worthley SG, Helft G, Fuster V, et al. High resolution ex vivo magnetic resonance imaging of in situ coronary and aortic atherosclerotic plaque in a porcine model. Atherosclerosis 2000; 150:321–329.
33. Fayad ZA, Fallon JT, Shinnar M, et al. Noninvasive in vivo high-resolution magnetic resonance imaging of atherosclerotic lesions in genetically engineered mice. Circulation 1998; 98:1541–1547.
34. Cai JM, Hatsukami TS, Ferguson MS, et al. Classification of human carotid atherosclerotic lesions with in vivo multicontrast magnetic resonance imaging. Circulation 2002; 106: 1386–1373.
35. Kerwin WS, Hooker A, Spilker M, et al. Quantitative magnetic resonance imaging analysis of neovasculature volume in carotid atherosclerotic plaque. Circulation 2003; 107:851–856.
36. Kramer CM, Cerilli LA, Berr SS, et al. MRI can distinguish plaque components including inflammation in abdominal aortic aneurysm. Circulation 2001; 104: 375–376.
37. Zhao XQ, Yuan C, Hatsukami TS, et al. Effects of prolonged intensive lipid-lowering therapy on the characteristics of carotid atherosclerotic plaques in vivo by MRI. Arterioscler Thromb Vasc Biol 2001; 21:1623–1639.
38. Corti R, Fuster V, Fayad ZA, et al. Lipid lowering by simvastatin induces regression of human atherosclerotic lesions. Circulation 2002; 106:2884–2887.
39. Greil GF, Stuber M, Botnar RM, et al. Coronary magnetic resonance angiography in adolescents and young adults with Kawasaki disease. Circulation 2002; 105(8):908–911.
40. Mavrogeni S, Papadopoulos G, Douskou M, et al. Magnetic resonance angiography is equivalent to X-ray coronary angiography for the evaluation of coronary arteries in Kawasaki disease. J Am Coll Cardiol 2004; 43(4):649–652.

41. Sato Y, Ishikawa K, Sakurai I, et al. Magnetic resonance imaging in diagnosis of right coronary arteriovenous fistula—a case report. Jpn Circ J 1997; 61(12): 1043–1046.

42. Heyne JP, Leder U, Pohl P, Kaiser WA. Imaging of coronary vascular abnormality with aneurysm and arteriovenous fistula using MRI bolus tracking. Radiologe 2001; 41(6):506–510.

43. Doyle M, Fuisz A, Kortright E, et al. The impact of myocardial flow reserve on the detection of coronary artery disease by perfusion imaging methods: an NHLBI WISE study. J Cardiovasc Magn Reson 2003; 5(3):475–485.

44. Lei T, Udupa JK, Saha PK, et al. 3D MRA visualization and artery-vein separation using blood-pool contrast agent MS-325. Acad Radiol. 2002 (Suppl 1): S127–S133.

45. Laurent S, Vander Elst L, Fu Y, Muller RN. Synthesis and physicochemical characterization of Gd-DTPA-B(sLex)A, a new MRI contrast agent targeted to inflammation. Bioconjug Chem 2004; 15(1):99–103.

46. Winter PM, Caruthers SD, Yu X, et al. Improved molecular imaging contrast agent for detection of human thrombus. Magn Reson Med 2003; 50(2):411–416.

47. Wickline SA, Lanza GM. Nanotechnology for molecular imaging and targeted therapy. Circulation 2003; 107(8):1092–1095.

48. Shechter G, Ozturk C, Resar JR, McVeigh ER. Respiratory motion of the heart from free breathing coronary angiograms, IEEE Transactions on Medical Imaging. (in press).

49. Uretsky BF, Thygesen K, Armstrong PW, et al. Acute Coronary Findings at Autopsy in Heart Failure Patients With Sudden Death Results From the Assessment of Treatment With Lisinopril and Survival (ATLAS) Trial. Circulation 2000; 102:611.

12

Myocardial Infarct Imaging

Jaime O. Henriquez and Mazda Motallebi

*Division of Cardiovascular Medicine, University of Southern California,
Los Angeles, California, U.S.A.*

Gerald M. Pohost

*Department of Medicine, Division of Cardiovascular Medicine,
Keck School of Medicine, University of Southern California,
Los Angeles, California, U.S.A.*

INTRODUCTION

Every year, approximately 800,000 people in the United States experience acute myocardial infarction (MI). Early recognition and treatment can improve mortality, reduce the size of myocardial injury, and preserve left ventricular (LV) function. Management of patients after acute MI also has long-term implications, including the possibility of ventricular aneurysm, reduced (frequently and severely reduced) ventricular function, heart failure, atrial and ventricular arrhythmia, and "sudden death." The amount of remaining viable myocardium provides a determinant of prognosis. Conversely, the amount of myocardial scar also provides a determinant of outcomes. Several imaging approaches provide a means to assess whether dysfunctional myocardium is alive (viable) or dead/scarred (nonviable). One of the first imaging approaches that allows assessment of myocardial viability was the radionuclide method. The two approaches include single photon methods (using thallium-201 and technetium-99m) as the radionuclides and positron emission tomography (PET) [using ^{18}F fluorodeoxyglucose (FDG) to detect the viable myocardium coupled with $^{13}NH_3$ or ^{82}Rb to evaluate myocardial perfusion]. It is most useful to assess myocardial perfusion or ventricular function, which is reduced in both viable ischemic myocardium and nonviable myocardium. Single photon emission computed tomography (SPECT) has been widely used for detection of myocardial ischemia and MI, since the early 1980s. SPECT has limited spatial resolution, making it difficult to determine the transmural extent and the presence of small territories of infarction. SPECT is also unable to provide high quality images of ventricular structure and function. Furthermore, imaging with SPECT to determine viability in segments with myocardial dysfunction requires follow-up imaging hours (up to 48 hours) after thallium administration. PET had been considered the "gold standard" imaging approach for the assessment of myocardial viability. However positron-emitting tracers are very expensive and technically difficult to produce, requiring a cyclotron or with the perfusion imaging agent ^{82}Rb, and an expensive generator. Also, the distribution of FDG is variably affected by the presence of diabetes. Finally, echocardiography has been a widely used approach for evaluating viability in asynergic myocardial segments by demonstrating improvement in wall motion during the infusion of low dose dobutamine. Cardiovascular magnetic resonance (CMR) imaging has become an important tool for identifying myocardial scar. This technique also is able to provide high-resolution images of cardiac morphology, function, and perfusion. The present chapter will describe the application of CMR imaging in acute and chronic MI.

CMR IMAGING OF MI

History of MI CMR Imaging

MI can be imaged using one of many approaches. The earliest CMR approach to image the heart was demonstrated in laboratory animals and used the paramagnetic contrast agent $MnCl_2$ to depict myocardial perfusion and infarction and used steady state free precession (SSFP) in order to determine the distribution of manganous chloride ($MnCl_2$) and thus the extent of MI (1). Unfortunately, the $MnCl_2$ contrast agent was toxic and the SSFP pulse sequence, at that time, was very sensitive to motion and led to blurring of the images. In the mid-1980s, spin echo CMR was used to detect the T2 changes associated with MI in the absence of a contrast agent (2). Such changes in T2 were related, in large part, to the accumulation of myocardial edema associated with MI and its reperfusion. The limitations of this technique included a long imaging time and low spatial resolution. Today, CMR allows imaging of acutely infarcted myocardium and/or myocardial scar, using the appearance of contrast enhancement typically observed 10 to 20 minutes after a gadolinium-based paramagnetic contrast agent injection (Fig. 1).

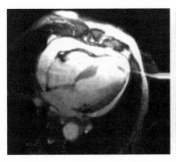
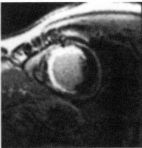

Figure 1   Contrast hyperenhancement in myocardial infarction. *Source*: Courtesy of Dr. Steven Wolff, Lenox Hill Heart and Vascular Institute of New York.

The Most Recent Technique for Demonstrating MI and Myocardial Scar: Delayed Enhancement

The contrast agent, gadolinium, shortens the proton T1 relaxation time, leading to an increase in signal intensity. Gadolinium accumulates in the interstitium of the infarcted tissue and allows visualization of the territory in which it localizes. In T1-weighted images, a bright signal is produced in the distribution of gadolinium. The shortened T1 relaxation signal in the infarct is maximally enhanced when inversion recovery preparation is used to reduce or null the signal in the noninfarcted myocardium. Segmented inversion recovery fast gradient echo (IR-FGRE) has been used as the pulse sequence of choice for demonstrating the location and size of the MI. With this sequence, the infarcted myocardium demonstrates intensity substantially greater than that of normal myocardium, generating excellent contrast, bright infarction or scar, and dim or nulled normal myocardial tissue (3,4). Recently, Kim et al. described in detail the procedure of image-delayed enhancement (DE). Their experience is based on the performance of DE imaging in almost 2000 patients (Fig. 2) (5).

The Technique for DE Imaging

The procedure is performed in a single examination lasting approximately 30 to 40 minutes. After placement of an intravenous (IV) catheter, the patient is positioned within the bore of the scanner (compared with 1.5 T, 3.0 T produces higher quality and more sensitive images). Scout images are obtained to delineate the short and long axis views of the ventricles. Cine images are obtained to evaluate morphology and contractile function, using an SSFP- or FGRE-based approach. Short axis slices (6 mm thickness and 4 mm gap) are acquired from the insertion of the mitral valve to the LV apex (7–10 slices). Two to three long axis slices are also depicted. Then, 0.1 to 0.15 mmol/kg of IV Gd-diethylenetriaminepentaacetic acid (DPTA)

(A)   (B)   (C)

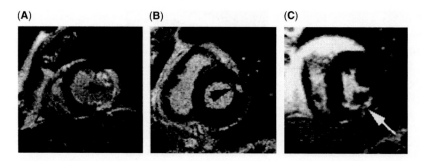

Figure 2 Cardiovascular magnetic resonance (CMR) delayed enhancement (DE) imaging after acute myocardial infarction (MI). (**A**) Transmural DE (*black arrow*) in a patient with a q-wave ST elevation MI two weeks after MI, (**B**) small anterolateral nontransmural enhancement (*black arrow*) six days after the MI, and (**C**) subendocardial DE of the inferior wall nine months after acute MI (*white arrow*). *Source*: Images courtesy of Dr. Raymond Kim and Dr. Robert Judd.

(or other gadolinium-based contrast agent with appropriate dose) is administered. One can image myocardial perfusion using the first-pass of this contrast agent (Chapter 9). Segmented IR-FGRE is used to obtain enhanced images at 10 to 15 minutes after contrast administration. Figure 3 illustrates the timing of the 2D segmented IR-FGRE pulse sequence. There is a time delay between the R wave and a nonselective 180° hyperbolic secant adiabatic inversion pulse. The inversion time (TI) is the interval between the inversion pulse and the center of the data acquisition window

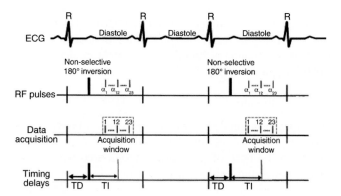

Figure 3 Timing diagram of two-dimensional segmented inversion-recovery fast gradient echo pulse sequence. Note that in this depiction, 23 lines of *k*-space are acquired every other heartbeat. *Abbreviations*: ECG, electrocardiogram; RF, radiofrequency; TD, trigger delay; TI, inversion time delay; α, shallow flip angle excitation. *Source*: From Ref. 5.

and is chosen such that the intensity of the noninfarcted (or scarred) myocardium is minimized. The acquisition window contains low flip angle FGRE acquisitions, with approximately 20 to 25 lines of k-space acquired per segment; and a flip angle of 20° to 30°. To allow adequate longitudinal relaxation (T1) between successive 180° pulses, inversion pulses and data acquisition are performed every other beat. Using this timing, breath-hold durations of 12 cardiac cycles are required for each image. Occasionally, it is necessary to perform imaging every third heart beat in the setting of tachycardia or every heart beat in the setting of a bradycardic rhythm.

The imaging parameters most frequently used by Kim et al. are shown in Table 1. The field of view (FOV) in both read and phase encode directions is minimized to improve spatial resolution. Typically, a FOV of 240 to 360 mm is used. If a repetition time of 8 msec is used and 23 lines of k-space are obtained, the acquisition time is 184 msec. The spatial resolution (in-plane) is $1.2 \times 1.2\,mm^2$ to $1.8 \times 1.8\,mm^2$ and a slice thickness of 6 mm is used to "optimize" signal-to-noise ratio, while avoiding significant partial volume effects.

Table 1 Typical Imaging Parameters

Parameter	Values
Gadolinium DTPA dose	0.10–0.15 mmol/kg
Field of view	300–380 mm
In-plane voxel size	$1.2–1.8 \times 1.2–1.8 \times 6\,mm^3$
Flip angle	20°–30°
Segments[a]	13–31
TI	Variable
Bandwidth	90–250 Hz/pixel
TE	3–4 msec
TR[b]	8–9 msec
Gating factor[c]	2
k-space ordering	Linear
Fat saturation	No
Asymmetric echo	Yes
Gradient moment refocusing[d]	Yes

[a]Fewer segments are used for higher heart rates.
[b]TR is generally defined as the time between RF pulses; however, scanner manufacturers occasionally redefine TR to represent the time from the ECG trigger (R wave) to the center or end of the data acquisition window (i.e., 100 msec less than the ECG R–R interval).
[c]Image every other heartbeat.
[d]Also known as gradient-moment nulling, gradient-moment rephrasing, or flow compensation.
Abbreviations: TI, inversion time; TE, echo time; TR, repetition time; RF, radio frequency; ECG, electrocardiogram; DTPA, diethylenetriaminepentaacetic acid.
Source: From Ref. 5.

The selection of the appropriate TI is essential. The TI controls the nulling of the signal in the noninfarcted, nonscarred myocardium and thus the difference in intensity between infarcted (contrast enhanced) and noninfarcted myocardium. An example of the inversion recovery curves and image intensity difference between normal and infarcted (or scarred) myocardium is shown in Figure 3. TI should be chosen to maximally reduce the signal or "null" the signal in normal myocardium. This will occur when the magnetization of normal myocardium reaches the zero intensity cross point. If the TI is set too short, the image intensity of normal myocardium is higher and contrast between infarcted and noninfarcted myocardium is less. If the TI is set too long, both infarcted and noninfarcted myocardium will have higher image intensities, and the relative contrast between infarcted and normal myocardium will be reduced. The optimal TI is estimated based on the amount of paramagnetic contrast agent used and the time after contrast agent administration. One or two test images with different inversion times are acquired to identify the optimal TI for the specific study. Another approach to optimizing the TI uses phase-sensitive reconstruction of inversion recovery data with a nominal TI and TI "scout" sequence. In general, TI requires no readjustment during a study. However, if imaging is performed at multiple points after administration of gadolinium (or comparable agent), TI should be gradually increased to compensate for the gradual washout of the contrast agent. It has been shown that when the TI is adjusted, the size of enhanced regions remains unchanged if imaging is performed between 10 and 30 minutes after agent administration (6).

Analysis of Contrast-Enhanced Myocardial Images

Kim et al. use a 17-segment model for reporting the results of the contrast-enhanced images. The extent of enhanced tissue within each segment is graded using a 5-point scale: 0 indicates no enhancement; 1 indicates, enhancement of 1% to 25%; 2 indicates 26% to 50%; 3 indicates 51% to 75%; and 4 indicates 76% to 100% (5). Planimetry is used to determine the (in plane) area of the enhanced territory and when multiplied by slice thickness (plus the interslice spacing), the mass is determined and expressed in grams. The basal portion of the slice is frequently used and the borders are usually well defined. Contrast enhancement strategies to improve border definition can also be applied.

Pitfalls of the Technique

The pitfalls of this technique (4) include patient-related issues and technical limitations. Image quality is degraded in patients with atrial fibrillation or frequent ventricular ectopy. Motion artifacts are generated in patients who are unable to hold their breath during image acquisition, Tissues and fluids within the FOV, which have long T1 relaxation times (e.g., pericardial effusion or cerebrospinal fluid), can result in ghosting artifacts. This can be corrected by application of a single nonselective saturation pulse 600 to 800 msec before the initial inversion pulse. Finally, if three-dimensional approaches are used, a gating factor of 1 (i.e., an acquisition for every heart-beat) is required in order to shorten breath hold to a tolerable duration.

DE Imaging: Clinical Considerations

The clinical basis for the detection of MI and/or scar is the localization of gadolinium contrast agent within the affected myocardium. During the first-pass of the paramagnetic contrast agent (e.g., Gd-DTPA), images depict passage through the cardiac chambers (right-sided chambers, left-sided chambers, and then myocardium). During the initial myocardial phase, areas of hypoenhancement are noted in the infarcted and underperfused territories (7,8). Images of the first-pass of contrast agent through the myocardium depict the regional distribution of myocardial perfusion. Over the course of 10 minutes or more, the contrast agent enters the infarcted territories as well as territories of myocardial scar, producing hyperenhance-ment. Enhancement of myocardial signal occurs over 10 to 30 minutes (even as early as 5 minutes) after contrast injection delineates nonviable myocar-dium including myocardial scar and acutely infarcted myocardium (9,10). When one compares delayed images demonstrating enhancement with the first-pass images demonstrating perfusion, the following can be concluded:

1. The zones of myocardium that are hypointense on the first-pass of contrast agent represent ischemic plus infarcted territories.
2. The zones of myocardium that are enhanced 10 minutes or later represent nonviable myocardium.
3. The zones of myocardium that were hypointense during first-pass but did not enhance on delayed imaging represent viable, but ischemic myocardium that is reversible with appropriate intervention.

Areas of DE can effectively identify the extent and location of MI (3,4). The transmural extent of myocardial enhancement defines the trans-mural extent of the infarcted myocardium. Thirty patients with their first acute MI were studied with gradient-echo imaging 10 to 15 minutes after contrast agent injection. Segmental wall thickening was evaluated by qualitative methods to determine myocardial segment dysfunction. The extent of enhancement was scored on the 5-point scale previously described: $1 = 0\%$; $2 = 1\%$ to 25%; $3 = 26\%$ to 50%; $4 = 51\%$ to 75%; $5 = 76\%$ to 100% enhancement. There was an inverse relationship between the extent of enhancement and the likelihood of improvement in dysfunctional myocar-dial segments (10). On a follow-up CMR study, dysfunctional myocardial segments with no enhancement (level 1) were 2.9, 14.3, and 20 times more likely to improve than segments with level 3, level 4, or level 5 enhancement, respectively.

Acute MI with DE Imaging

In MI, there are several patterns observed by DE CMR imaging. A common pattern is a homogeneous zone of enhanced myocardium. Again, the ischemic territory is visualized using both first-pass and delayed contrast imaging.

A second pattern is observed in more severe MI. In this pattern, the center of the infarct is hypointense on delayed contrast images, 10 minutes or more after injection. This hypointense area is surrounded by an enhanced territory, which is surrounded by a territory of ischemia, which, in turn, is surrounded by normal myocardium. The central area of hypointensity occurs as a result of microvascular obstruction, which prevents the contrast agent from reaching the central territory of the infarct. This microvascular obstruction is also responsible for the phenomenon of "no reflow." The no reflow phenomenon does not allow territories of myocardium to be reperfused by intervention.

The presence of the pattern of microvascular obstruction has a deleterious affect on prognosis. Because the endocardium is kept viable by the blood within the left ventricle, the subendocardium is the territory that gets the least amount of blood in general, because of its exposure more directly to the pressures within the left ventricle. The subepicardium is exposed to less pressure from the left ventricle and, therefore, is better perfused and is less likely to demonstrate the phenomenon of microvascular obstruction.

A third pattern is the least severe MI. In this pattern, there is considerable viable myocardium and only a small territory of nonviable tissue.

In acute MI, tissue injury and recovery after reperfusion is not homogeneous. The regions identified by histological evaluation include a central necrotic area, a surrounding rim of tissue at risk with variable degrees of ischemia, and normal myocardium. The areas of DE after paramagnetic contrast agent administration on T1-weighted images delineate MI and scar. In laboratory animals, a significant inverse correlation has been found between the distribution of defects on T1-weighted contrast enhanced images and on triphenyltetrazolium chloride (TTC) or comparable histological staining (correlation coefficient $r^2 = 0.95$). In studies that do not use contrast agents, T2-weighted imaging can also delineate MI. However, such images tend to overestimate infarct size, since the area of increased T2 depicted as increased images intensity includes both infarcted nonviable edematous myocardium and noninfarcted viable edematous myocardium (11). Thus the areas with increased intensity on T2-weighted images represent injured, but not necessarily necrotic myocardium, including both viable and nonviable myocardium (12).

Few studies have assessed the changes noted on CMR within the first 24 hours after an ischemic event. Schulz-Menger et al. assessed eight patients with hypertrophic obstructive cardiomyopathy after septal artery embolization, with a T2-weighted spin echo sequence to visualize myocardial edema (13). Myocardial scarring was evaluated using the delayed contrast enhancement approach with T1-weighted acquisitions up to 20 minutes after an IV gadolinium bolus. No relevant signal intensity changes were visualized in T2-weighted images within one hour of embolization. However, at 24 hours after the intervention, there was T2 signal increase in the territory supplied by the "embolized" artery, i.e., the infarct area. In the T1-weighted images, the signal intensity between septal and remote myocardium was increased as early as one hour after septal embolization. Using CMR to generate a combination image of regional contractile function, regional myocardial perfusion, and infarcted myocardium, Kwong et al. studied the accuracy of CMR for detecting possible acute coronary syndromes in an emergency department (14). The average patient was away from the emergency department for 58 ± 10 minutes and most had their CMR study before they underwent a second troponin measurement. Qualitative CMR readings displayed enhancement consistent with MI with a sensitivity of 84% and a specificity of 85%.

Quantitative T1 mapping has also been used to identify injured myocardium without using contrast agents. T1 mapping consists of pixel-by-pixel calculation of T1 values (15). This technique provides quantitative images and provides T1 values rather than relative signal intensities. A recent study using T1 mapping in patients with acute MI used an inversion recovery–prepared FGRE sequence to image. The most important finding was significant T1 prolongation in infarcted areas ($18\% \pm 7\%$) compared to remote myocardium. However, the extent of the prolonged T1 region involved the central infarct and peri-infarct myocardium (15). This technique is faster than T2 mapping and does not require the use of a contrast agent (that increases the cost of the study). Accordingly, this approach may become a screening tool during an acute MI.

Viability in MI After Reperfusion

After reperfusion of MI, regional wall motion is frequently diminished in a process known a "stunning." The differentiation between stunned (viable) and normal myocardium is challenging because both lack DE. Dog and rat models of stunning have demonstrated no DE in stunned myocardial tissue (4,16). Segments with myocardial stunning have been found to have abnormal wall thickening, which differentiates them from normal myocardium. Absence of TTC uptake correlates well with contrast-enhanced segments on delayed imaging. In addition, cine magnetic resonance demonstrating akinesis/dyskinesis and little, if any, wall thickening and wall thinning suggests infarction in contrast to stunning.

CMR has many advantages for myocardial viability imaging over other imaging modalities. In addition to DE, segmental wall thickening and the fractional change in the length of the myocardium between end systole and end diastole has been used to predict viability using CMR. At rest, LV end diastolic wall thickness of less than 5.5 mm is suggestive of a histological transmural scar. The ability of CMR to delineate nonviable myocardium was recently compared to that of PET. The thickness of viable myocardial segments on delayed enhancement CMR was correlated with FDG defects on PET (17). FDG uptake greater than 50% of that of the normal myocardium is thought to predict functional recovery after revascularization (12,18). Schwaiger and coworkers found a specificity and sensitivity of CMR in identifying transmural infarcts of 0.86 and 0.94, respectively (19). PET has been considered a "gold standard" for identifying viable myocardium. However, CMR may provide a more accurate representation of infarcted or scarred tissue, especially in the subendocardial location (19,20). In a study looking at dogs with MI, CMR was compared with SPECT. SPECT was only able to detect 28% of segments with subendocardial defects, while CMR detected 92% of segments with subendocardial defects. This same study then compared SPECT to CMR in humans, and SPECT failed to detect defects in 47% of the segments found to have a subendocardial infarct with CMR (20). It is clear that subendocardial MI can be detected with CMR more accurately than with other noninvasive modalities.

CMR spectroscopy has also been used to differentiate between myocardial scar and myocardial ischemia. The intracellular sodium (^{23}Na) content has been observed to be elevated in nonviable myocardium using CMR spectroscopy (21). In addition to sodium, ^{31}P CMR spectroscopy demonstrates very low levels of adenosine triphosphate (ATP) and absence of creatine phosphate in recently infarcted myocardium. In myocardial scar, the same is true but the ATP is further reduced.

MYOCARDIAL ENHANCEMENT IN PATHOLOGIES NOT ASSOCIATED WITH CORONARY ARTERY DISEASE

Other pathologies have demonstrated DE after contrast agent administration. Patients with both dilated and hypertrophic cardiomyopathies have demonstrated DE, presumably related to the presence of associated fibrosis. The enhancement patterns with dilated cardiomyopathy (DCM) are more diffuse in contrast to those in patients with heart failure associated with MI. With MI, the scar is confluent for each of the territories associated with the given coronary occlusion. With DCM, the DE pattern is generalized and not localized, but, as with MI, the wall is thinned. In hypertrophic cardiomyopathy (HCM), the pattern is again diffuse and the myocardial wall is thick.

EVALUATION OF ANATOMY IN MI

CMR is capable of detecting structural abnormalities in the setting of MI. Prior to coronary angiography, CMR can demonstrate anomalous origins of the coronary arteries (22). Complications of MI, including wall rupture, pericardial effusion (e.g., associated with Dressler's syndrome), and valvular dysfunction can also been visualized with CMR (23,24). Lesser et al. have suggested that CMR has the ability to define patients at risk for myocardial rupture (25).

CONCLUSIONS

CMR has proven to be a valuable modality for the identification of MI in the acute and chronic setting and also for excluding MI or myocardial scar for the definition of myocardial viability. New sequences and higher magnetic fields (i.e., 3 Tesla) leading to faster acquisition and improved spatial resolution have made CMR an important approach for the diagnosis, prognosis, and understanding of MI. CMR is now viewed as the "gold standard" for the detection of infarcted and/or scarred myocardium by contrast enhancement and for the myocardium that does not enhance, representing viable MI. Furthermore, due to its high resolution, CMR has proven to be a sensitive means for the diagnosis of transmural and subendocardial MI. With its ability to safely and accurately image structure, perfusion, metabolism, and function, CMR provides the most comprehensive assessment of the ventricular myocardium available by any technology—noninvasive or invasive.

REFERENCES

1. Goldman MR, Brady TJ, Pykett IL, et al. Quantification of experimental myocardial infarction using nuclear magnetic resonance imaging and paramagnetic ion contrast enhancement in excised canine hearts. Circulation 1982; 66(5):1012–1016.
2. Wesbey G, Higgins CB, Lanzer P, Botvanick E, Lipton MJ. Imaging and characterization of acute myocardial infarction in vivo by gated nuclear magnetic resonance. Circulation 1984; 69(1):125–130.
3. Simonetti OP, Kim RJ, Fieno DS, et al. An improved MR imaging technique for the visualization of myocardial infarction. Radiology 2001; 218(1):215–223.
4. Kim RJ, Fieno DS, Parrish TB, et al. Relationship of MRI delayed contrast enhancement to irreversible injury, infarct age, and contractile function. Circulation 1999; 100(19):1992–2002.
5. Kim RJ, Shah DJ, Judd RM. How we perform delayed enhancement imaging. J Cardiovasc Magn Reson 2003; 5(3):505–514.
6. Mahrholdt H, Wagner A, Holly T, et al. Reproducibility of chronic infarct size measurement by contrast-enhanced magnetic resonance imaging. Circulation 2002; 106:2322–2327.
7. Rochitte CE, Lima JA, Bluemke DA, et al. Magnitude and time course of microvascular obstruction and tissue injury after acute myocardial infarction. Circulation 1998; 98(10):1006–1014.

8. Lima JA, Judd RM, Bazille A, Schulman SP, Atalar E, Zerhouni EA. Regional heterogeneity of human myocardial infarcts demonstrated by contrast-enhanced MRI. Potential mechanisms. Circulation 1995; 92(5):1117–1125.

9. Wu KC, Rochitte CE, Lima JA. Magnetic resonance imaging in acute myocardial infarction. Curr Opin Cardiol 1999; 14(6):480–484.

10. Beek A, Harald P, Rossum AC, et al. Delayed contrast-enhancement magnetic resonance imaging for the predication of regional functional improvement after myocardial infarction. J Am Coll Cardiol 2003; 42:895–901.

11. Dymarkowski S, Ni Y, Miao Y, et al. Value of T2-weighted magnetic resonance imaging early after myocardial infarction in dogs: comparison with bis-gadolinium-mesoporphyrin enhanced T1-weighted magnetic resonance imaging and functional data from cine magnetic resonance imaging. Invest Radiol 2002; 37(2):77–85.

12. Bonow RO, Dilsizian V, Coucolo A, et al. Identification of viable myocardium in patients with chronic coronary artery disease and left ventricular dysfunction: comparison of thallium scintigraphy with reinjection and PET imaging with ^{18}F-flurodeoxyglucose. Circulation 1991; 83:26–37.

13. Schulz-Menger J, Gross M, Messroghli D, Uhlich F, Dietz R, Friedrich MG. Cardiovascular magnetic resonance of acute myocardial infarction at a very early stage. J Am Coll Cardiol 2003; 42(3):513–518.

14. Kwong RY, Schussheim AE, Rekhraj S, et al. Detecting acute coronary syndrome in the emergency department with cardiac magnetic resonance imaging. Circulation 2003; 107(4):531–537.

15. Messroghli DR, Niendorf T, Schulz-Menger J, Dietz R, Friedrich MG. T1 mapping in patients with acute myocardial infarction. J Cardiovasc Magn Reson 2003; 5(2):353–359.

16. Saeed M, Wendland MF, Takehara Y, Masui T, Higgins CB. Reperfusion in irreversible myocardial injury: identification with nonionic MR contrast medium. Radiology 1992; 182:675–683.

17. Knuesel PR, Nanz D, Wyss C, et al. Characterization of dysfunctional myocardium by positron emission tomography and magnetic resonance. Circulation 2003; 108:1095–1100.

18. Baer FM, Voth E, Schneider CA, et al. ^{18}F-fluorodeoxyglucose in patients with coronary disease: a functional and morphological approach to the detection or residual myocardial viability. Circulation 1995; 9:1006–1015.

19. Klein C, Nekolla S, Bengel F, et al. Assessment of viability with contrast-enhanced magnetic resonance imaging. Comparison with positron emission tomography. Circulation 2002; 205:162–167.

20. Wagner A, Mahrholdt H, Holly T, et al. Contrast-enhanced MRI and routine single photon emission computed tomography (SPECT) perfusion imaging for detection of subendocardial myocardial infarcts: an imaging study. Lancet 2003; 361:374–379.

21. Horn M, Weidensteiner C, Scheffer H, et al. Detection of myocardial viability based on measurement of sodium content: a ^{23}Na-NMR study. Magn Reson Med 2001; 45:756–764.

22. Lee J, Choe YH, Kim HJ, Park JE. Magnetic resonance imaging demonstration of anomalous origin of the right coronary artery from the left coronary sinus with acute myocardial infarction. J Comput Assist Tomogr 2003; 27(2):289–291.

23. Chiu C, So N, Lam W, Chan K, Sanderson J. Combined first-pass perfusion and viability study at MR imaging in patients with non-ST segment-elevation acute coronary syndromes: feasibility study. Radiology 2003; 22:717–722.
24. Paelinck B, Dendale P. Images in clinical medicine. Cardiac tamponade in Dressler's syndrome. N Engl J Med 2003; 348(23):e8.
25. Lesser J, Johnson K, Lindberg J, Reed J, Virmani R, Schwartz R. Myocardial rupture, microvascular obstruction and infarct expansion elucidated by cardiac magnetic resonance. Circulation 2003; 108:116–117.

13

Cardiomyopathies

Uzma Iqbal

Cardiology and Internal Medicine, Syracuse, New York, U.S.A.

Anthony R. Fuisz

Cardiac MRI Laboratory, Washington Hospital Center, Washington, D.C., U.S.A.

DEFINITION

The cardiomyopathies are a group of chronic progressive diseases in which the dominant feature is direct involvement of the heart muscle associated with cardiac dysfunction.

CLASSIFICATION

Based on morphology, physiology, and etiology they can be divided into four main types: dilated, hypertrophic, restrictive, and arrhythmogenic right ventricular dysplasia (ARVD). The cardiomyopathies that do not fall into any of these categories are placed in the unclassified section.

Current cardiovascular magnetic resonance (CMR) techniques have much to offer in the evaluation of cardiomyopathies. In most ways the promises made by the "one-stop shop" ideal have been realized in this area of cardiac pathology. Magnetic resonance imaging's ability to combine high-resolution imaging of the heart, viability imaging using delayed hyperenhancement imaging, tissue characterization, and coronary angiography have allowed patients with left ventricular (LV) dysfunction to be characterized completely in one noninvasive sitting. This chapter will focus on how to evaluate the patient with presumed cardiomyopathy (CM) using cardiovascular MRI.

Classification of the Cardiomyopathies

Disorder	Description

Dilated cardiomyopathy
Dilatation and impaired contraction of the left or both ventricles caused by familial/ genetic, viral and/or immune, alcoholic/toxic, or unknown factors, or is associated with recognized cardiovascular disease

Hypertrophic cardiomyopathy
Left and/or right ventricular hypertrophy, often asymmetrical, which usually involves the interventricular septum. Mutations in sarcoplasmic proteins cause the disease in many patients (Fig. 1)

Restrictive cardiomyopathy
Restricted filling and reduced diastolic size of either or both ventricles with normal or near-normal systolic function; is idiopathic or associated with other disease (e.g., amyloidosis, endomyocardial disease)

Arrhythmogenic right ventricular dysplasia
Progressive fibrofatty replacement of the right, and to some degree left, ventricular myocardium. Familial disease is common

Unclassified cardiomyopathy
Diseases that do not fit readily into any category. Examples include systolic dysfunction with minimal dilatation, mitochondrial disease, and fibroelastosis

PERFORMING THE STUDY AND POSTPROCESSING

The first consideration with imaging patients for presumed CM is basic safety issues. This patient group, more commonly than others, will have implanted devices such as pacemakers and cardiac defibrillators. While there is some data to say that imaging patients with these devices is not as risky as it was thought to be (1), the prudent approach is to avoid the use of CMR in these patients unless a convincing case can be made that justifies the risk. Patients must also be able to remain nearly flat for 15 minutes. Supplemental oxygen can be used, but decompensated congestive heart failure or florid pulmonary edema can make scanning difficult to impossible. Because breath-hold durations maybe be difficult for these patients, accurate gating is essential. In patients with frequent ectopy or recurrent patterns of grouped beating, gating with the peripheral pulse unit may be preferable. One must realize in this case, however, that the diastolic and systolic frames will be in different locations in the resulting image sequence.

In many ways, the basic cardiovascular magnetic resonance (CMR) sequences to evaluate for CM are the same as those used for a standard cardiac function study (2,3). One approach is to follow a scout with axial T1-weighted images covering the heart and great vessels. These can be used to identify the left and right ventricle, and provide for measurements of the left atrium, pulmonary arteries, and thoracic aorta. Two-chamber (2-ch) and

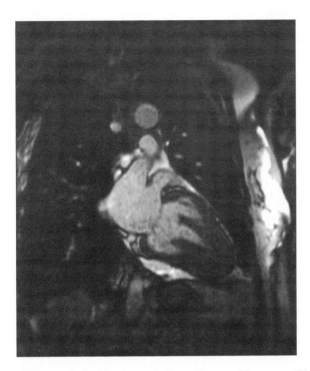

Figure 1 Apical hypertrophy in a 45-year old woman. This image is a single phase of a cine BFFE breath-hold.

four-chamber (4-ch) cine MRIs, preferably using breath-hold techniques are planned from the axial images. Short-axis images are then acquired, making sure to completely cover the ventricle from apex to base. Another approach is to use available fluoro or real-time CMR sequences to establish the geometry of the various needed sequences and then follow with diagnostic images.

For the cine images, the number of phases chosen should reflect a temporal resolution of less than 30 msec, and extend as close as possible to the entire R-R interval. Techniques that allow the duration of the breath-holds to be minimized like SENSE are especially useful in this patient population. More recent cine techniques that use retrospective gating are helpful in that the entire R-R interval is covered.

A slice thickness of 6 to 8 mm is usually sufficient, and an interslice gap that is chosen is a compromise between the desire to collect the most data possible and the number of breath-holds that patients can tolerate (10–12 slices). Free breathing techniques using standard and rapid GRE sequences can also be used, but in the patient who can tolerate them, BFFE/Fiesta/True FISP techniques are preferable for the increase in myocardium to blood pool contrast they provide.

After the basic functional exam as described above, other sequences can be done to add to the evaluation of the patient. One of the most useful in this population is a phase velocity mapping sequence prescribed perpendicular to the mid-portion of the thoracic aorta, and configured to measure blood flow through the aorta. This sequence provides the physician with accurate information about actual forward flow of blood, as opposed to the stoke volume measurements available after processing the short-axis views using Simpson's rule. Many patients with a dilated CM, regardless of etiology, will have some degree of mitral regurgitation, making the direct measurement of aortic forward flow important information. The lack of sensitivity to turbulence seen in most modern cine sequences also makes this especially useful, because mitral regurgitation may be difficult to detect otherwise.

RF tagging can also be performed if later detailed measurements of regional function are planned. The intricacies of this analysis and the time involved in performing it limit its use to research applications except in a few cases.

The careful observer of the initial images may already have surmised the diagnosis or cause of the CM. Thinning of the ventricular walls to a thickness less than 6 mm, or a subtle decrease in signal on BFFE images can demonstrate areas of previous infarction. Marked variation in regional wall motion can also help distinguish ischemic CM from nonischemic CM.

It is still useful, however, to pursue delayed hyperenhancement imaging in these patients, again looking for evidence of previous MI. The diagnosis of ischemic CM automatically leads to consideration of revascularization and so viability imaging is also important. Delayed hyperenhancement images at 10 and 20 minutes in short-axis, 2-ch and 4-ch orientations should be performed. Keep in mind that the inversion delay is a function of time from injection (should get longer to get optimal nulling of normal muscle as time from contrast injection increases) and, at least in some sequences, a function of heart rate (faster heart rate means shorter delay time for optimal images) (Table 1) (Fig. 2).

Changes to delay time should be made in 10-minute intervals to avoid overshooting the perfect time. Studies have shown that 10-minute views may lead to infarct size overestimation (4), because of the peri-infarct edema

Table 1 Effects of Different Parameters on Optimal Inversion Time

Variable	Ti
Heart rate	Slower = increase Ti
	Faster = decrease Ti
Dose of Gad	Less = longer Ti
Time from injection	Longer = increase Ti

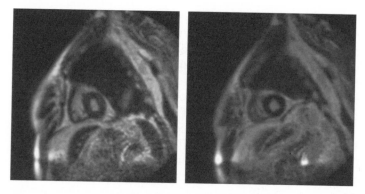

Figure 2 Note the slightly inhomogeneous nulling of the left ventricle muscle in the first image. The second is the same sequence with a 25 msec longer inversion delay.

sequestering some of the gadolinium (Fig. 3). Twenty-minute images allow time for this gadolinium to leave the peri-infarct zone. A practical clinical approach is to obtain images at 10 minutes, and proceed to 20-minute views only if an infarct is present, or in patients where recent myocardial infarction (MI) is suspected. It is helpful to have a timer to set for 10 or 20 minutes to allow reliable imaging at a fixed time point after injection. With a little experimentation, the optimal delay time can be arrived upon, and this will allow good image quality in at least 85% of future patients with a minimum of guessing and redo acquisitions. Another approach that can be used is to deliberately overshoot the optimal Inversion Time (TI), and reacquire the same until the heart's ideal TI lengthens match the chosen one. Some platforms may have sequences designed to generate a series of images with

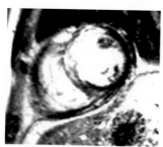

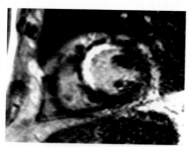

Delayed hyper-enhancement
images in a patient 5 hours
post TPA, presalvage PTCA

Same patient, same slice 7
weeks later. Note the rim of
variable epicardial muscle not
easily seen before

Figure 3 Perfusion and viability studies showing overestimation of perfusion defect after Gd infusion, with delayed images showing area of viable myocardium.

different TI delays to allow a quick determination of TI when it is otherwise lost. These are most useful when patients have inadvertently received a different dose of gadolinium secondary to a failed intravenous for example.

In addition to acquiring short-axis images, acquiring long-axis images are very helpful. On some platforms, it is possible to acquire the whole heart in a single breath-hold using a three-dimensional (3D) sequence. If you have access to this, performing three breath-holds and acquiring the whole heart in short-axis, 2-ch and 4-ch orientations is ideal. This coverage allows the comparison of a defect seen in short-axis with the same area on another 3D set, helping to establish real defects from artifact. No matter what technique is used, setting up your sequence to allow easy rescanning with a different TI is important.

Finding an area of hyperenhancement is not the end of the story, however. The location of the area (endocardial, mid-wall or epicardial), correlation to a vascular territory, and overall image quality and nulling are all-important features. All hyperenhancement does not represent MI.

The ventricle that is dilated and poorly functioning due to coronary artery disease may not have evidence of previous infarction, and so a full evaluation should include at least an attempt to evaluate for the presence of coronary artery disease (CAD), in the event a coronary computed tomography or invasive angiogram has not already been performed. Navigator-assisted coronary magnetic resonance angiography (MRA) has been shown to be effective in ruling out three-vessel disease (5). In motivated patients (in sinus rhythm), good quality images are achievable more often that not. In this population, the important findings are usually significant proximal disease, areas that lie within the abilities of commercially available imaging sequences. Patients with severe ventricular dysfunction also have less motion of their hearts in general, and seem to be better candidates for coronary imaging.

An alternative to coronary imaging is to perform CMR perfusion imaging, using adenosine or dypiridimole and a first-pass imaging technique. While faster and in some ways less technically demanding than coronary imaging to perform, these images are certainly more difficult to interpret, and should be used only by experienced CMR reviewers. Combining perfusion images with coronary imaging of the suspect vessel or vessels may be the best and most thorough approach.

In the case of reduced LV function without any evidence of delayed hyperenhancement, care should be taken before pronouncing the ventricle "viable." The presence of significant multivessel disease is required to explain marked LV functional decline in the absence of infarct. The patient with 60% to 70% coronary lesions and no evidence of previous MI but markedly decreased LV function should be approached with caution. It is certainly possible for an underlying CM to coexist with mild to moderate CAD. It is possible to perform detailed imaging of left and right ventricular function, perfusion imaging, using adenosine and delayed hyperenhancement imaging, all within a 45-minute imaging session.

After the images are acquired, left and right ventricular ejection fractions, stroke volumes, and overall chamber volumes are calculated. The difficult part, especially with newer imaging sequences, is what to include in the tracing of the endocardial border. BFFE/FIESTA/True FISP techniques provide better endocardial border definition, but provide the endocardial border tracer with many options. Should every little trabeculation be included or just ignored? Should the papillary muscles be included or ignored? In the case where aortic forward flow measurements are being performed with a phase velocity sequence, the best results are obtained when the endocardial surface is most accurately traced, and papillary muscles accounted for. In this case (and in the absence of mitral regurgitation), differences of 2 to 5 mL between the measured stroke volume and aortic forward flow can be achieved. If only a reasonably accurate ejection fraction is needed, this is not necessary. Because many of the patients with a CM may return for further imaging, consistency or a notation in the report as to the method used is crucial.

Finally, it is also important to accurately describe the degree of hyperenhancement as a percentage of wall thickness, and also make note of the overall wall thickness. Making a determination of viability based on the percentage of wall thickness scar fails to take into account the shrinkage of infarcts that can be seen over time. It makes little sense that a segment with a subendocardial infarction is becoming more likely to recover because the scar portion shrinks and the resulting percentage of scar decreases. Making note of both the scar percentage and the overall thickness (or more simply the thickness of viable muscle) combines the two ways to determine viability from static images and will likely reflect the best overall method for viability determination (6). For infarcts involving 50% of wall thickness, adding dobutamine imaging may yield additional data (7).

DILATED CARDIOMYOPATHY

Dilated CM is characterized primarily by systolic dysfunction, four Chamber enlargement, and ventricular dilatation out of proportion to wall thickness (Fig. 4). This can be further divided into ischemic versus nonischemic based on etiology.

ISCHEMIC CARDIOMYOPATHY

The most common form of CM is the ischemic CM. As mentioned above, CMR techniques allow regional and global function assessments, viability determinations, and in many cases, determining the presence or absence of epicardial coronary disease. CMR techniques can even allow assessments of ischemia at the cellular level using spectroscopy techniques (8).

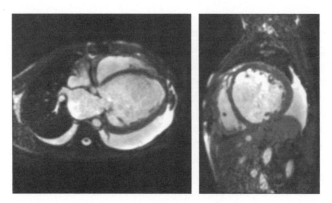

Figure 4 This patient has a presumed HIV-related cardiomyopathy. The LVEDD is over 11 cm.

CMR techniques are also well suited to identifying common complications of MI.

The most basic use of CMR techniques in the ischemic CM population is the simple calculation of the ejection fraction because therapies (ace-inhibitor use, and defibrillator use) are based on ejection fraction cut-offs. In many patients, especially those with difficult acoustic windows and regional wall motion abnormalities, CMR-derived ejection fractions may be significantly different from visual estimates or semiquantitative values derived from standard transthoracic echocardiograms.

Once the ejection fraction is measured, delayed hyperenhancement images are the next most useful sequences (Figs. 5–8). After injecting the double dose of gadolinium, look at the 2-ch and 4-ch views again. If there is any question of thrombus, repeat these sequences just after the injection of gadolinium. In this early phase (a few minutes after the injection), the myocardium will be enhanced as well as the blood, leaving thrombus dark and easy to distinguish from the adjacent muscle.

In some patients with infarctions, a central area of dark "muscle" is sometimes seen on the delayed hyperenhancement images. This "island" of viable muscle is the result of dense obstruction of flow in the center of the infarct (microvascular obstruction) and is not viable. If there is a doubt, reimaging in 5 to10 minutes will show that the "island" is getting smaller. "Viable" muscle is rarely surrounded by scar on all sides.

VIRAL CARDIOMYOPATHIES

Aside from accurate measurement of ventricular function that may be important both in terms of diagnosis and defining response to treatment, CMR techniques can, in some cases, provide further details. Patterns of enhancement following gadolinium have been shown to diagnose myocarditis, and

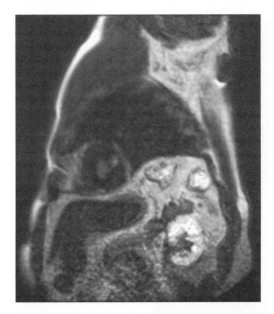

Figure 5 Small infarction in patient presenting with unstable angina. This technique can help identify the culprit vessel when the ECG is not helpful precath.

also provide information about the timing of the infection (9). Early work by Dr. D. Ian Paterson (personal communication) has shown a patchy pattern of enhancement using a standard delayed hyperenhancement technique in patients with presumed viral CM. This pattern generally resolves in patients that have resolution of the CM, and it becomes more generalized in patients that have prolonged functional abnormalities. Distinguishing this

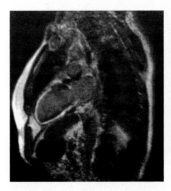 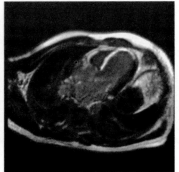

Figure 6 This patient has suffered both an anterior and inferior infarction, with a preserved LCX territory.

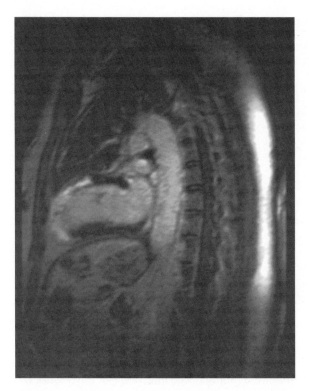

Figure 7 Transmural infarction of the anterior wall and apex resulting from a LAD occlusion.

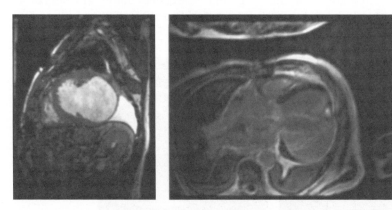

Figure 8 Lateral-wall aneurysm related to failure of an LCX bypass graft. Note the delayed hyperenhancement images show a severely displaced portion on the basal lateral wall to be viable. The nonviable portion of the aneurysm was successfully resected.

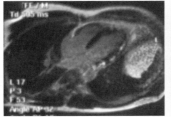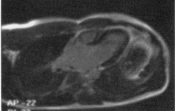

Figure 9 Initial images in a patient with presumed viral cardiomyopathy. Second image is the same patient five months later. The EF has improved from 40% to 60% in the interval.

pattern from more conventional ischemia-related disease can be done by noting the location of the hyperenhancement in the myocardial wall. Hyperenhancement related to infarction always includes the endocardial surface, while the hyperenhancement associated with myocarditis is seen in the midwall and the epicardial portions of the muscle, often sparring the endocardial surface. This pattern is also patchy, and does follow expected vascular territories (Fig. 9) (10–12).

As mentioned previously, navigator-based 3D coronary MRA protocols have been shown to be effective in ruling out three-vessel disease. Patients with marked decreases in systolic function and dilated CM may be well served by using coronary MRA as an alternative to diagnostic angiography (Fig. 10).

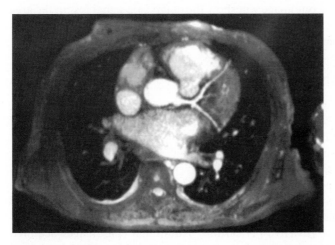

Figure 10 This patient had a dilated cardiomyopathy with an ejection fraction of 13%. Renal insufficiency and a history of severe anaphylaxis to contrast media made coronary magnetic resonance angiography preferable. This soap-bubble reformat of the three-dimensional data set shows the widely patent left main, LAD, and LCX.

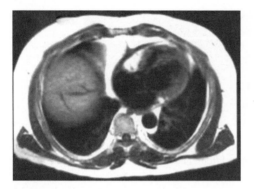

Figure 11 T2-weighted image showing a metastatic pheochrocytoma, located just above the RCA. This tumor had been detected by MIBG imaging, but the cardiovascular magnetic resonance data allowed surgeons to anticipate the necessary RCA bypass to remove it.

ENDOCRINE CARDIOMYOPATHIES

Pheochromocytoma has particular signal characteristics that that can be used to identify tumors in cases of suspected catecholamine-induced CM (Fig. 11).

INFILTRATIVE CARDIOMYOPATHIES

The dilated CM seen in hemochromatosis is perhaps the easiest to characterize. Often the first scout image will show the diagnostic signal loss in the area of the liver due to the iron deposition there. Myocardium may similarly demonstrate signal characteristics that appear to be metallic artifact.

RESTRICTIVE CARDIOMYOPATHIES

Restrictive CM is characterized by biatrial enlargement, enlarged venae cavae, normal to small-sized ventricular chamber, normal pericardial thickness, and diastolic dysfunction.

The pathophysiology is endomyocardial scarring that usually affects one or both ventricles and restricts filling.

For CMR, a common referral is the patient with suspected restrictive CM versus constrictive pericarditis (Table 2). The standard T1-weighted axial images are usually all that is necessary to document the thickened pericardium seen in constrictive pericarditis. Additional cine images acquired with RF tagging, especially in a 4-ch orientation, can show either the normal "sliding" at the epicardial pericardial border, most easily seen adjacent to the basal portions of the ventricle, or deformation of the grid lines extending into the tissue that is outside the pericardium. This deformation of gridlines

Table 2 Constrictive vs. Restrictive Cardiomyopathy

	Constrictive	Restrictive
Atrial size	Normal/mildly enlarged	Enlarged
Pericardial thickness	Usually 2–3 times normal	Normal
Tagged long axis images	May show evidence of adhesion	Normal sliding at epicardial/pericardial border
Wall motion	Septal bounce	Delayed filling

is because of adhesions across the pericardium, providing a visual representation of the additional work the heart must do with this pathology (Fig. 12). While "constrictive" physiology has been described in patients without thickened or abnormal pericardium, CMR, in this instance, can be seen as providing anatomical data that is useful in treatment. Identifying the patient with constrictive/restrictive symptoms and a markedly thickened pericardium with adhesions identifies a population with a potentially treatable process. Patients with marked symptoms but normal pericardium and no adhesions are much less likely to benefit from a thoracotomy and pericardial stripping.

The CM associated with amyloid is a restrictive one. For most patients, the appearance of systolic dysfunction associated with amyloid is a harbinger of poor outcome. The primary distinguishing aspects by CMR are the marked thickness of the ventricular walls with decreased systolic function (contrasting with HCM where systolic function is usual normal to supranormal) with a low voltage ECG. Atrial walls are sometimes thickened as well, though this can be a subtle finding. Patterns of enhancement with gadolinium have been reported, but these findings are, in general, nonspecific (Fig. 13).

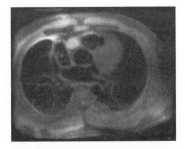

Figure 12 Note the thickened pericardium in this patient with presumed restrictive cardiomyopathy. Tagged images slowed evidence of adhesions. Patient went on to have pericardial stripping and improvement in symptoms.

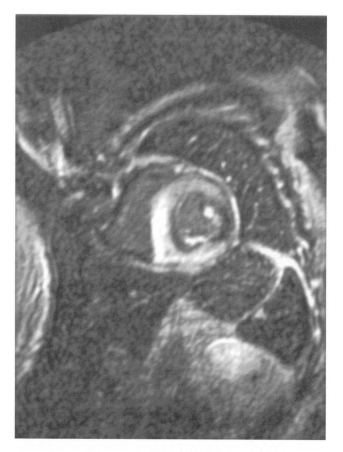

Figure 13 Delayed hyperenhancement images in a patient with amyloid cardiomyop-athy. Enhancement pattern is opposite of what is expected in ischemic heart disease, with nonenhancing endocardial borders. Interestingly the lateral wall, the most nor-mal in thickness, has the least hyperenhancement.

SARCOIDOSIS

In patients with sarcoidosis, granulomas are seen in the heart in 20% to 30% of the patients, though they are suspected clinically in only 5%.

CMR findings are those nonspecific findings associated with inflam-mation and edema-higher signal intensity in T2-weighted images and patchy enhancement following gadolinium injection (13,14).

While these findings are not diagnostic of sarcoid, they can assist in the diagnosis or add additional information to the patient's evaluation.

RADIATION-INDUCED CARDIOMYOPATHY

Some patients with presumed radiation-induced CM (nonischemic CM with a history of chest radiation and no other explanation) may demonstrate linear hyperenhancement in the left ventricle, especially in the midwall portions. This likely represents fibrosis, and can be confirmed by follow-up imaging that shows no change in appearance.

GENETIC CARDIOMYOPATHIES

Hypertrophic Cardiomyopathy

The hallmarks of hypertrophic obstructive cardiomyopathy are marked ventricular hypertrophy, small chamber volumes, systolic cavity obliteration, and diastolic dysfunction. The interventricular septum is typically more prominently involved than the LV free wall.

CMR techniques can be used to determine ventricular mass, and precisely define the location and subtype (15).

The approach is similar to other cardiomyopathies. Axial images, and 2-ch and 4-ch images are acquired. As in transthoracic echocardiography, a left ventricular outflow tract (LVOT) view is helpful, and may demonstrate narrowing of the LVOT with systole. Turbulence arising from the septal prominence that forms during systole, as well as systolic anterior motion of the mitral valve can be appreciated.

Delayed hyperenhancement images are also useful. Patients without history of "infarction" may have areas of hyperenhancement. This technique can also be used after septal ablation therapy to determine the volume of the septum that has been altered (16).

Noncompaction CM is another rare form of congenital CM well demonstrated by CMR techniques. CMR images give the ability to clearly see the epicardial border, and so make clear trabeculations that have pits that extend almost the full thickness of the LV wall. Noncompaction cardiomyopathies can involve large areas of the ventricle or be limited (17–19).

NEUROMUSCULAR CARDIOMYOPATHIES

Tako-Tsubo Cardiomyopathy

Tako-Tsubo CM is most commonly seen in older women, usually involving the distal portions of the left ventricle. Unusual cases sometimes show spared apical function, but midventricle severe hypokinesis. The initial views are often easily mistaken for a large LAD infarct. Viability images however show no infarct, and follow-up imaging at a later time point usually shows near complete recovery. The cardiac CMR findings though are difficult to

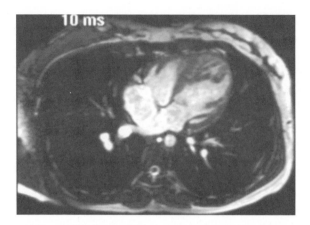

Figure 14 Thirty-five-year-old mother of one with newly diagnosed "cardiomyopathy," actually congenitally corrected transposition. Note the orientation of the AV valves and the prominent trabeculation in the apex of the systemic but morphologic right ventricle.

distinguish from those of a patient with transient LAD ischemia, and so care should be taken in the diagnosis in the absence of angiographic data.

Postpartum

CMR techniques are useful in documenting ejection fraction, and possible recovery (Fig. 14). The ability to reliably follow ejection fraction and detect small changes makes CMR ideal for long-term follow-up. Remember that standard gadolinium-based agents are secreted into breast milk if the patient is nursing.

ARRHYTHMOGENIC RIGHT VENTRICULAR DYSPLASIA

ARVD is a primary disorder of the right ventricle characterized by partial or total replacement of muscle by adipose or fibrous tissue.

The exact incidence of ARVD is not known but it appears to be more common in southern Italy accounting for 12.5% of all cases. It is an important cause of sudden death in young adults.

The exact etiology is not known. The disease is often familial with autosomal dominant inheritance and variable penetrance. The gene defects have been mapped to chromosomes 14 and 1.

The diagnosis of ARVD is based on major and minor criteria of the Task Force of Working Group of Myocardial and Pericardial Disease of the Scientific Council on Cardiomyopathies of the International Society and Federation of Cardiology. A definitive diagnosis of ARVD is based on histological demonstration of transmural fibro-fatty replacement of right ventricular myocardium at either necropsy or surgery. This is difficult because of the segmental nature of the disease and also because the interventricular septum is rarely involved resulting in false negative results.

Because ARVD is a difficult topic for the CMR reader, it will be covered separately in Chapter 14.

OTHER ENTITIES

Because CMR is often used in difficult diagnostic cases, some patients referred for evaluation of CM based on initial imaging tests may indeed have another diagnosis completely.

The referral for a dilated right ventricle/right ventricular CM may in fact be due to a previously unseen sinus venosus atrial septal defect or anomalous pulmonary venous return. Previously undiagnosed entities like congenitally corrected transposition may present as patients with CM. The superior imaging abilities of CMR make these cases easier to define and diagnose.

CONCLUSIONS

In view of its three dimensional coupled with its high resolution capabilities, CMR has become known as the gold standard for determination of LV function, and as a result has become the method of choice for assessing the severity of the dilated cardiomyopathies. By virtue of its ability to evaluate function, perfusion, viability, coronary vasculature and metabolism, CMR has can provide the appropriate classification for patients with heart failure due to cardiomyopathy. The cardiomyopathic pathophysiological class (dilated, hypertrophic, restrictive and ARVC/ARVD) are readily established using CMR. Function is preserved or variably depressed; volumes vary from reduced (hypertrophic or certain restrictive CMs) or variably increased; myocardial mass is variably increased and morphology is frequently characteristic. Viability through contrast enhancement imaging provides further evaluation of the dilated cardiomyopathies by identifying myocardial scar related to epicardial coronary artery disease ("ischemic cardiomyopathy") as opposed to those that are not. For the nonischemic types, the morphological pattern by CMR can characterize particular etiologies. CMR is extremely useful for diagnosing, prognostication, and following patients with cardiomyopathy.

REFERENCES

1. Edward TM, James AC, Frank GS, Christopher CP, Fair R, Jenkins K. Magnetic resonance imaging and cardiac pacemaker safety at 1.5-Tesla. J Am Coll Cardiol 2004; 43(7).
2. Martin ET, Fuisz AR, Pohost GM. Imaging cardiac structure and function. In: Cardiology Clinics, Cardiac Magnetic Resonance Imaging. Philadelphia: WB Saunders, 1998:135–160.

3. Blackwell GG, Cranney GB, Pohost GM. Cardiomyopathies. MRI: Cardio-vascular System. Gower Medical Publishing, 1992:8.1–8.11.

4. Saeed, Maythe, Lund, et al. Magnetic resonance characterization of the peri-infarction zone of reperfused myocardial infarction with necrosis-specific and extracellular nonspecific contrast media. Circulation; 103(6):871–876.

5. Kim WY, et al. Coronary magnetic resonance angiography for the detection of coronary stenoses. N Engl J Med 2001; 345:1863–1869.

6. Kim RJ, Wu E, Rafael A, et al. The use of contrast-enhanced magnetic resonance imaging to identify reversible myocardial dysfunction. N Engl J Med 2000; 343(20):1445–1453.

7. Wellnhofer E, Olariu A, Klein C, et al. Magnetic resonance low-dose dobuta-mine test is superior to SCAR quantification for the prediction of functional recovery. Circulation 2004; 109(18):2172–2174. [Epub 2004 Apr 26.].

8. Steven BD, den Hollander Jan A, et al. Abnormal myocardial phosphorus-31 nuclear magnetic resonance spectroscopy in women with chest pain but normal coronary angiograms. N Engl J Med 2000; 342:829–835.

9. Friedrich MG, Strohm O, Schulz-Menger J, Marciniak H, Luft FC, Dietz R. Contrast media–enhanced magnetic resonance imaging visualizes myocardial changes in the course of viral myocarditis. Circulation 1998; 97:1802.

10. Dill T, Ekinci O, Hansel J, Kluge A, Breidenbach C, Hamm CW. Delayed contrast-enhanced magnetic resonance imaging for the detection of autoimmune myocarditis and long-term follow-up. J Cardiovasc Magn Reson 2005; 7(2):521–523.

11. Hunold P, Schlosser T, Vogt FM, et al. Myocardial late enhancement in contrast-enhanced cardiac MRI: distinction between infarction scar and non-infarction-related disease. Am J Roentgenol 2005; 184(5):1420–1426.

12. Abdel-Aty H, Boye P, Zagrosek A, et al. Diagnostic performance of cardio-vascular magnetic resonance in patients with suspected acute myocarditis: comparison of different approaches. J Am Coll Cardiol 2005; 45(11): 1815–1822.

13. Vignaux O, Dhote R, Duboc D, et al. Clinical significance of myocardial mag-netic resonance abnormalities in patients with sarcoidosis: a 1-year follow-up study. Chest 2002; 122(6):1895–1901.

14. Smedema JP, Snoep G, van Kroonenburgh MP, et al. The additional value of gadolinium-enhanced MRI to standard assessment for cardiac involvement in patients with pulmonary sarcoidosis. Chest 2005; 128(3):1629–1637.

15. Maier SE, Fischer SE, McKinnon GC, Hess OM, Krayenbuehl HP, Boesiger P. Evaluation of left ventricular segmental wall motion in hypertrophic cardiomyop-athy with myocardial tagging. Circulation; 86(6):1919–1928.

16. Van Dockum, Willem G Beek, Aernout M Cate, et al. Early onset and progression of left ventricular remodeling after alcohol septal ablation in hypertrophic obstruc-tive cardiomyopathy. Circulation; 111(19):2503–2508.

17. Bax JJ, Atsma DE, Lamb HJ, et al. Noninvasive and invasive evaluation of non-compaction cardiomyopathy. J Cardiovasc Magn Reson 2002; 4(3):353–357.

18. Petersen SE, Selvanayagam JB, Wiesmann F, et al. Left ventricular non-compaction: insights from cardiovascular magnetic resonance imaging. J Am Coll Cardiol 2005; 46(1):101–105.

19. Pujadas S, Bordes R, Bayes-Genis A. Ventricular non-compaction cardiomyop-athy: CMR and pathology findings. Heart 2005; 91(5):582.

14

Electrophysiologic Disorders

Szilard Voros

Cardiovascular MRI and CT, Fuqua Heart Center of Atlanta, Piedmont Hospital, Atlanta, Georgia, U.S.A.

VENTRICULAR TACHYCARDIA, SYNCOPE AND SUDDEN CARDIAC DEATH

Clinical Perspective

In the hand of the electrophysiologist, cardiovascular magnetic resonance (CMR) can be helpful in patients presenting with ventricular arrhythmias, syncope, or sudden cardiac death. The most common cause of cardiomyopathy and ventricular arrhythmias is ischemic heart disease or coronary artery disease, which is described in detail elsewhere in this text. This section focuses on patients presenting with ventricular tachycardia, syncope, or unexplained sudden cardiac death, in whom ischemia has been ruled out as a cause. The most important entities to evaluate in this setting are hypertrophic cardiomyopathy (HCM), arrhythmogenic right ventricular cardiomyopathy (ARVC), and anomalous coronary arteries (typically in young persons).

Hypertrophic cardiomyopathy is a genetically determined condition, characterized by asymmetrical left ventricular hypertrophy in the absence of increased afterload, caused by myocardial disarray due to the underlying genetic abnormality. CMR is excellent in the diagnosis of HCM, since it is able to identify left ventricular hypertrophy and when present its hemodynamic consequences, such as mid-cavity obliteration and systolic anterior motion of the mitral valve. In addition, the most important CMR feature of HCM is the presence of delayed contrast enhancement in the myocardium

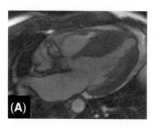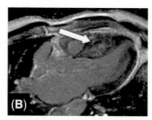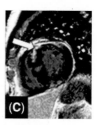

Figure 1 Diastolic still frame from an SSFP cine image, showing profound septal hypertrophy (**A**). Inversion recovery late contrast-enhanced image with phase-sensitive reconstruction in the horizontal long axis view reveals the presence of delayed contrast enhancement in the ventricular septum, identifying the area of myofiber disarray (*arrow*) (**B**). Mid-ventricular short axis view using the same technique shows a typical pattern of delayed contrast enhancement in the ventricular septum at the right ventricular insertion points (*arrow*) (**C**). *Abbreviation*: SSFP, steady-state free precession.

in a noncoronary distribution. The most common pattern is the presence of delayed enhancement in the septum; typically at the insertion point of the right ventricle (RV) to the left ventricle (LV) (Fig. 1) (1).

Nonischemic right ventricular arrhythmias typically occur in the setting of arrhythmogenic right ventricular cardiomyopathies. In 1995, the World Health Organization (WHO) and International Society and Federation of Cardiology Task Force devised new definitions and a new classification system to describe cardiomyopathies and included arrhythmogenic right ventricular cardiomyopathies as a major category (Table 1) (2). ARVC include a heterogeneous group of disorders and it is clear that there is a spectrum of diseases within this category, with progressively more severe features from a genetic, epidemiologic, morphologic, and prognostic perspective (Table 2) (3).

Arrhythmogenic right ventricular dysplasia (ARVD) is a rare but important form of right ventricular cardiomyopathy, characterized by progressive fibrofatty replacement of the right ventricular myocardium, initially with regional and later with global right and some left ventricular involvement (2). It is responsible for a significant portion of sudden cardiac death in young persons. ARVD is a progressive disease, which may eventually lead

Table 1 World Health Organization/International Society and Federation of Cardiology Task Force on the Definition and Classification of Cardiomyopathies

Dilated cardiomyopathy
Hypertrophic cardiomyopathy
Restrictive cardiomyopathy
Arrhythmogenic right ventricular cardiomyopathy
Unclassified cardiomyopathies

Table 2 Different Forms of Arrhythmogenic Right Ventricular Cardiomyopathy

Isolated RV dysplasia
Pure Form of ARVD
Naxos disease
Venetian cardiomyopathy
Noncoronary RV precordial ST-segment elevation
RV outflow tract tachycardia
Benign extrasystoles
Uhl's anomaly
Mitral valve prolapse
Nonarrhythmogenic forms of ARVD
Dysplasia with major LV involvement
Pure biventricular dysplasia
Dysplasia complicated by myocarditis

Abbreviations: ARVD, arrhythmogenic right ventricular dysplasia; LV, left ventricle; RV, right ventricle.

to overt congestive heart failure and sudden death. Despite this, our experience with this disorder is quite limited and it is based on a small number of patients. For example, the current classification of ARVCs is based on about 250 patients with 72 histological samples collected over a period of 23 years in eight countries (3).

Since most of the information on ARVD had been gathered by many different investigators around the globe in different patient populations using different methodologies, the definition of the disease had to be standardized. The most commonly accepted criteria were suggested by McKenna and colleagues in 1994 (Table 3) (4).

It is estimated that the prevalence of ARVD in the general population is one in 5000. However, this number is much higher in younger patients; the prevalence is reported to be 5% in patients with sudden cardiac death under age 65 and 20% in patients under age 30 (5). Furthermore, there is some significant geographic clustering with 20% of patients with sudden cardiac death in the Veneto region of Italy reported as having had ARVD. Finally, ARVD is responsible for 3% to 4% of sudden cardiac death in young athletes (5).

Magnetic resonance imaging (MRI) has been used to evaluate ARVD since 1989, when Casolo et al. described the first report of CMR in a patient with angiographically diagnosed ARVD (6). Initial reports of accuracy of CMR to establish the diagnosis of ARVD appear higher than the true accuracy seen in subsequent clinical practice. This is probably due to the fact that patients in the initial series either had known ARVD or had a very high pretest likelihood of disease based on clinical predictors, and CMR performed very well in those populations. One of the difficulties in comparing

Table 3 Diagnostic Criteria for Arrhythmogenic Right Ventricular Dysplasia

Global of regional dysfunction and structural alterations[a]
Major
    Severe dilatation and reduction of RV ejection fraction with no (or only
        mild) LV impairment
    Localized RV aneurysms (akinetic or dyskinetic areas with diastolic
        bulging)
    Severe segmental dilatation of the RV
Minor
    Mild global RV dilatation or ejection fraction reduction with normal LV
    Mild segmental dilatation of the RV
    Regional RV hypokinesia
Tissue characterization of walls
Major
    Fibrofatty replacement of myocardium on endomyocardial biopsy
Repolarization abnormalities
Minor
    Inverted T-waves in right precordial leads (V2 and V3) (people aged
        more than 12 yrs; in the absence of right bundle branch block)
Depolarization/conduction abnormalities
Major
    Epsilon waves or localized prolongation (>110 msec) of the QRS
        complex in right precordial leads (V1 to V3)
Minor
    Late potentials (signal-averaged ECG)
Arrhythmia
Minor
    Left bundle branch block type ventricular tachycardia (sustained and
        non-sustained) (ECG, Holter, exercise testing)
    Frequent ventricular extrasystoles (more than 1000/24 hr) (Holter)
Family history
Major
    Familial disease of confirmed at necropsy or surgery
Minor
    Familial history of premature sudden death (<35 yr) due to suspected
    RV dysplasia
    Familial history (clinical diagnosis based on present criteria)

Note: Requirements to fulfill positive diagnosis of arrhythmogenic right ventricular dysplasia
(one of the three): 1. Two major criteria; 2. One major plus two minor criteria; 3. Four minor
criteria.
[a]Detected by echocardiography, angiography, magnetic resonance imaging or radionuclide
scintigraphy.
Abbreviations: ECG, electrocardiogram; LV, left ventricle; RV, right ventricle.

different reports on the frequency of ARVD is the difference in pretest likelihood in the referral population.

Patients with known ARVD. Initial experience with CMR in ARVD was derived from patients who had known ARVD, as defined by clinical criteria, right ventricular angiography, or endomyocardial biopsy. Most of these early examinations were done on 0.5 to 1.5 T imaging systems, using gated spin echo and gradient echo cine sequences. Common MRI findings of ARVD are derived from these reports and include right ventricular structural abnormalities [RV enlargement, RV wall thinning, right ventricular outflow tract (RVOT) dilatation], right ventricular functional abnormalities (global and focal RV wall motion abnormalities, impaired diastolic relaxation), and areas of increased signal intensity within the right ventricular myocardium, suggesting fibrofatty replacement (6–8). These abnormalities are considered to be "classic" findings in ARVD.

Patients with suspected ARVD. Midiri et al. evaluated 30 consecutive patients in whom ARVD was suspected on clinical grounds (9). Clinical suspicion was based on the presence of ventricular tachycardia with left bundle branch block (LBBB) morphology, T-wave inversions in the right precordial leads, right ventricular wall motion abnormalities observed on echocardiography or angiography, or unexplained right ventricular failure. The CMR examination included T1-weighted spin echo sequences in the four-chamber and short axis orientation and gradient echo cine images for functional assessment. It is important to point out that the authors had five prespecified criteria for the MRI diagnosis of ARVD and divided patients into four categories based on the number of prespecified criteria such as highly probable, probable, dubious, and negative. CMR diagnosis for ARVD was highly probable in eight patients (27%), probable in four (13%), dubious in seven (23%), and negative in 11 (37%) patients. The authors concluded that CMR is a very effective tool in the evaluation of ARVD in patients in whom the disease is suspected on clinical grounds.

Patients with documented right ventricular tachycardia. Klersy et al. reported 21 patients in abstract form; 19 had sustained ventricular tachycardia and two were asymptomatic relatives (10). They noted fatty infiltration of the right ventricle in 17 patients (81%) and in most cases these areas corresponded to the origin of the arrhythmia. In another abstract, White et al. reported 17 patients with documented ventricular tachycardia, in whom ARVC was suspected (11). Based on WHO Task Force criteria, the diagnosis was confirmed in seven patients (41%). Interestingly, 12 patients had CMR features suggestive of ARVC.

Characteristic findings in ARVD were derived from observational and descriptive studies from patients who were diagnosed with the disease based on clinical or histologic criteria, but these features have never been formally validated against a standardized reference standard. Nevertheless, generally accepted features associated with ARVD are summarized in

Table 4, including imaging sequences, useful views, and quantitative measurements (Fig. 2).

The diagnostic accuracy of CMR in ARVD has not been firmly established. To our knowledge, there is only one report in the literature

Table 4 Typical Cardiovascular Magnetic Resonance Features of Arrhythmogenic Right Ventricular Dysplasia in the Literature

Abnormality	Sequence	Views	Quantification
Structural abnormalities			
RV enlargement	Spin echo	AX, 2-C, 4-C, SAX, RV-LAX	
	Gradient echo cine	AX, 2-C, 4-C, SAX, RV-LAX	AP-EDD > 42 mm (4-C)[a]
RVOT dilatation	Spin echo	RVOT view	> 1.5 × aortic bulb or > LVOT
	Gradient echo cine	RVOT view	> 1.5 × aortic bulb or > LVOT
Functional abnormalities			
RV wall thinning	Spin echo	AX, 2-C, 4-C, SAX, RV-LAX	
	Gradient echo cine	AX, 2-C, 4-C, SAX, RV-LAX	
RV wall motion abnormality Hypokinesis Akinesis Dyskinesis (diastolic bulging)	Gradient echo cine	AX, 2-C, 4-C, SAX, RV-LAX	
Impaired RV relaxation	Gradient echo cine Time–volume Curves		
Tissue characterization			
High signal intensity	Spin echo	AX, 2-C, 4-C, SAX, RV-LAX	
	Gradient echo cine	AX, 2-C, 4-C, SAX, RV-LAX	

[a]The anteroposterior end-diastolic dimension of the right ventricle is measured perpendicular to the line connecting the RV apex and the middle of the tricuspid valve in the four-chamber view. *Abbreviations*: 2-C, two-chamber view; 4-C, four-chamber view; AP-EDD, anteroposterior end-diastolic dimension; AX, axial; CMR, cardiovascular magnetic resonance imaging; LAX, long axis; LVOT, left ventricular outflow tract; RV, right ventricle; SAX, short axis.

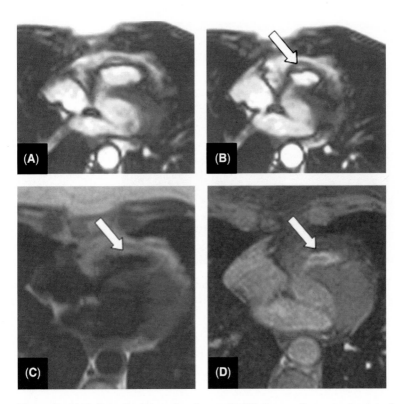

Figure 2 End-diastolic (**A**) and end-systolic (**B**) frames from steady-state free precession cine imaging shows dyskinesis of the anterior portion of the right ventricular outflow tract (RVOT) (*arrow*) (**B**). T1-weighted spin echo image shows fatty replacement of the anterior portion of the RVOT (*bright signal; arrow*) (**C**). The presence of fat is confirmed by signal drop out in the same area on gradient echo fat-suppressed imaging (*arrow*) (**D**). *Abbreviation*: RVOT, right ventricular outflow tract tachycardia.

(in abstract form) with a formal assessment of the accuracy of CMR in patients with suspected ARVC (11). White et al. evaluated 17 patients with documented ventricular arrhythmias, presumably originating from the right ventricle. Seven of the 17 patients were found to have ARVC based on WHO criteria. All 17 patients underwent conventional right ventricular angiography and electrocardiogram (ECG)-gated spin echo CMR examination. Using the WHO criteria as the reference standard, the sensitivity and specificity of MRI were 86% and 40%, respectively. In contrast, the sensitivity and specificity of angiography were 100% and 100%, respectively. Furthermore, the presence or absence of increased signal intensity in the myocardium had no incremental diagnostic value on CMR.

Finally, anomalous coronary arteries need to be ruled out in young persons presenting with unexplained ventricular tachycardia, syncope or sudden

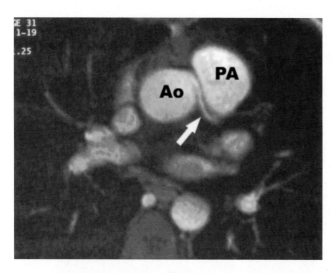

Figure 3 Anomalous left coronary artery arising from the right coronary cusp, coursing between the aorta and pulmonary artery. *Abbreviations*: Ao, aorta; PA, pulmonary artery.

cardiac death. CMR has been shown to be superior to conventional angiography in delineating the proximal course of the coronary arteries (Fig. 3).

CMR Approach

In patients presenting with unexplained ventricular tachycardia, syncope, and sudden cardiac death, the CMR examination is directed toward the identification of an anatomic substrate of the arrhythmia. An integrated CMR approach that is designed to identify the most important entities is outlined below. This approach will identify the presence of myocardial scar due to ischemic cardiomyopathy, dilated nonischemic cardiomyopathy, and hypertrophic cardiomyopathy; it will identify the presence of arrhythmogenic right ventricular cardiomyopathy and can diagnose anomalous coronary arteries. In general, steady-state free precession (SSFP) cine images are used to evaluate global and regional left ventricular and right ventricular function. Regional wall motion abnormalities of the right ventricle are the most important feature in the recognition of ARVC. The presence of fatty or fibrofatty infiltration of the myocardium can be recognized by high signal intensity on T1-weighted spin echo approaches. Furthermore, the presence of intramyocardial fat is confirmed by visualizing signal drop out on fat-suppressed pulse sequences. Finally, inversion recovery fast low-angle shot (FLASH)-based or SSFP-based images with magnitude image and phase image reconstruction are used to identify myocardial scarring.

An example of a commonly used protocol for patients with unexplained ventricular tachycardia, syncope, or sudden cardiac death is outlined below:

1. Multi-planar localizer pulse sequences.
2. Axial Half-fourier single-shot (HASTE) image stack to cover the entire heart (typically in two breath-holds).
3. SSFP cine images

   a. Two-chamber (vertical) long axis orientation
   b. Four-chamber (horizontal) long axis orientation
   c. Anatomical short axis stack from base to apex
      i. Alternatively, some CMR experts prefer true axial cine images rather than anatomical short axis images of the left and right ventricles.

   d. Three-chamber long axis orientation
   e. Right ventricular long axis orientation

4. T1-weighted spin echo pulse sequence without fat suppression in the anatomical short axis stack (matching slices with the SSFP cine short axis stack)

   a. Alternatively, some CMR experts prefer true axial images rather than anatomical short axis images of the left and right ventricles.

5. Fat-suppressed imaging pulse sequence in the anatomical short axis stack (matching slices with the SSFP cine short axis stack)

   a. Alternatively, some CMR experts prefer true axial images rather than anatomical short axis images of the left and right ventricles.

6. Fat-suppressed gradient echo imaging pulse sequence in a parallel stack at the aortic root, parallel to the aortic valve to cover the origin and the proximal course of the coronary arteries. This is only performed in young patients with sudden cardiac death or syncope.
7. Delayed (late) contrast enhancement images

   a. Two-chamber (vertical) long axis orientation
   b. Four-chamber (horizontal) long axis orientation
   c. Anatomical short axis stack from base to apex
      i. Alternatively, some CMR experts prefer true axial cine images rather than anatomical short axis images of the left and right ventricles.

   d. Three-chamber long axis orientation
   e. Right ventricular long axis orientation

Important technical considerations regarding this approach are outlined below.

Multiplanar localizer pulse sequences. This multiplanar pulse sequence typically utilizes single-shot SSFP approaches to obtain three to four slices in each of the major anatomical planes. These images are used for subsequent slice positioning.

Axial HASTE image stack to cover the entire heart (typically in two breath-holds). This axial stack of images is traditionally obtained at the start of most CMR examinations. The purpose is to provide a quick overview of the major anatomic landmarks of the heart and these images are also used for subsequent planning and slice positioning. Depending on the heart rate, these images are typically T2-weighted black blood images and can also be used for some tissue characterization.

SSFP cine images. The SSFP cine images are the most important ones for the evaluation of left and right ventricular function. These images can usually reveal the presence of hypertrophic cardiomyopathy or ARVC if present. Hypertrophic cardiomyopathy can be recognized by the asymmetric septal hypertrophy, systolic anterior motion of the mitral valve and by the presence of intracavitary turbulence. When present, intracavitary turbulence can be better visualized by gradient echo cine pulse sequences, using relatively long time-to-echo (6–8 ms). The most important features of ARVC are global or regional RV wall motion abnormalities. These can be readily recognized by the experienced reader on SSFP cine images. We believe that the presence of RV wall motion abnormalities is more important in the diagnosis of ARVC than the presence of fat in the myocardium. Our usual approach is to acquire images in the anatomical planes (vertical long axis, horizontal long axis, three-chamber view, and anatomical short axis stack). However, some CMR experts prefer the more traditional approach of acquiring axial cine images. From a technical standpoint, the most important consideration is to use the highest flip angle that is allowed given the energy deposition constraints. This will ensure the highest signal-to-noise ratio for these images.

Trouble-shooting for SSFP cine images. Adequate gating is critical for good-quality images. If there are multiple premature beats present, which are common in this particular patient population, real-time SSFP cine images might be considered, realizing the loss in both spatial and temporal resolution. Some authors have used beta-blockers prior to CMR to minimize premature beats.

T1-weighted spin echo pulse sequence without fat suppression in the anatomical short axis stack (matching slices with the SSFP cine short axis stack). Alternatively, some CMR experts prefer true axial images rather than anatomical short axis images of the left and right ventricles. These images are directed toward the identification of the sine qua non of ARVC, which is fibrofatty infiltration. This imaging approach is excellent for the detection of fat, since it appears as areas of bright signal intensity. It is crucial to recognize that intramyocardial fatty infiltration can occur in entities other than ARVC and we require the presence of regional or global RV wall motion abnormalities in order to make the diagnosis of ARVC. The presence of fat can further confirm this.

From a technical perspective it is important to optimize blood nulling by optimizing repetition time. This can be achieved by using a table or a formula to determine optimal repetition time as a function of heart rate. Another important consideration is to achieve the best resolution possible, since the detection of fat in the thin-walled RV can be at the edge of maximum achievable spatial resolution. This can be optimized by using significant rectangular field of view and by the use of saturation bands to avoid wrap.

Finally, these pulse sequences are typically very sensitive to ECG gating. It cannot be emphasized enough how critical it is to have reliable ECG gating for these images. In the presence of significant arrhythmias, single-shot approaches may be utilized.

Fat-suppressed imaging pulse sequence in the anatomical short axis stack (matching slices with the SSFP cine short axis stack). Alternatively, some CMR experts prefer true axial images rather than anatomical short axis images of the left and right ventricles. To obtain these images, the traditional approach has been to repeat the T1-weighted black blood spin echo sequences outlined above, with the addition of a fat saturation pulse. However, in our experience, that is not as reliable as some other approaches. Instead, our laboratory currently utilizes a gradient echo approach with strong fat suppression, which has been developed for coronary artery imaging. This seems to work extremely well for this purpose. We repeat matching slices with the cine images and with the T1-weighted spin echo images.

From a technical standpoint, it is important to utilize a trigger delay for this acquisition to ensure imaging in mid-diastole.

Fat-suppressed gradient echo imaging pulse sequence in a parallel stack at the aortic root, parallel to the aortic valve to cover the origin, and the proximal course of the coronary arteries. These images are obtained in "young" patients with syncope or sudden cardiac death, when anomalous coronary arteries might be suspected based on clinical grounds. We typically use the same gradient echo–based fat-suppressed pulse sequence outlined above. Slices are prescribed based on the three-chamber view and the aortic outflow tract view, to prescribe a parallel stack of slices just over the aortic valve and parallel to the valve, to cover the origin and the proximal course of the coronary arteries. We typically obtain 5–7 cm thick slices with 50% overlap to maximize the spatial localization of the coronary arteries. Again, from a technical standpoint it is important to utilize a trigger delay for this acquisition to ensure imaging in mid-diastole, when the coronary arteries are relatively motion free.

Delayed (late) contrast enhancement images in the standard anatomical planes (horizontal long axis, vertical long axis, and short axis stack). Alternatively, some CMR experts prefer true axial images rather than anatomical short axis images of the left and right ventricles. These images are obtained approximately 10 to 15 minutes after the injection of 0.2 mM/kg gadolinium-diethylenetriamike pentaacetic acid (DTPA)–based contrast agent. The traditional approach has been the use of a gradient echo–based double inversion recovery pulse sequence with optimal inversion time (TI). Optimal inversion time is then determined by the use of a "TI-scout." This is either an SSFP-based or a gradient echo–based sequence, with a progressively increasing inversion time (from about 50 to 600–800 ms every 50–75 ms). Images are then reviewed and optimal TI is chosen based on the image with maximum nulling of the signal in normal myocardium. This TI is then utilized to perform the delayed contrast enhancement sequences. The challenge of this method is that considerable experience is required to determine the optimal TI.

Recently, a new approach has been introduced to overcome the difficulty of manually determining optimal TI. This method relies on the reconstruction of phase images rather than magnitude images and is relatively independent of inversion time. These images are critical in the identification of nonischemic cardiomyopathy, ischemic cardiomyopathy, hypertrophic cardiomyopathy, and ARVC. It is important to point out that identifying delayed contrast enhancement in the right ventricular wall is somewhat controversial. The thin wall of the RV poses a challenge in identifying delayed contrast enhancement, since there only might be two or three pixels across the wall of the right ventricle. Furthermore, it has been suggested that optimal TI for the right ventricle might be slightly different from that of the left ventricle. Optimal TI in the RV has been reported to be in the 200–250 ms range, compared to 250–300 ms range for the LV.

PULMONARY VENOUS IMAGING

Clinical Perspective

Atrial fibrillation is one of the most common clinical problems in cardiology today and nonpharmacologic approaches are becoming more widespread for its treatment. Current ablation approaches focus on the isolation of the pulmonary venous focus from the rest of the atrium with the use of radiofrequency ablation catheters. One of the important potential complications of this approach is pulmonary vein stenosis, manifesting in dyspnea and hemoptysis. In order to avoid these potential complications, it is important to know the size of the pulmonary veins prior to ablation. CMR and cardiovascular CT have been utilized for this purpose and they have been compared to intracardiac echocardiography. CMR can also be used after pulmonary vein ablation if patients present with signs and symptoms of pulmonary vein stenosis.

CMR Approach

The CMR examination of the pulmonary veins is typically designed to provide cine images of the individual pulmonary veins for functional evaluation and to provide an magnetic resonance angiograpahy (MRA) for accurate measurements. SSFP or gradient echo–based cine images can identify turbulent flow in pulmonary vein stenosis. High-resolution MRA of the left atrium and of the pulmonary veins is used to obtain accurate measurements.

Several studies have examined the interstudy variability of pulmonary venous measurements between cardiovascular CT, CMR, and intracardiac echocardiography. Although there were some systematic differences in measurements, reproducibility with the same imaging modality is very high.

Our typical approach is outlined below:

1. Multiplanar localizer pulse sequences.
2. Axial HASTE image stack to cover the entire heart (typically in two breath-holds).
3. SSFP cine images.

    a. Two-chamber (vertical) long axis orientation
    b. Four-chamber (horizontal) long axis orientation
    c. Anatomical short axis stack from base to apex if volumetric determination of ejection fraction is needed. If not, one might only perform three short axis slices (basal, mid, and apical)
    d. Three-chamber long axis orientation
    e. Axial cine images to cover the left atrium
    f. Double-oblique cine images through each of the pulmonary veins

4. Gradient echo cine images. These are obtained only if turbulence is suspected due to pulmonary vein stenosis on the basis of the SSFP cine images.
5. 3D-gadolinium–enhanced MRA in a coronal slab to include the left atrium and all pulmonary veins; timing of bolus if for the left atrium.

Important practical and technical considerations are outlined below.

Multiplanar localizer pulse sequences. These images are utilized to plan subsequent imaging planes.

Axial HASTE image stack to cover the entire heart (typically in two breath-holds). This axial stack of images is traditionally obtained at the start of most CMR examinations. The purpose is to provide a quick overview of the major anatomic landmarks of the heart and these images are also used for subsequent planning and slice positioning. Depending on the heart rate, these images are typically T2-weighted black blood images and can also be used for some tissue characterization.

SSFP cine images. If the volumetric determination of ejection fraction is not necessary, we obtain the vertical and the horizontal long axis view of the heart with three representative short axis slices (basal, mid, and apical). With the latest parallel imaging approaches we can easily obtain three short axis slices in one breath-hold. After this, we typically obtain axial SSFP cine

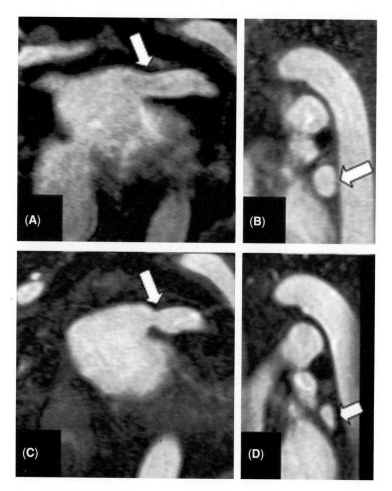

Figure 4 Pulmonary vein stenosis. Normal-sized left superior pulmonary vein before pulmonary vein isolation for atrial fibrillation in a coronal view (*arrow*) (**A**) and in a cross-sectional view (*arrow*) (**B**). Mild stenosis is seen on follow-up examination three months after the procedure in the same views [coronal (**C**) and cross-sectional (**D**)].

images of the left atrium to cover the pulmonary veins. Once the pulmonary veins are identified on these axial images, double-oblique slices are prescribed through each of the major pulmonary veins. These images can identify pulmonary vein stenosis and might reveal turbulent flow as a result of the stenosis. If turbulence is identified, we obtain gradient echo cine images in the same slices as outlined below.

Gradient echo cine images. These are obtained only if turbulence is suspected due to pulmonary vein stenosis on the basis of the SSFP cine images. Gradient echo–based cine images are better suited for the identification of turbulence as a result of spin dephasing. For this reason, we perform gradient echo cine images in double oblique orientations through the pulmonary veins to identify turbulent flow as a result of stenosis.

From a technical perspective, relatively long time to echo is used to best assess turbulence [time-to-echo (TE 6–8 ms)].

3D–gadolinium–enhanced MRA in a coronal slab to include the left atrium and all pulmonary veins; timing of bolus if for the left atrium. The 3D–gadolinium–enhanced MRA is the most important tool for precise measurements of the pulmonary veins in a 3D fashion. Our laboratory uses a coronal 3D slab to include the left atrium and the pulmonary veins; slice thickness is typically about 1.25 mm. Either a timing bolus or a bolus tracking approach can be utilized, as long as the acquisition is correctly timed for the left atrium. This allows for best delineation of the left atrium and the pulmonary veins. Similar to other MRA approaches, first a non contrast–enhanced "mask" is obtained, which is used for subtraction after the contrast-enhanced data set has been acquired (Fig. 4).

CONCLUSIONS

CMR's usefulness extends into the realm of the electrophysiologist in defining the anatomic substrate for arrhythmias. The chapter emphasizes the major cardiomyopathy associated with malignant arrhythmias: ARVC/ARVD. Using CMR's ability to image regional and global RV (and LV) function, regional wall motion to assess the extent of aneurysmal dilation and the extent of lipid infiltration and involvement, CMR provides the most comprehensive method to detect and determine the extent of ARVC/ARVD. For management of atrial fibrillation, the identification and size of the pulmonary veins can be readily assessed before and after of ablative therapy for atrial fibrillation. Again, CMR is an enormous asset to the electrophysiologist to diagnose and evaluate the hearts of patients with arrhythmias.

REFERENCES

1. Choudhury, L, Mahrholdt H, Wagner A, et al. Myocardial scarring in asymptomatic or mildly symptomatic patients with hypertrophic cardiomyopathy.

2. Report of the 1995 World Health Organization/International Society and Federation of Cardiology Task Force on the definition and classification of cardiomyopathy. Circulation 1996; 93:841–842.

3. Fontaine G, Fontaliran F, Frank R. Arrhythmogenic right ventricular cardiomyopathies. Clinical forms and main differential diagnoses. Circulation 1998; 97:1532–1535.

4. McKenna WJ, Thiene G, Nava A, et al. Diagnosis of arrhythmogenic right ventricular dysplasia/cardiomyopathy. Br Heart J 1994; 71:215–218.

5. Gemayel C, Pelliccia A, Thompson PD. Arrhythmogenic right ventricular cardiomyopathy. J Am Coll Cardiol 2001; 38:1773–1781.

6. Casolo GC, Poggese L, Boddi M, et al. ECG-gated magnetic resonance imaging and right ventricular dysplasia. Am Heart J 1989; 113:1245–1248.

7. Wichter T, Aufferman W, Breithardt G, Borggrefe M, Bongartz G, Peters PE. Magnetic resonance imaging in arrhythmogenic right ventricular disease. Eur Heart J 1989; 10(suppl D):83.

8. Aufferman W, Wichter T, Breidhardt G, et al. Arrhythmogenic right ventricular disease: MR imaging vs angiography. Am J Roentgenol 1993; 161:549–555.

9. Midiri M, Fiazzo M, Brancato M, et al. Arrhythmogenic right ventricular dysplasia; MR features. Eur Radiol 1997; 7:307–312.

10. Klersy C, Raisaro A, Salerno J, et al. Arrhythmogenic right and left ventricular disease: evaluation by computed tomography and nuclear magnetic resonance imaging. Eur Heart J 1989; 10(suppl D):84–88.

11. White JB, Kay N, Plumb VJ, Epstein AE. Relative utility of magnetic resonance imaging and right ventricular angiography to diagnose arrhythmogenic right ventricular cardiomyopathy. PACE 2002; 24:587.

15

The Pericardium and Pericardial Disease

Lynne Hung

Department of Medicine, Division of Cardiovascular Medicine,
LACUSC Medical Center, Keck School of Medicine, University of Southern
California, Los Angeles, California, U.S.A.

ANATOMY OF THE PERICARDIUM

The pericardium is composed of an outer fibrous layer and an inner serous membrane. The serous sac is divided into (a) a visceral pericardium, which consists of one layer of mesothelial cells and is closely applied to the epicardial surface of the heart and (b) a parietal pericardium, which lines the inside of the fibrous layer and extends to cover portions of the proximal great vessels. A potential space can exist between the serosal layers and may normally contain about 15 to $50 \, cm^3$ of fluids. This pericardial fluid is an ultrafiltrate of plasma, with protein content about one-third that of plasma. The posterior pericardial reflection about the pulmonary veins and inferior vena cava forms an inverted U-shaped pocket called the oblique pericardial sinus.

A variety of diseases can exist within the pericardium. A multitude of infections (i.e., viral, bacterial, myobacterial, or fungal) can occur in the pericardium and produce local inflammations. Patients with uremia, myocardial infarction (Dressler's syndrome), or surgical pericardiotomy performed during cardiac surgery (postpericardiotomy syndrome) can develop pericarditis.

MAGNETIC RESONANCE IMAGING AND THE PERICARDIUM

Imaging of the pericardium has been a challenging task (Table 1). Transthoracic echocardiography is widely used to provide both functional and

Table 1 Modalities for Evaluating the Pericardium

	Advantages	Disadvantages
Transthoracic echocardiography	Noninvasive Readily available	Operator dependent Body habitus may interfere with acoustic window Limited views
Transesophageal echocardiography	Wider field of views than TTE	Invasive
CT	Excellent spatial resolution Wide field of view	Difficult to differentiate between pericardial thickening and fibrous from high protein content of pericardial effusion Contrast injection required
Electron beam X-ray CT	Rapid acquisition	Same problems as traditional CT
Cardiac magnetic resonance imaging	Fast, high-resolution multiplane images No contrast injection	Not readily available in all medical centers Patients with medical devices (i.e., pacemakers) will be a problem

Abbreviations: CT, computed tomography; TTE, transthoracic echocardiography.

anatomical informations. However, it is unreliable for assessing pericardial thickness in the absence of pericardial fluid. It is operator dependent and provides limited views. Acoustic windows are suboptimal in many patients with obesity, emphysema, or large pleural effusion. Transesophageal echocardiography may overcome some of these problems, but it is invasive. X-ray computed tomography (CT) has the advantage of excellent spatial resolution, a wide field of views, and can accurately detect pericardial effusion, thickness, as well as calcifications. However, the pericardium is often not visualized laterally due to the absence of fat between the heart and the adjacent lung. It may be difficult to differentiate between pericardial thickening and fibrous or high protein content pericardial effusion on CT scan. CT scan is often undesirable because of poor tissue contrast, requires injection of contrast medium, and acquires images only in the axial planes. Electron beam X-ray CT enables rapid acquisition of images but still has the disadvantages of CT scans.

Unlike echocardiography and CT scan, cardiac magnetic resonance imaging (CMR) can provide fast, high-resolution multiplane images that is synchronized with the cardiac cycle. CMR provides excellent images of the entire pericardium without injection of intravenous contrast or ionizing radiation. CMR can visualize the pericardium with either gated spin echo (SE) or gradient echo technique (1). The normal pericardium is identified on T1-weighted SE–MRI as a line of low signal intensity that is located between the high signal of pericardial fat on the outside and the epicardial fat on the inside (2). The visibility of this pericardial band can vary depending on the amount of epicardial and pericardial fat. On SE–MRI, some parts of the pericardium, particularly the region overlying the right atrium and the posterolateral wall of the left ventricle, may not be identifiable because of its paucity of epicardial fat (3). The low signal intensity of the pericardium itself is due to its fibrous structure and lack of fluid. Small quantities of pericardial fluid posterior to the aorta in the superior pericardial recess of the transverse sinus or anterior to the aorta in the preaortic recess are considered normal. The normal pericardial thickness is approximately 2 mm, although values of up to 4 mm are not necessarily pathologic (4). Care must be taken when measuring the pericardial thickness because overestimation can occur when measurements are taken too close in proximity to the diaphragm and may not be visible when it is contiguous with the lung. One study suggests that the most sensitive area for measuring pericardial thickness is anterior or lateral to the right ventricle when in a transverse plane and in a three-chamber view (i.e., right atrium, right ventricle, and left ventricle) (5).

PERICARDIAL EFFUSION

CMR imaging is very sensitive for identifying generalized or localized pericardial effusions. Accumulation of more than 50 cm^3 of fluid in the pericardial space is abnormal (Figs. 1A and B).

Pericardial effusion may be hemorrhagic, chylous, or serous. Transudative fluids usually produce low signal intensity on T1-weighted and high signal intensity on T2-weighted SE or gradient-echo images. Whereas hemorrhagic or proteinaceous effusion have increased signal on T1- and T2-weighted SE–MRI (6). Both the pericardium and the pericardial adhesions, as seen in effusions from uremic patients, have greater signal intensity than normal pericardium. Rapid CMR acquisition allows for volumetric determination of the pericardial effusion by use of Simpson's rule. Moderate effusions are often associated with a pericardial space anterior to the right ventricle of >5 mm.

Furthermore, cine MRI can detect cardiac tamponade in patients showing diastolic collapse of the right-sided and even left-sided cardiac chambers.

CONSTRICTIVE PERICARDITIS

It is often difficult to distinguish between constrictive pericarditis and restrictive cardiomyopathy because both can impair diastolic filling and thus can have similar clinical presentations and overlapping hemodynamic profiles at cardiac atherization (Fig. 2).

(A)

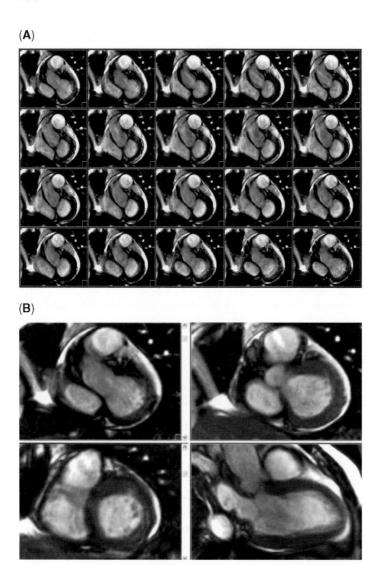

(B)

Figure 1 (**A**) Pericardial effusion. This is a 65-year-old male with chest pain and prior mediastinal surgery has a moderate-sized effusion that partially covers the origin of the main pulmonary artery and aorta (images from FIESTA cine exam). (**B**) Pericardial effusion. This is same as shown in (**A**), but the image is enlarged for viewing. The pericardial effusion is circumferential. *Source*: Courtesy of Patrick M. Colletti, MD, University of Southern California.

Constrictive pericarditis results from progressive pericardial fibrosis, leading to impaired filling of the ventricles during diastole. Pericardial thickening of >4 mm on SE–MRI is considered evidence of pericardial constriction

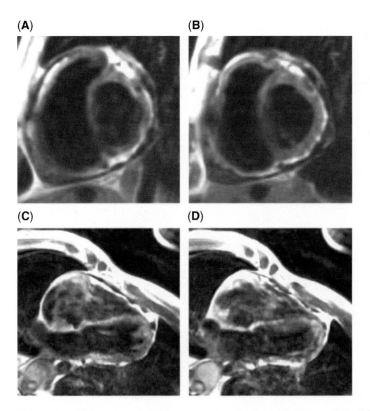

(A) **(B)**

(C) **(D)**

Figure 2 (*Figure continued on next page*) Constrictive pericarditis. This is a 33-year-old patient who presented with shortness of breath. His CMR is consistent with constrictive pericarditis. Double inversion horizontal long-axis views (**A** and **B**) and short-axis (**C** and **D**) views demonstrate nodular pericardial thickening. Short-axis diastolic (**E**) and systolic (**F**) cine SSFP views demonstrate diastolic septal straightening. Note the dilated middle hepatic vein. Horizontal (**G**) and vertical (**H**) long-axis systolic SSFP views show left and right atrial and hepatic vein dilatation. *Source*: Courtesy of Patrick Colletti, MD, University of Southern California.

when correlate clinically (7). Pericardial thickening from fibrosis may be difficult to differentiate from inflammation. One helpful feature is that the thickening associated with an inflammatory process usually shows a change from the normal low-intensity signal to a medium- or high-intensity signal.

Calcification may appear as focal areas of decreased signal with irregular borders.

Compared to CT scan, CMR has the advantage of obtaining views in multiple planes and assessing left ventricular function, but lacks the ability to clearly detect calcifications.

The presence of pericardial thickening by itself does not indicate constrictive pericarditis.

(E)   (F)

(G)   (H)

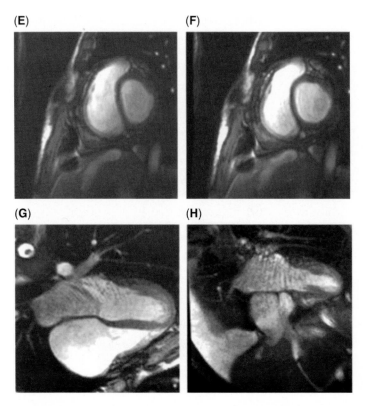

Figure 2 (*Continued*)

In constrictive pericarditis, the inferior vena cava, hepatic veins, and right atrium may be greatly dilated, whereas the right ventricle may be normal or elongated. SE–MRI has been reported to have a sensitivity of 88%, specificity of 100%, and a diagnostic accuracy of 93% when axial and coronal images were taken to diagnose constrictive pericarditis (8). In chronic constriction, the thickened pericardium is of lower signal intensity compared with that in acute pericarditis.

CONGENITAL ABSENCE OF THE PERICARDIUM

Congenital absence of the pericardium may be complete or partial. Complete absence of the pericardium is benign and patients are usually asymptomatic. However, partial absence of the pericardium may be associated with herniation of the left atrial appendage, the entire left atrium, or both of the ventricles through the defect, which may lead to life-threatening cardiac strangulation or compression of the coronary arteries. Cardiac MRI has been helpful in showing the leftward protrusion of the left atrial appendage or the main pulmonary artery, as well as lung that insinuates between the aorta and pulmonary artery and between the base of the heart and left hemidiaphragm. Because of the serious nature of this disease, elective surgery is recommended in patients who may or not be symptomatic from partial absence of the pericardium when detected by cardiac MRI.

PERICARDIAL CYST

CMR has been useful in detecting pericardial cyst. It is a mesothelial cyst that may exist in either cardiophrenic angle, most commonly in the right, of asymptomatic patients.

They are unilocular and are usually filled with clear, simple fluid composed of low protein concentration, and nonhemorrhagic. These cysts are paracardiac mass with low signal intensity on T1-weighted and high signal intensity on T2-weighted SE–MRI (9). With prolongation of the echo time, there generally is a progressive increase in signal intensity of fluids within the pericardial cyst.

MALIGNANCY OF THE PERICARDIUM

Malignancies involving the pericardium are rare and are most due to direct invasion or metastasis. The most common metastasis is usually from the lung, breast, lymphoma, or esophagus. Primary tumors of the pericardium include mesothelioma, lipoma, and sarcoma. High-resolution imaging such as CMR imaging enable tissue planes to be clearly delineated and the wide field of view allows the extent of tumor spread to be determined.

CONCLUSIONS

CMR is unique in its ability to image the pericardium. A major capability of CMR is its ability to allow determination of the etiology in patients with restrictive syndromes. The thickened pericardium in patients with constrictive pericarditis versus restrictive cardiomyopathy is easily seen on CMR study and pericardial thickness can be measured. Accordingly, surgically remediable constriction is identified and treatment strategy determined. Other uses of CMR in pericardial disease are described.

REFERENCES

1. Gutierrez FR, Brown JJ, Mirowitz SA., eds. Cardiovascular Magnetic Resonance Imaging. Mosby Year Book, 1992:104–111.
2. Bluemke DA, Halefoglu AM. Cardiac disease in the adults: MR evaluation. Crit Rev Diagnost Imaging 1999; 40(4):203–249.
3. Martin E, Fuisz A. Imaging cardiac structure and pump function. In: Reichek, ed. Cardiology Clinics. Saunders Co, 1998:141–144.
4. Pohost G, O'Rourke R, Berman D, Shah P, eds. Imaging in cardiovascular disease. Lippincott Williams and Wilkins, 2000:409–410

5. Sechtem U, Tscholakoff D, et al. MRI of the normal pericardium. Am J Roentgenol 1986; 147:239–244.
6. Smith WHT, Beacock DJ, et al. Magnetic resonance evaluation of the pericardium. Br J Radiol 2001; 74:384–392.
7. Frank H, Globits S. Myocardial and pericardial MRI evaluation. J Magn Reson Imaging 1999; 10(5):617–626.
8. Masui T, Finck S, et al. Constrictive pericarditis and restrictive cardiomyopathy: evaluation with MR imaging. Radiology 1992; 182:369–373.
9. Vick GW, Rokey R. Cardiovascular magnetic resonance evaluation of the pericardium in health and disease. In: Manning WJ, Pennell DJ, eds. Cardiovascular Magnetic Resonance. Churchill Livingstone, 2002:355–363.

16

Cardiac and Paracardiac Masses

Vikas K. Rathi

*Division of Cardiology, Cardiovascular MRI Lab, Allegheny General Hospital,
Drexel University College of Medicine, Philadelphia, Pennsylvania, U.S.A.*

INTRODUCTION

Although very rare cardiac tumors can be elusive, and accurate early diagnosis is essential for effective patient management. In recent years, development in various imaging techniques and specifically advances in the field of cardiovascular magnetic resonance (CMR) imaging has significantly enhanced the accurate diagnosis and management of patients with cardiac and paracardiac masses.

The greatest advantage of CMR over various imaging modalities is its unique ability to characterize tissue composition based on the inherent T1 and T2 relaxation properties of the tissue. This ability to perform tissue characterization combined with excellent temporal and spatial resolution, a large field of view, multiplanar 3D imaging, as well as the ability to clearly demonstrate the surrounding vasculature, lymph nodes, and mediastinal structures makes CMR an ideal technique for the evaluation of cardiac and paracardiac masses (1,2). An additional advantage of CMR is its ability to clearly depict the pericardium. The pericardial effusions and thickening due to inflammation, fibrosis, or malignant involvement are well demonstrated on CMR images (3). Together, all these characteristics permit accurate staging and surgical planning. Imaging techniques such as echocardiography lack the ability to characterize tissue and have a very limited field of view. Like CMR, computed tomography (CT) scanners offer a wide field of view and 3D imaging capabilities. However, they have the drawback of using high doses of ionizing radiation and nephrotoxic contrast agents, and they lack the ability to assess the myocardial function.

On routine clinical CMR imaging, the axial nonbreathold spin echo (SE) T1-weighted images offer good detail about the location, morphology, and characteristics of normal and pathologic tissue. Occasionally, thin slice breathold images are obtained to further characterize the pathology. Steady-state free precession (SSFP) cine images in axial and multiple double oblique planes are acquired to differentiate abnormal tissue from contractile myocardium. These images are also helpful to evaluate valvular function in cases where the mass lesion is adjacent or attached to the valve apparatus. The above imaging sequences as well as the T2-weighted and fat saturation (triple inversion recovery) sequences form an integral part of the cardiac mass evaluation. Differential signal change between T1- and T2-weighted images yield information regarding the tissue composition of these abnormal masses. Fat-containing tissue is bright on T1-weighted but loses signal on T2-weighted or triple inversion recovery images. Water-containing cysts show low signal intensity on T1-weighted and high signal on T2-weighted images. Acute and subacute hemorrhage is bright on T1- and T2-weighted images. Tissues with dysmorphic calcification, chronic hemorrhage, thrombus or dense fibrous tissue have low signal intensity on T1- and T2-weighted images. Table 1 enlists common primary cardiac neoplasms and their tissue characteristics based on T1 and T2 relaxation properties.

Newer techniques such as myocardial tagging are also useful to differentiate cardiac masses from the contractile myocardium and can give information about the extent and mechanism of invasion into normal structures (4). In addition, gadolinium (Gd)-based contrast agents further adds to the superiority of CMR for the identification, characterization, and risk stratification of both benign and malignant tumors (5).

While pursuing the diagnosis of cardiac neoplasms, one has to keep a watchful eye and knowledge of the common mediastinal structures and masses (Table 2), which may aid in the diagnosis of the cardiac or paracardiac tumors. A diligent effort should be made to look for any abnormal mediastinal masses, lymphadenopathy or pulmonary paranchymal lesions on all cases referred for CMR evaluation of cardiac neoplasms. At our center, we have often discovered masses in the vicinity of heart, which were either related to the cardiac neoplasm as the primary tumor (Fig. 1) or were entirely a separate neoplasm (Fig. 2).

CARDIAC NEOPLASMS

Cardiac neoplasms are classified as primary or metastatic. The metastatic cardiac masses are 20 to 40 times more common than primary tumors. The annual incidence of primary cardiac tumors is approximately 0.001% to

Table 1 Characteristics of Common Cardiac Neoplasms

Primary cardiac tumors	Predilection	T1-W signal	T2-W signal	Gd enhancement	Main feature
Myxoma	LA	Iso	High	++	Stalk
Rhabdomyoma	LV	Iso	High	+	Intramural
Fibroma	IVS	Iso/Low	Low	+/−	Circumscribed
Lipoma	LA/RA	High	Low	−	Obese females
Fibroelastoma	AV	Iso	Iso	−	Small (<1 cm)
Hemangioma	LV	Iso	High	+++	Vascular caverns
Paragangliomas	LA roof	Low	High	+/−	Catecholamine secreting
Angiosarcoma	RA	Iso	High	+++	Sunray or cauliflower enhancement
Pericardial Mesothelioma	Pericardium	Iso	High	+	Pericardial origin

Note: (+) and (−) indicate degree of enhancement after gadolinium contrast administration.
Abbreviations: LA, left atrium; RA, right atrium; IVS, interventricular septum; LV, left ventricle; Iso, isointense compared to myocardium; Gd, gadolinium contrast enhancement.

Table 2 Common Nonneoplastic and Neoplastic Masses in Mediastinum

Medias-tinum	Boundaries	Normal Contents	Non-neoplastic Masses	Neoplastic Masses
Anterior	Anterior—sternum; posterior—pericardium, heart and brachiocephalic vein	Thymus gland Fat Lymph nodes	Thymus cyst Lymphangioma or cystic hygroma Intrathoracic goiter	Thymoma Thymic carcinoma Thyroid carcinoid Thymolipoma Germ cell tumor Parathyroid adenoma Mesenchymal tumors Lipoma or Liposarcoma Fibroma or Fibrosarcoma
Middle	Pericardium	Heart Ascending aorta Transverse aorta Brachiocephalic vessels Vena cavae Pulmonary arteries Pulmonary veins	Aortic aneurysm and pseudoaneurysm Mediastinal cyst Foregut cysts Bronchogenic cysts Esophageal duplication cyst Neuroenteric cyst Pericardial cyst	Primary cardiac neoplasms Primary mediastinal lymphoma Hodgkins Non-Hodgkins Tracheal tumors

Posterior	Trachea	Left atrial appendage aneurysm	Neurogenic tumors
Anterior—heart, pericardium and Trachea; posterior—vertebral bodies and paravertebral gutters	Bronchi	Esophagocele	Peripheral nerve tumors
	Lymph nodes	Hiatal hernia	Schwannoma and Neurofibroma
	Descending thoracic aorta	Meningocele	Malignant tumor of nerve sheath origin
	Esophagus	Pancreatic pseudocyst	Sympathetic ganglia tumor
	Azygous veins		Ganglioneuroma
	Autonomic ganglia		Ganglioneuroblastoma
	Nerves		Neuroblastoma
	Thoracic duct		Mesenchymal tumors or soft tissue tumors
	Lymph nodes		
	Fat		

(A)   **(B)**

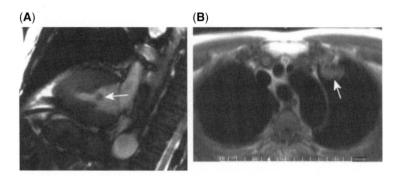

Figure 1 A 66-year-old male with history of recurrent transient ischemic attacks and amaurosis fugax of right eye was referred for cardiovascular magnetic resonance imaging (CMR) evaluation. On steady-state free precession cine images a mobile 8.9 × 9.6 mm mass was seen attached to the tip of the anteroseptal papillary muscle and chordae (**A**). On T1- and T2-weighted images, the mass was isointense and was thought to be thrombus or papillary fibroelastoma. A 2.4×2.0 cm left anterior apical pulmonary density was also seen on the CMR examination (**B**). Interestingly, surgical evacuation of the left ventricular mass and open biopsy of the apical lung mass were reported to be of identical histology revealing adenocarcinoma of lung metastasized to left ventricle.

0.28% and is classified as benign or malignant neoplasm (6). The primary benign cardiac tumors are more common and include myxoma, fibroma, rhabdomyoma, lipoma, fibroelastoma, hemangioma, and paragangliomas. The primary malignant cardiac neoplasms are generally sarcomas (angiosarcomas, rhabdomyosarcomas, fibrosarcoma, osteosarcoma), mesotheliomas, or lymphomas.

It is important to take into consideration certain characteristics of these neoplasms to facilitate the differential diagnosis. In a retrospective data analysis on 55 cardiac neoplasms diagnosed by CMR, Hoffmann et al. showed that malignant lesions (primary or secondary) were common on right side of the heart (7). In addition, specific but less sensitive markers of malignancy were tumor infiltration of adjacent compartments, size > 5 cm, and the presence of pericardial or pleural effusions. Inhomogeneous tumor composition was the strongest predictor of the tumor pathology. Indeed, all the inhomogeneous tumors located in the right heart with concurrent pericardial effusion were malignant, whereas all homogenous tumors located in the left heart without pericardial effusion were always benign.

MYXOMA

Myxomas are the most common of the primary benign cardiac tumors in adults and constitute nearly 50% of all histologically benign tumors of the

(A)

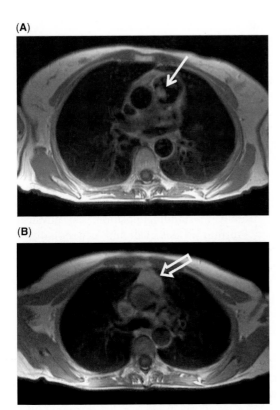

(B)

Figure 2 A 62-year-old female with past history of benign tumor of ovaries and multiple uterine fibroids presented with history of palpitations and was evaluated by transesophageal echocardiogram, which showed a pedunculated mass on the pulmonic valve. This was further evaluated by a cardiovascular magnetic resonance imaging examination. On spin echo and gradient–recalled echo cine images a mobile pedunculated 1.5 × 1.5 cm mass attached to the posterior leaflet of the pulmonic valve was identified, freely moving in systole and diastole (*arrow*) (**A**). The signal characteristics on T1- and T2-weighted images were consistent with fibroelastoma, which was later confirmed on histology. Interestingly, a 1.5 × 3.2 cm mass was also identified in the anterior mediastinum (*block arrow*) (**B**). The signal characteristics and location were suggestive of a thymoma, which was indeed confirmed on histology. This case illustrates two separate histological tumors in and around the vicinity of heart.

heart. Seventy-five percent are located in the left atrium. Table 3 shows the chamber predilection for the cardiac myxomas in adults.

A female predominance is reported and the presentation is usually in middle age. Most patients present with a triad of constitutional, embolic, or obstructive manifestations. The constitutional symptoms are nonspecific and are rarely helpful in prospective diagnosis. The embolic phenomenon

Table 3 Myxoma Predilection (%)

Left atrium	75
Right atrium	15–20
Right ventricle	3–4
Left ventricle	3–4

is produced by extensively myxoid and polypoid lesions. Systemic embolization is frequent since most myxomas are located in the left atrium. The most
common sites of embolization are central nervous system, coronary arteries,
aorta, kidney, spleen, and extremities. The signs and symptoms may also
mimic the clinical picture of mitral or tricuspid stenosis because of the
obstructed filling of ventricle, usually in standing position. On physical
examination, usually a cardiac murmur is detected and occasionally a
characteristic "tumor plop" may be heard.

Myxomas most commonly occur as sporadic lesions but are also known
to be familial or as part of Carney syndrome (8). Sporadic lesions most
commonly occur in the left atrium, are single, and their estimated risk of developing a second myxoma after complete excision is 1% to 2%, whereas the
familial myxomas are often multicentric, found in atypical locations and carry
a 12% to 22% recurrence rate after excision. The Carney complex is an autosomal dominant disorder typified by cardiac, cutaneous, and mammary
myxomas, spotty skin pigmentation, endocrine over-reactivity, psommoma-
tous melanotic schwannoma, primary pigmented nodular adrenal disease, and
testicular neoplasms (particularly large cell calcifying sertoli cell tumor) (9).

Most myxomas originate from the border of the fossa ovalis, but may
arise from elsewhere within the atria. True myxomas arise only from the mural
endocardium, attached by a broad base. Seventy-five percent of these are
pedunculated and are usually polypoid and friable. A myxoma is a soft, gelati-
nous, mucoid mass with areas of hemorrhage, thrombosis, or calcification.
These lesions vary from 1 to 15 cm in diameter, with most measuring 5 to 6 cm.

CMR provides unimpeded visualization of the atria, atrial septum,
and the ventricles. The SE, SSFP, and post-Gd contrast sequences are helpful in characterization of these tumors. The signal intensity and outline of
cardiac myxomas depend on the tumor composition. On T1-weighted
images, the myxomas are isointense relative to the adjacent myocardium
(Fig. 3A). CMR can differentiate tissue composition making it possible to
identify hemorrhage, thrombosis, fat, calcification, necrotic foci, and cysts
in the myxomas. Fatty infiltration within the myxoma will appear bright
on T1-weighted and dark on fat saturation or T2-weighted images. On
T1- and T2-weighted images, intratumoral areas of subacute hemorrhage
appear bright, while an area of calcification and hemosiderin deposition
has low signal intensity (10). Myxomatous components appear low in signal
intensity on T1-weighted and high on T2-weighted images (Fig. 3B). At

(A)   (B)

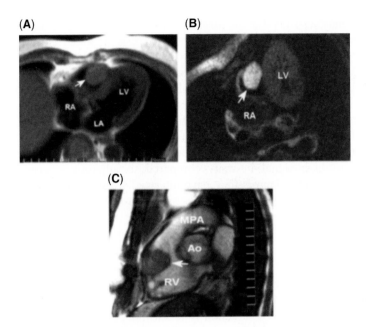

(C)

Figure 3 A 75-year-old male with right ventricular myxoma (uncommon). (**A**) T1-weighted SE axial image demonstrate an isointense circumscribed homogenous mass attached to the right ventricular free wall (*arrow*) with a broad base (uncommon). On T2-weighted sequence, the mass is bright confirming myxomatous composition (*arrow*) (**B**). A right ventricular outflow tract steady-state free precession image from same patient shows the broad-based attachment of the mass to the right ventricular free wall (*arrow*) (**C**). *Abbreviations*: Ao, aorta; LA, left atrium; LV, left ventricle; MPA, main pulmonary artery; RA, right atrium; RV, right ventricle.

times the surface of the tumor is surrounded by slow flow, which gives a larger appearance to the tumor size on SE images than on SSFP where it appears isointense to the myocardium (Fig. 3C). After Gd administration, myxomas may or may not increase in intensity depending upon the extent of vascularity (5).

RHABDOMYOMA

It is the most frequent cardiac tumor in infants and children and is debated to be a hematoma rather than a true neoplasm. Rhabdomyomas are the most frequent tumor found at fetal echocardiography, comprising 17 of 19 fetal tumors found in a series of 14,000 fetal echocardiograms (11). It frequently regresses spontaneously by the age of two years.

These tumors most often involve ventricular myocardium and are usually multiple and occur with equal frequency in both the right and left ventricle. They may also involve the atria but not the valves. About one-third of the patients have associated tuberous sclerosis in which case it is termed as "Bourneville's" tuberous sclerosis (12). Usually, it manifests due to chamber obstruction, tachyarrhythmia, AV block, heart failure, pericardial effusion, or sudden death. Grossly they appear as firm, well-circumscribed lobulated nodules. Mostly, they are intramural and solitary, but multiple small lesions have been documented (rhabdomyomatosis).

On CMR they manifest as solid masses located in the ventricular myocardium. On T1-weighted images they appear well circumscribed and isointense to high signal intensity compared to adjacent myocardium, and on T2-weighted images they have intermediate signal intensity. Gd enhancement pattern of the tumor is similar to the surrounding myocardium (5).

FIBROMA

Cardiac fibromas are the second most common neoplasm in children. Mean age of presentation is 13 years. Common clinical manifestations are due to invasion or compression of the conduction system leading to life-threatening arrhythmias and sudden death. Other manifestations are due to obstruction of the outflow tract and heart failure. Fibromas are almost always solitary, well circumscribed, round, firm, and rubbery tumors located intramurally with protuberance into the chamber cavity (Fig. 4). Tumor calcification is common, but cyst, hemorrhage, or necrosis is rare. Over 50% of the cardiac fibromas occur in the left ventricle and predominantly involve the

(A)   **(B)**

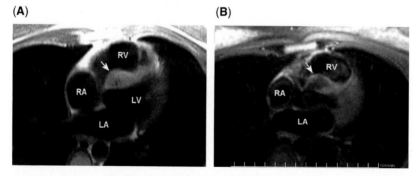

Figure 4   A 44-year-old female being followed for past eight years for right ventricular mass arising from the interventricular septum. T1-weighted spin echo (SE) axial image demonstrating isointense, homogenous mass projecting from the upper interventricular septum into the right ventricle (*arrow*) (**A**). On T2-weighted SE axial image the mass remains isointense to myocardium with central dark area, confirming a dense fibroma (**B**). *Abbreviations*: RV, right ventricle; RA, right atrium; LV, left ventricle; LA, left atrium.

interventricular septum and anterior wall. However, they are seen with decreasing frequency in right ventricle and rarely the atria. When localized in the apex of the left ventricle, fibromas need to be differentiated from other apical masses such as thrombus, eosinophilic cardiomyopathy, endomyocardial fibrosis, lipoma, rhabdomyoma, and malignant tumors. Timely excision is required, as risk of sudden death is significant. Patients with Gorlin syndrome are at increased risk of cardiac fibroma. This syndrome is characterized by multiple nevoid basal cell carcinoma of the skin, odontogenic keratocysts of the mandible, bifid ribs, and a tendency for neoplastic growth in several organ systems (13).

The affected myocardium usually demonstrates regional wall motion abnormalities with a focal bulge or irregularity (Fig. 4). On T1-weighted images the tumor appears homogenous and isointense or hypointense relative to the surrounding myocardium (Fig. 4A). Similarly, on T2-weighted images it is hypointense or remains isointense (Fig. 4B). After gadolinium administration the tumor demonstrates little or no contrast enhancement because of the dense fibrous tissue and diminished vascularity. Findings include a heterogeneous enhancement pattern with a lower-intensity nonenhancing central area that represents the dense fibrous core, which is surrounded by a peripheral rim of hyperenhancement that has been described in the literature (14).

LIPOMA

Lipomas account for 14% of benign cardiac tumors in adults and have similar characteristics to lipomas elsewhere in the body (15). Because of their common location in atria, they must be differentiated from the cases of lipomatous hypertrophy of interatrial septum. This is defined as the deposition of fat in the atrial septum at the level of the fossa ovalis measuring ≥2 cm in transverse diameter. This fatty infiltration characteristically spares the fossa ovalis, a feature that can be very well demonstrated by CMR (Fig. 5A). Lipomas are encapsulated, whereas lipomatous hypertrophy of the interatrial septum is non-encapsulated and the term is actually a misnomer because it is caused by increase in the number of adipocytes, not hypertrophy. On histologic sections, lipomatous hypertrophy demonstrates myocytes distributed throughout the mass, which is uncommon in lipomas. Also, lipomatous hypertrophy is more common than cardiac lipomas and most cases are incidentally diagnosed in obese female patients on echocardiography.

The heart is occasionally dilated in patients with cardiac lipoma. T1-weighted SE images demonstrate homogenously high signal intensity compared with surrounding myocardium (Fig. 6A). This signal intensity decreases with the fat saturation sequences or T2-weighted sequences (Fig. 6B). On Gd administration, these tumors do not uptake contrast agent.

(A) **(B)**

(C)

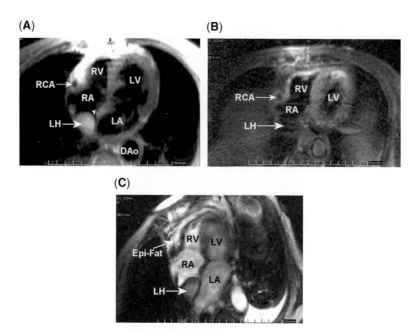

Figure 5 An 83-year-old female with lipomatous hypertrophy of the interatrial septum. T1-weighted spin echo axial image demonstrate the selective thickening and brightness of the septum secundum and posterior wall of the right atrium, suggestive of lipomatous hypertrophy of interatrial septum (**A**). Note that fossa ovalis is spared (*arrow head*). Triple inversion recovery images show the nulling of fatty septum (**B**). Steady-state free precession four-chamber cine image shows the bright septum secundum (**C**). *Abbreviations*: DAo, descending aorta; LA, left atrium; LH, lipomatous hypertrophy of interatrial septum; LV, left ventrical; RA, right atrium; RCA, right coronary artery; Epi-Fat, epicardial fat.

PAPILLARY FIBROELASTOMA

Papillary fibroelastoma, also known as papilloma of the valves or papillary fibroma is the most common tumor of the cardiac valves (16). They are the second most common primary benign cardiac tumors in adults. They have no predilection for gender and are seen most commonly over 50 years of age. Usual presentation is by chest pain, transient ischemic attacks, or stroke due to embolic phenomena. Though located on valvular surface they typically do not cause valvular dysfunction.

They most commonly involve the left-sided heart valves with slight predilection for the aortic rather than the mitral valve. Though less common on right side, when seen, the tricuspid valve is more commonly involved than the pulmonic valve. They are usually small, solitary, and occur away from the valvular free margins.

Besides tissue characterization, CMR SSFP or gradient echo cine images offer accurate multiplanar information of the valvular function. This

(A) **(B)**

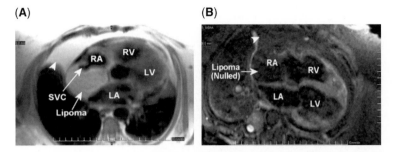

Figure 6 A 55-year-old female with echogenicity in right atrium on a transthoracic echocardiogram was diagnosed as lipoma by cardiovascular magnetic resonance imaging. T1-weighted spin echo axial image show a large circumscribed, encapsulated, homogenous mass in the right atrium (**A**). On this sequence the signal intensity of lipoma is similar to that of the anterior extrapericardial fat (*arrow head*) (**A**). Also note that the SVC is compressed by lipoma. On triple inversion recovery image, the fatty lipoma as well as the anterior extrapericardial fat is dark (**B**). *Abbreviations*: LA, left atrium; LV, left ventricle; RA, right atrium; RV, right ventricle; SVC, superior vena cava.

enables 3D visualization of the valves, which is critical in evaluation of fibroelastomas that are generally very small (<1 cm), and due to the dynamic nature of the valves accompanied by surrounding flow they can easily be over-looked (17). If located on pulmonic valve they can be missed or obscured by other imaging modalities such as transesophageal echocardiogram. CMR well visualizes the pulmonic valve and on SSFP images they are seen as mobile pedunculated masses, rarely with an attached thrombus. The SE images dem-onstrate an isointense tumor on both T1- and T2-weighted images (Fig. 2). On SSFP cine images, the signal intensity is low compared to the surrounding blood and myocardium and Gd contrast uptake is variable.

HEMANGIOMA

Hemangiomas are vascular tumors composed of a network of capillaries and caverns, and rarely occur in the heart. They are typically diagnosed on coronary angiography representing a characteristic tumor blush. Most favored location is the lateral wall of the left ventricle followed by the anterior wall of the right ventricle and the interventriclular septum. Cardiac hemangiomas are also described to be associated with Kasabach–Merritt syndrome, which manifests as widespread systemic hemangiomas associated with recurrent thrombocytopenia. It is important to distinguish true heman-giomas from arteriovenous malformations not uncommon in and around heart. Most arteriovenous malformations communicate with the cardiac chambers by one or two aberrant vessels; however, occasionally serpiginous collection of such aberrant vessels can mimic as a hemangioma (Fig. 7).

(A)

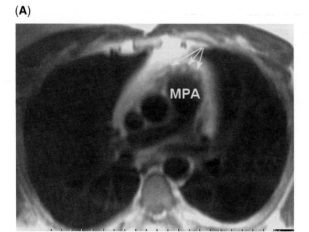

(B)

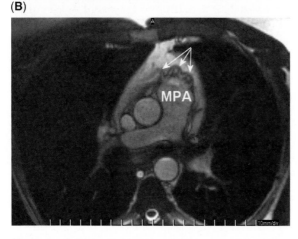

Figure 7 A 38-year-old male with history of chest pain was evaluated by coronary angiogram, which showed an aberrant vessel originating from the circumflex coronary artery with unknown termination. A right heart cathetrization with oxygen saturation was not performed, as patient underwent allergic reaction to the contrast agent while performing procedure. A cardiovascular magnetic resonance imaging (CMR) evaluation was performed, which showed two aberrant vessels originating from the left circumflex and terminated in a very tortuous and serpentine collection of vessels with three communicating ostia into the main pulmonary artery at the level just above the pulmonic valve. A collection of these vessels anterior to the main pulmonary artery (MPA) (*arrows*) may mimic a hemangioma mass (**A** and **B**). A CMR phase velocity mapping was performed on pulmonary artery and ascending aorta to evaluated pulmonary and systemic flow ratio ($Q_p:Q_s$) for shunt calculation which was 1.17:1.

On T1-weighted images hemangiomas have intermediate signal intensity compared to the surrounding myocardium and T2-weighted images allow clear delineation with high signal intensity. Because blood flow is slow in hemangiomas, after gadolinium administration, there will be high signal intensity due to longer persistence of contrast in these channels.

PARAGANGLIOMAS

Primary cardiac paragangliomas are usually intrapericardial, located over the base of the heart, but can be found anywhere in the cardiac chambers. They arise form the cardiac paraganglial cells and majority of them produce catecholamines. Most paragangliomas are located on the roof of left atrium, which is the major site of vagus nerve distribution and also the intrinsic chrommafin cells. Most tumors are flat based with poor margins.

CMR helps in preoperative evaluation and precise localization of these tumors (18). On T1-weighted images the tumor is hypointense, but on T2-weighted images there is marked increase in signal intensity (19). Gadolinium administration may give further information on tumor vascularity.

MALIGNANT TUMORS OF THE HEART

Primary cardiac malignancies are rare with few noninvasive references as to their pathology. Most of these malignancies are sarcomas arising from the myocardium or pericardium. Available data from the series published by Armed Forces Institute of Pathology on cardiac tumors indicated angiosarcoma as the most common primary malignant cardiac tumor with rhabdomyosarcoma, undifferentiated sarcoma, fibrosarcoma, malignant fibrous histiocytoma, leiomyosarcoma, and osteosarcoma following down the list of rare tumors (6,20). Although recent reports have cited the role of CMR in diagnosis and accurate delineation of the malignant tumors, the data largely remains limited to few tumors.

ANGIOSARCOMA

Lymphangiosarcoma and hemangiosarcoma are grouped under angiosarcoma, both arise from the endothelium of the lymphatics or blood vessels, respectively. Cardiac angiosarcomas are mostly hemangiosarcomas unless specified. They are very aggressive and bear poor prognosis.

Angiosarcoma occurs slightly more frequently in middle-aged males. It more frequently arises from the right atrium and presentation is often due to the compression of right-side chambers or obstruction of the tricuspid valve. Patients present with dyspnea, peripheral edema, or cardiac cachexia. Involvement of the pericardium is not uncommon and patients commonly present with cardiac tamponade.

Angiosarcomas are heterogeneous masses with a broad base and carry intermediate signal intensity on T1-weighted images interspersed with focal areas of increased signal intensity representing hemorrhagic foci. The mass may be well defined and protruding or diffusely infiltrative into the pericardium. The pericardial involvement usually leads to a hemorrhagic pericardial effusion, which on T1-weighted axial images will be of intermediate-to-high signal intensity. Such effusion should be further interrogated with T2-weighted images where it will be of high signal intensity if it is acute or subacute, whereas an intermediate-to-low signal intensity will be seen if it is chronic. Single oblique radiofrequency tissue tags are important to distinguish between the adherent and nonadherent pericardium. Signal intensity of the tumor on T2-weighted images is higher than the T1-weighted images. Kim et al. described these signal intensity patterns as "cauliflower appearance" and Yahata et al. described "sunray appearance" of contrast enhancement pattern of the vascular channels (21,22).

RHABDOMYOSARCOMA

Rhabdomyosarcoma is the most common primary cardiac malignancy in children and infants. The signal characteristics of the tumor are inconsistent and depend upon the stromal and vascular content of the tumor. Most rhabdomyomas exhibit isointensity compared to surrounding myocardium on T1-weighted images and high intensity on T2-weighted images (23). In contrast to rhabdomyoma, on Gd administration these tumors show increased contrast uptake compared to the myocardium.

RARE CARDIAC SARCOMAS

Many other cardiac sarcomas are so rare that they do not merit description in separate headlines. Most of these tumors are malignant fibrous histiocytomas, undifferentiated sarcomas, osteosarcomas, fibrosarcomas, liposarcomas, leiomyosarcomas, lymphomas, and Kaposi sarcomas.

Malignant fibrous histiocytoma commonly occur in the left atrium, and on T1-weighted images has intermediate signal intensity compared to the myocardium and high signal intensity on T2-weighted images (21,24).

Primary liposarcomas of the heart are extremely rare tumors. They commonly arise from the right ventricle but may arise from anywhere within heart including valves. Most liposarcomas metastasize by the time of diagnosis. On T1-weighted imaging, liposarcomas have lower signal intensity than the subcutaneous fat or lipomas and appear inhomogeneous because of areas of necrosis and hemorrhage (25).

Osteosarcomas commonly arise from the left atrium. Their gross and microscopic features are influenced by the basic nature of the cells forming these tumors. Most tumors are formed by osteoblasts or chondroblasts. Calcification of these tumors is not uncommon and most tumors are stone hard. On T1-weighted images, the signal intensity depends upon the amount of calcification. More calcified tumors have lower signal intensity on T1- and T2-weighted images.

Cardiac leiomyosarcomas are smooth muscle sarcomas that may arise from the smooth muscles of subendocardium, pulmonary veins, or arteries. They predominantly arise from the left atrium. On T1- and T2-weighted images they show intermediate and high signal intensity, respectively, compared to the surrounding myocardium (26).

Primary cardiac lymphoma is non-Hodgkin's lymphoma of the heart and or pericardium. Most are B-cell lymphomas. They have been reported to be commonly originating from the right atria. Versluis et al. showed high sensitivity for the CMR diagnosis of the primary cardiac lymphoma, which is isointense on T1- and T2-weighted images with heterogeneous contrast enhancement in most of the patients after Gd administration (27).

Malignant Mesothelioma of the Pericardium

Malignant pericardial mesothelioma are very rare tumors with an incidence of less than 0.0022% in 500,000 autopsy cases studied by Cohen JL in 1976 (28). Salcedo et al. reported incidence of malignant pericardial mesothelioma of 15% of all malignant tumors (29).

Most patients present with the history of general fatigue, chest pain, and progressively worsening dyspnea. Other clinical features may mimic effusive pericarditis, cardiac tamponade, and constrictive pericarditis. CMR provides substantial information about the tumor location and outlines the extent of the tumor. Mesotheliomas of the pericardium involve both parietal and visceral pericardium rarely infiltrating the myocardium. In such cases, resection of the tumor and involved pericardium is the treatment of choice.

Mesotheliomas may be seen as pericardial thickening and an associated pericardial effusion is often visible on multislice SE axial or coronal images. Larger tumors are visualized as mass occupying the pericardial space. Most literature has reported isointensity or slightly higher intensity of these tumors compared to surrounding myocardium on T1-weighted images (Fig. 8A and E) (30,31). Their signal intensity is similar to subcutaneous fat or even higher on T2-weighted images (Fig. 8B). On Gd administration, the margins of the tumor can be defined (Fig. 8C).

Metastatic Cardiac Tumors

Metastatic tumors of the heart are 20 to 40 times more common than the primary cardiac tumors. Direct extension and hematogenous spread are the two most common modes of cardiac involvement. Venous extension and lymphatic spread of the metastases to the heart are relatively rare.

Bronchial and the breast carcinoma directly invade heart and pericardium (Fig. 9). Esophageal carcinoma and mediastinal tumors may also involve cardiac structures by direct extension. CMR plays an important role in such neoplasms by accurately identifying the pericardial involvement, which is critical in surgical planning. The initial manifestations are due to pericardial effusion or tamponade. Mediastinal lymphomas commonly involve the pericardium and occasionally the heart.

Tumors may involve cardiac structures through growth along and within the blood vessels. Table 4 enlists all the tumors with venous extension to heart.

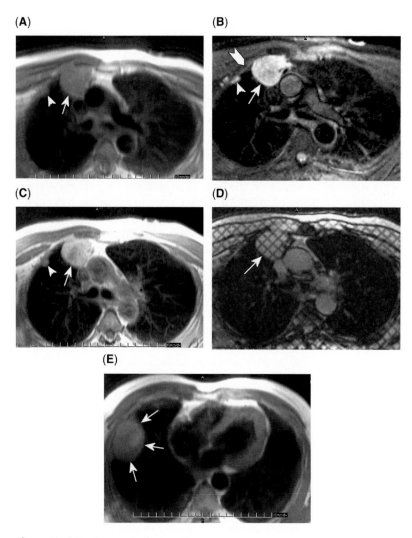

Figure 8   (*Caption on facing page*)

The intra-abdominal and pelvic tumors grow into the inferior vena cava (IVC) and extend into the right atrium (32,33). These mass lesions can be observed on CMR as filling defect of IVC opening into the right atrium (Fig. 10). These tumors may also cause severe obstruction of the IVC and the tricuspid valve and may actually protrude into the right ventricle through the valve. Thyroid and thymal tumors extend into the right atrium through the superior vena cava and lung carcinomas often use pulmonary veins to reach the left atrium (34). CMR distinguishes the size, shape, and the extension of these tumors. On CMR the tumor embolus or extension can be differentiated from the thrombus or the primary tumor of the heart.

Tumors that metastasize by hematogenous route are renal cell carcinoma bronchial carcinoma, breast carcinoma, malignant melanoma, lymphoma, and leukemia. Glancy and Roberts reported that 64% of the malignant melanoma metastasizes to heart (35). The melanotic melanoma metastases are hyperintense on T1- and T2-weighted images due to the iron-containing melanin component (36). These tumors also enhance after gadolinium administration.

CARDIAC PSEUDOMASSES

Cardiac pseudomasses are structures in or around the vicinity of heart mimicking as tumor or tumor-like structures. There are innumerable such structures classified under the broad list of pseudomasses. For clinical significance, cristae terminalis, pericardial cyst, thrombus, valvular vegetations, perivalvular abscess, aneurysms, or pseudoaneurysms will be discussed further.

Cristae terminalis also known as the terminal crest of the right atrium or taenia terminalis is present inside the cavity of right atrium corresponding to the sulcus terminalis groove on the external surface of the right atrium.

Figure 8 (*Figure on facing page*) A 67-year-old male with known pleural mesothelioma was referred for cardiovascular magnetic resonance imaging (CMR) evaluation to rule out pericardial invasion. On spin echo T1-weighted images, a large right anterior isointense mass measuring 4.7 × 4.3 cm was seen (*arrow*) (**A**). A second mass measuring 4.0 × 5.4 cm was seen in the right lateral pleural surface (*arrows*) (**E**). Multiple small lesions were also seen scattered in other parts of the pleura (*arrow head*) (**A, B,** and **C**). On T2-weighted images these masses were hyperintense (**B**) and on gadolinium (Gd) contrast images the tumors partially enhanced with central hypoperfusion (**C**). There was no invasion of the pericardium and the fat plane between the pleura and the tumor was intact. Tissue tagging was performed to illustrate disease-free pericardium (**D**). Also, CMR was very helpful in identifying adjacent periosteal invasion of the ribs (*block arrow*) (**B**), which was not evident on the preceding CT scan. The T1, T2 and post-Gd characteristics of the mesothelioma of pericardium would be similar to this case owing to identical cell cytology.

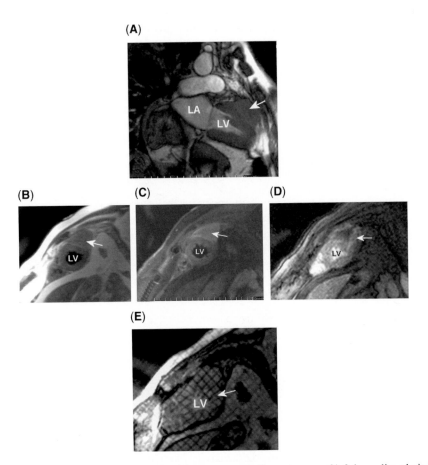

Figure 9 A 69-year-old male with squamous cell carcinoma of left lung directly infiltrating into the left ventricular wall. Two-chamber steady-state free precession cine image demonstrating direct invasion (*arrow*) of the lung carcinoma into the anterior wall of the left ventricle (LV) (**A**). T1-weighted spin echo short axis image showing the isointense signal characteristic of this mass in comparison to the LV myocardium (**B**). T2-weighted images show the mass as an slightly bright intensity compared to the LV myocardium (**C**). Gd contrast injection showed equal signal enhancement of the mass (*arrow*) and the myocardium indicating absence of necrotic core (increased signal intensity) (**D**). Tagging grid overlayed on the short axis image shows deformation of the tag margins crossing the mass border with the LV myocardium diagnostic of infiltration into the myocardium (**E**). *Abbreviations:* LA, left atrium; LV, left ventricle.

The cristae terminalis is a smooth ridge that extends from the opening of superior venae cava to the opening of inferior venae cava into the right atrium. It separates the trabeculated surface of the right atrial appendage from the smooth posterior wall and appears isointense to myocardium on

Table 4 Tumors with Venous Extension to the Heart

Renal cell carcinoma
Uterine leiomyoma
Wilms tumor
Adrenocortical carcinoma
Pheochromocytoma
Endometrial carcinoma
Hepatocellular carcinoma
Thyroid carcimoma
Lung carcinoma

(A)

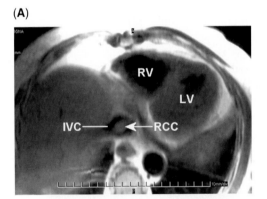

(B)

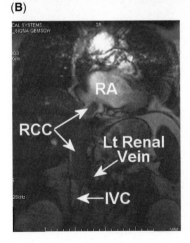

Figure 10 A 78-year-old male with venous metastasis of renal cell carcinoma (RCC) into the right atrium. T1-weighted spin echo axial image show the inferior venae cava (IVC) opacified by the extension of RCC (**A**). Coronal steady-state free precession cine images showing the RCC extending from left kidney into the left renal vein and inferior vena cava to finally enter the right atrium (**B**).

T1- and T2-weighted images (Fig. 11A and B) (37). The ridge appears dark on SSFP images (Fig. 11C) and does not enhance on Gd contrast administration.

A pericardial cyst is a commonly encountered paracardiac mass. These are the most common benign tumors of the pericardium with peak incidence in fourth decade of life. They are most commonly located at the right cardiophrenic angle, rarely communicating with the pericardium via a diverticulum. Most pericardial cysts grow to be large in size but rarely do they cause hemodynamic compromise by chamber obstruction. On CMR images they appear to have a very thin capsule with homogenous appearance (Fig. 12). The serous fluid with large water content gives them a low signal intensity on T1-weighted images and intensely bright on T2-weighted images (Fig. 12A to D) (38). The cyst may appear brighter on T1-weighted images if the protein content is high (39).

Cardiac thrombi should always be considered for differential diagnosis of the cardiac masses, as they account for most of the cases of pseudomasses. Virtually, any cardiac chamber with slow and disrupted laminar flow and associated wall motion abnormality is prone to develop thrombus. They are most commonly seen in the left ventricle with severe

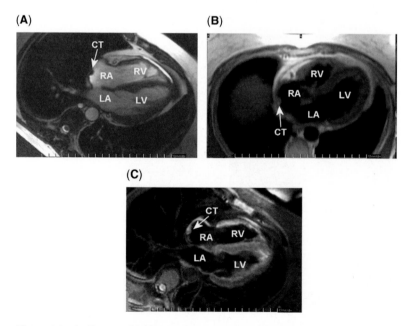

Figure 11 A 47-year-old female with normally appearing cristae terminalis. (**A**) Four-chamber steady-state free precession cine image showing the cristae terminalis (CT) located at the junction of the right atrial appendage and the posterior wall of the right atrium. (**B** and **C**) are T1- and T2-weighted images, respectively, showing the isointense nodular cristae terminalis on the inside of the right atrium. *Abbreviations*: CT, cristae terminalis; LA, left atrium; LV, left ventricle; RA, right atrium; RV, right ventricle.

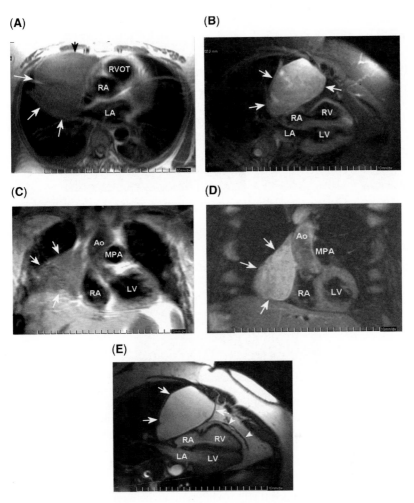

Figure 12 A 50-year-old female with pericardial cyst seen at the typical location of right cardiophrenic angle. T1-weighted spin echo image shows relative low intensity of the well-demarcated, homogenous cyst (**A** and **C**). T2-weighted axial images show the bright cystic fluid (**B** and **D**). Steady-state free precession four-chamber cine image demonstrating the clear separation of pericardium (*arrow heads*) from the pericardial cyst (*arrows*) (**E**). *Abbreviations*: Ao, aorta; LA, left atrium; LV, left ventricle; MPA, main pulmonary atrium; RA, right atrium; RV, right ventricle; RVOT, right ventricular outflow tract.

regional or global dysfunction or in left atrial appendage in patients with atrial fibrillation. The signal intensity of the thrombus is variable and depends upon the chronicity, calcification, and presence of deoxyhemoglobin and/or hemosiderin. Most thrombi have intermediate to slightly high signal intensity on T1-weighted images, which further increases on T2-weighted images

(A) (B)

(C)

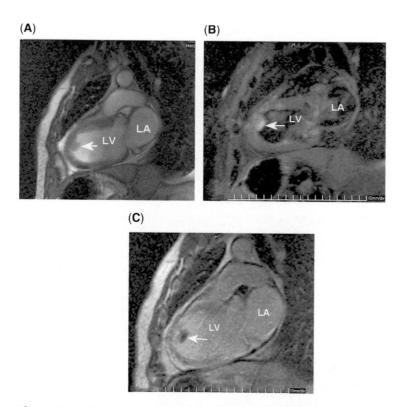

Figure 13 A 63-year-old male with left ventricular thrombus in a patient with apical akinesia. Two-chamber steady-state free precession cine image shows apical density attached to the myocardium (**A**). On T2-weighted image the thrombus is brighter compared to the myocardium (**B**). The thrombus did not uptake the gadolinium contrast agent as shown in this image (**C**). *Abbreviations*: LA, left atrium; LV, left ventricle.

(Fig. 13B) (40). At times it is difficult to differentiate between the slow flow and the stationary thrombus, in which case SSFP images are helpful. On SSFP images, the thrombus has low signal and the slow flowing blood will appear white (Fig. 13A). After Gd administration thrombus can be clearly delineated as a dark signal compared to the bright blood pool and myocardium due to lack of uptake of contrast in the thrombus (Fig. 13C). Newer techniques such as phase velocity imaging can be used to differentiate between the moving blood and stationary tissue such as thrombus. Rumancik et al. described the approach of using phase imaging by showing no phase shift in thrombus in comparison to a phase shift in slow flow (41).

Vascular aneurysms and pseudoaneurysms are commonly encountered in the vicinity of the heart and occasionally are mistaken as masses. Sinus of valsalva aneurysm, ascending aortic aneurysm or pseudoaneurysm, and rarely coronary aneurysms can masquerade as a mass (Fig. 14). Their

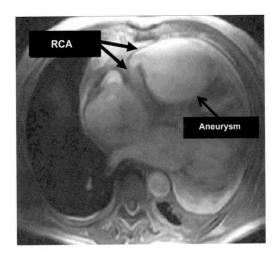

Figure 14 A 74-year-old male with 10-week history of increasing shortness of breath and chest pressure sought evaluation at outside hospital where a coronary angiogram showed an ambiguous mass with right coronary artery (RCA) feeding into it and a CT scan confirmed the findings of anterior mediastinal mass. Patient was then evaluated by cardiovascular magnetic resonance imaging and gradient–recalled echo cine images demonstrated a giant $7 \times 9 \times 9$ cm RCA aneurysm that was partially compressing the right ventricle. The RCA aneurysm was resected and the patient recovered well. *Abbreviation*: RCA, right coronary artery.

visualization on SE images should be confirmed on SSFP cine images, where it is easy to identify the flow as well as the entry and exit point of the blood. Turbulence is seen as a filling defect on SSFP images. Gadolinium contrast injection with 3D volume rendered postprocessing is sometimes used to finalize the diagnosis.

Valvular vegetations like Lambl excrescences, Libman–Sacks endocarditis, and bacterial endocarditis can be diagnosed on CMR. These vegetations may not be seen on SE images but are clearly visible on SSFP images. The bright blood on SSFP images provides contrast to low-to-intermediate signal intensity of these vegetations.

Perivalvular abscesses are common in cases of prosthetic valve endocarditis. CMR is ideal for evaluation of perivalvular abscesses by virtue of its high spatial resolution and simultaneous evaluation of the valvular function on SSFP cine images, but may be limited by the metallic valve artifact if it is a small abscess. The aortic valve ring is the most frequently involved. Abscesses on T1-weighted images have low signal intensity as compared to high signal intensity on T2-weighted images. These abscesses have been described to increased signal intensity after Gd administration owing to their inflammatory pathology (42).

CONCLUSION

The field of cardiovascular diseases is now armed with the power of CMR imaging where we not only can assess the morphology, function, perfusion, and myocardial metabolism but also distinctly characterize the tissue. The use of noniodinated and nonnephrotoxic gadolinium contrast agents has greatly enhanced the imaging experience. Newer fibrin avid contrast agents are under trial, which will further increase the specificity of identifying thrombus- and fibrin-rich masses. CMR can be used as a confirmatory imaging modality after evaluation by echocardiography or CT scans, as well as a destination diagnostic modality for patients who need follow-up to track tumor progression or reoccurance after therapy. Finally, the greatest advantage of CMR is in its confidence in making the noninvasive tissue diagnosis of cardiac masses and its pivotal role in surgical planning.

REFERENCES

1. Freedberg RS, Kronzon I, Rumancik WM, Liebeskind D. The contribution of magnetic resonance imaging to the evaluation of intracardiac tumors diagnosed by echocardiography. Circulation 1988; 77(1):96–103.
2. Lund JT, Ehman RL, Julsrud PR, Sinak LJ, Tajik AJ. Cardiac masses: assessment by MR imaging. AJR Am J Roentgenol 1989; 152(3):469–473.
3. Sechtem U, Tscholakoff D, Higgins CB. MRI of the abnormal pericardium. AJR Am J Roentgenol. 1986; 147(2):245–252.
4. Bouton S, Yang A, McCrindle BW, Kidd L, McVeigh ER, Zerhouni EA. Differentiation of tumor from viable myocardium using cardiac tagging with MR imaging. J Comput Assist Tomogr 1991; 15(4):676–678.
5. Semelka RC, Shoenut JP, Wilson ME, Pellech AE, Patton JN. Cardiac masses: signal intensity features on spin echo, gradient-echo, gadolinium-enhanced spin echo, and TurboFLASH images. J Magn Reson Imaging 1992; 2(4):415–420.
6. McAllister HA Jr. Primary tumors and cysts of the heart and pericardium. Curr Probl Cardiol 1979; 4(2):1–51; Review.
7. Hoffmann U, Globits S, Schima W, et al. Usefulness of magnetic resonance imaging of cardiac and paracardiac masses. Am J Cardiol 2003; 92(7):890–895.
8. Carney JA. The Carney complex (myxomas, spotty pigmentation, endocrine overactivity, and schwannomas). Dermatol Clin 1995; 13(1):19–26. Review.
9. Carney JA, Gordon H, Carpenter PC, Shenoy BV, Go VL. The complex of myxomas, spotty pigmentation, and endocrine overactivity. Medicine (Baltimore) 1985; 64(4):270–283.
10. Masui T, Takahashi M, Miura K, Naito M, Tawarahara K. Cardiac myxoma: identification of intratumoral hemorrhage and calcification on MR images. AJR Am J Roentgenol 1995; 164(4):850–852.
11. Holley DG, Martin GR, Brenner JI, et al. Diagnosis and management of fetal cardiac tumors: a multicenter experience and review of published reports. J Am Coll Cardiol 1995; 26(2):516–520.

12. Bass JL, Breningstall GN, Swaiman KF. Echocardiographic incidence of cardiac rhabdomyoma in tuberous sclerosis. Am J Cardiol 1985; 55(11):1379–1382.

13. Coffin CM. Congenital cardiac fibroma associated with Gorlin syndrome. Pediatr Pathol 1992; 12(2):255–262.

14. Funari M, Fujita N, Peck WW, Higgins CB. Cardiac tumors: assessment with Gd-DTPA enhanced MR imaging. J Comput Assist Tomogr 1991; 15(6):953–958.

15. McAllister HA Jr., Fenoglio JJ Jr. Tumors of the Cardiovascular System. In: Hartmann WH, ed. Atlas of Tumor Pathology. Washington, D.C.: Armed Forces Institute of Pathology, 1978.

16. Edwards FH, Hale D, Cohen A, Thompson L, Pezzella AT, Virmani R. Primary cardiac valve tumors. Ann Thorac Surg 1991; 52(5):1127–1131.

17. al-Mohammad A, Pambakian H, Young C. Fibroelastoma: case report and review of the literature Heart 1998; 79(3):301–304. Review.

18. Conti VR, Saydjari R, Amparo EG. Paraganglioma of the heart. The value of magnetic resonance imaging in the preoperative evaluation. Chest 1986; 90(4):604–606.

19. Varghese JC, Hahn PF, Papanicolaou N, Mayo-Smith WW, Gaa JA, Lee MJ. MR differentiation of phaeochromocytoma from other adrenal lesions based on qualitative analysis of T2 relaxation times. Clin Radiol 1997; 52(8):603–606.

20. Burke A, Virmani R. Tumors of the heart and great vessels. In: Atlas of Tumor Pathology. 3rd series, fasc 16. Washington, D.C.: Armed Forces Institute of Pathology, 1996.

21. Kim EE, Wallace S, Abello R, et al. Malignant cardiac fibrous histiocytomas and angiosarcomas: MR features. J Comput Assist Tomogr 1989; 13(4):627–632.

22. Yahata S, Endo T, Honma H, et al. Sunray appearance on enhanced magnetic resonance image of cardiac angiosarcoma with pericardial obliteration. Am Heart J 1994; 127(2):468–471.

23. Villacampa VM, Villarreal M, Ros LH, Alvarez R, Cozar M, Fuertes MI. Cardiac rhabdomyosarcoma: diagnosis by MR imaging. Eur Radiol 1999; 9(4): 634–637.

24. Mahajan H, Kim EE, Wallace S, Abello R, Benjamin R, Evans HL. Magnetic resonance imaging of malignant fibrous histiocytoma. Magn Reson Imaging 1989; 7(3):283–288.

25. Dooms GC, Hricak H, Sollitto RA, Higgins CB. Lipomatous tumors and tumors with fatty component: MR imaging potential and comparison of MR and CT results. Radiology 1985; 157(2):479–483.

26. Lo FL, Chou YH, Tiu CM, et al. Primary cardiac leiomyosarcoma: imaging with 2-D echocardiography, electron beam CT and 1.5-Tesla MR. Eur J Radiol 1998; 27(1):72–76.

27. Versluis PJ, Lamers RJ, van Belle AF. Primary malignant lymphoma of the heart: CT and MRI features. Rofo Fortschr Geb Rontgenstr Neuen Bildgeb Verfahr 1995; 162(6):533–534. Review.

28. Cohen JL. Neoplastic pericarditis. Cardiovasc Clin 1976; 7(3):257–269.

29. Salcedo EE, Cohen GI, White RD, Davison MB. Cardiac tumors: diagnosis and management. Curr Probl Cardiol 1992; 17(2):73–137.

30. Kaminaga T, Yamada N, Imakita S, Takamiya M, Nishimura T. Magnetic resonance imaging of pericardial malignant mesothelioma. Magn Reson Imaging 1993; 11(7):1057–1061.

31. Gossinger HD, Siostrzonek P, Zangeneh M, et al. Magnetic resonance imaging findings in a patient with pericardial mesothelioma. Am Heart J 1988; 115(6): 1321–1322.
32. Nguyen BD, Westra WH, Zerhouni EA. Renal cell carcinoma and tumor thrombus neovascularity: MR demonstration with pathologic correlation. Abdom Imaging 1996; 21(3):269–271.
33. Choh JH, Gurney R, Shenoy SS, Upson J, Lajos TZ. Renal-cell carcinoma; removal of intracardiac extension with aid of cardiopulmonary bypass. N Y State J Med 1981; 81(6):929–932.
34. Gandhi AK, Pearson AC, Orsinelli DA. Tumor invasion of the pulmonary veins: a unique source of systemic embolism detected by transesophageal echocardiography. J Am Soc Echocardiogr 1995; 8(1):97–99.
35. Glancy DL, Roberts WC. The heart in malignant melanoma. A study of 70 autopsy cases. Am J Cardiol 1968; 21(4):555–571.
36. Mousseaux E, Meunier P, Azancott S, Dubayle P, Gaux JC. Cardiac metastatic melanoma investigated by magnetic resonance imaging. Magn Reson Imaging 1998; 16(1):91–95.
37. Mirowitz SA, Gutierrez FR. Fibromuscular elements of the right atrium: pseudomass at MR imaging. Radiology 1992; 182(1):231–233.
38. Vinee P, Stover B, Sigmund G, et al. MR imaging of the pericardial cyst. J Magn Reson Imaging 1992; 2(5):593–596.
39. Murayama S, Murakami J, Watanabe H, et al. Signal intensity characteristics of mediastinal cystic masses on T1-weighted MRI. J Comput Assist Tomogr 1995; 19(2):188–191.
40. Dooms GC, Higgins CB. MR imaging of cardiac thrombi. J Comput Assist Tomogr 1986; 10(3):415–420.
41. Rumancik WM, Naidich DP, Chandra R, et al. Cardiovascular disease: evaluation with MR phase imaging. Radiology 1988; 166(1 Pt 1):63–68.
42. Furber A, Geslin P, Le Jeune JJ, et al. Value of MRI with injection of gadolinium in the diagnosis of mitral ring abscess. Apropos of a case. Arch Mal Coeur Vaiss 1997; 90(3):399–404.

17

The Aorta and Great Vessels

Agostino Meduri

Department of Radiology, Catholic University of Rome, Rome, Italy

THE NORMAL AORTA

The thoracic aorta consists of an ascending segment, the arch, and a descending segment. The aortic root is the most proximal portion of the aorta, which is formed by the aortic valve, the annulus, and the aortic sinuses where the aorta has the largest diameter. The coronary arteries arise from the left and right sinuses of Valsalva. The ascending aorta is about 5 cm in length. The aortic diameter becomes mildly larger at the junction of the ascending aorta with the arch (bulb of the aorta). The proximal part of the aortic arch gives rise to the innominate artery, the left carotid, and the left subclavian artery. The most frequent variations of the origin of the great vessels are the common origin of the innominate and left carotid artery, and the separate origin of the left vertebral artery between the left carotid and left subclavian artery. The innominate artery divides in the uppermost portion of the mediastinum; the visualization of four vessels immediately cranial to the arch is frequently associated with an aortic arch anomaly. The junction of the arch with the descending aorta is called aortic isthmus. It extends from the left subclavian artery to the ligamentum arteriosus and is slightly narrower than the proximal and distal segments. The descending aorta is mildly dilated immediately after the ligamentum arteriosus (aortic spindle). The major branches of the descending thoracic aorta are the intercostal and bronchial arteries. The abdominal aorta gives rise to the celiac axis, the

Table 1 Normal Aortic Diameters

Aortic valve sinus	2.98 ± 0.46 cm
Ascending aorta	3.09 ± 0.41 cm
Ascending aorta proximal to the innominate artery	2.94 ± 0.42 cm
Proximal aortic arch	2.77 ± 0.37 cm
Distal aortic arch	2.61 ± 0.41 cm
Aortic isthmus	2.47 ± 0.40 cm
Descending aorta (diaphragmatic level)	2.43 ± 0.35 cm

superior and inferior mesenteric arteries, and the renal arteries. At the iliac bifurcation, it divides into the common iliac arteries.

The aortic diameter tapers progressively and smoothly so that the ascending aorta is larger than the arch and the descending aorta (Table 1) (1). Aortic size is dependent on age, and the ascending aorta dimensions increases more than the area of the arch or of the descending aorta (2).

TECHNIQUES

CMR has emerged as a valuable tool for evaluating both congenital and acquired diseases of the aorta. CMR has the advantages that it can image in multiple planes, evaluate valvular competency, quantify flow, does not use ionizing radiation, nor require iodinated contrast media (3–5).

The morphological study of the aorta is based on the family of spin echo (SE) images that are most widely used to visualize aortic anatomy (6). On SE images, circulating blood in the aortic lumen presents as an absence of signal due to the wash-out phenomenon (dark blood); however, slow flowing blood, excited by both the 90° and 180° pulses, produces signal appearing gray or white in the image (7). The high spatial resolution and contrast between the lumen and vessel wall are ideal for depicting anatomic details and allow for the evaluation of mural pathology. Standard SE T1-weighted images are acquired with an echo time of 20–30 msec, whereas TR is equal to the RR interval time. Slice thickness is 5–8 mm in the high-resolution matrix.

Black-blood fast SE sequences acquire images in a single breath hold (16 heart beats/image) with reduced imaging time, eliminating respiratory, and motion artifacts (8,9). A double-inversion preparation pulse is used to null the signal of flowing blood. The first pulse is not slice-selective and inverts the magnetization in the whole tissue volume, while the second pulse is slice-selective and restores the signal in the slice to be imaged. At a specific inversion time, signal of blood entering the slice is nulled, therefore it appears "black." Fast SE sequences make it possible to acquire high-quality T2-weighed images (TE = 80–100 msec) allowing tissue characterization to be performed which is helpful in evaluating patients with graft infection or aortitis. CMR is insensitive to calcium so that atheromatic calcifications or the displacement of intimal calcifications are not detected.

Parallel imaging allows a significant decrease in the imaging time, as k-space is only partially explored and the final images are reconstructed by integrating signals from the different elements of the phased-array coil.

T1-weighted gradient echo (GRE) with fat saturation (GRE-FS) pre and postcontrast provides an overview of the aorta and surrounding structures and is useful in evaluating luminal and intramural pathologies.

The functional/dynamic study is performed with cine techniques. In these images, blood in laminar flow through the plane appears hyperintense (bright). This technique is particularly useful in distinguishing thrombosis (hypointense) from slow flow (high intensity, variable during the cardiac cycle).

Turbulent flow causes loss of coherence of the spins and is detected as a "black" area of signal void. Several technical parameters have an effect on the conspicuity of the signal void phenomenon. The most important is the echo time and the turbulent area is more evident with longer TEs.

GRE cine sequences acquire multiple images per cardiac cycle that can be displayed in cine mode. Conventional GRE sequences use TE of 8–14 msec, TR of 20–40 msec, and low flip angles. The conventional GRE sequences are time-consuming (3–4 min for 1–2 slices) and the images are often degraded by respiratory motion artifacts.

Fast GRE sequences shorten the acquisition time so that 20–30 images per cardiac cycle can be acquired during a breath hold. Using fast GRE, it is therefore possible to perform a more complete study and generate images free from breathing artifacts. Echo times range from 3 to 8 sec, with TRs of 7–12 msec.

Steady–state free precession (SSFP) is bright-blood imaging pulse sequences that use fully balanced gradients to rephase the transverse magnetization at the end of each TR interval. These sequences produce high SNR images at very short sequence times. The resulting signal intensity is independent of TR and related to T2/T1 ratio. Therefore, tissues with high T2/T1 ratios (such as blood, cerebral-spinal fluid, water, and fat) display high signal, whereas signal is reduced from tissues with low T2/T1 ratios (such as muscle and myocardium). The sequence can be implemented as a cine or a multi-slice technique. Images are acquired during a single breath hold. Additionally, the sequence can be acquired as multi-slice during free breathing to allow a rapid examination in acute or non-cooperative patients. Contrast between flowing blood and the aortic wall is optimal because blood's high signal is dependent only from its T2/T1 ratio and not from inflow phenomena (11). Therefore, signal is bright even when the imaging plane is parallel to the flow direction.

Magnetic resonance angiography (MRA) is a revolutionary tool in vascular imaging. It permits angiographic assessment of the thoracic aortic anatomy and accurately images branch vessels. Angiographic images can be obtained with time of flight, phase contrast, and 3D dynamic contrast-enhanced MRA (CE-MRA) sequences (11).

In time-of-flight sequences, the stationary tissue signal is suppressed, whereas the inflowing blood does not become saturated and appears hyper-intense. If the blood vessel has a course parallel to the imaging plane or in the case of slow flow, blood may become saturated and its signal is then suppressed (12).

Phase-contrast MRA relies on the phase shift that blood experiences when flowing along a magnetic gradient. To determine flow in all directions, it is necessary to repeat the sequence changing the axis of the magnetic gradient and thus increasing the imaging time.

Excellent results are obtained with CE-MRA (13–16). This 3D T1-weighed GRE sequence is acquired during a bolus infusion of paramagnetic contrast that reduces T1 shortening with high signal contrast of the opacified blood vessels (17,18). Three-dimensional images offer a unique perspective of vascular anatomy. CE-MRA has proven useful in diagnosing abnormalities obscured by slow or turbulent flow in the SE and cine GRE images, as well as for the study of complicated small vessel anomalies.

High magnetic fields and gradient strength allow very short TR and TEs so that 3D images can be acquired during the arterial phase and in a single breath hold. Timing of the bolus to achieve maximum contrast within the arteries allows suppression of the venous enhancement. Optimal timing is obtained by observing the transit time of a test bolus of 2 ml of contrast or by using a pulse sequence designed to sense the arrival of contrast and triggers the angiographic sequence (19). Most reproducible results require an automatic bolus injector; $20-40\,cm^3$ of Gd-DTPA are injected at a rate of $2.5-5\,ml/sec$.

Source images must be evaluated directly or through multiplanar reformatting. In maximum intensity projection (MIP), post-processed images of only the highest signal intensity voxels are displayed, thus creating good visualization of the vascular structures. Volume 3D reconstruction produces three-dimensional images of the vessels. The entire data set is used to select only the desired anatomical structures that can be displayed from different points of view. Major indications of MRA are the study of aneurysms, penetrating ulcers, dissection, congenital anomalies, and patency of bypass grafts.

Flow velocity mapping can be used to assess blood flow within the aorta and its branches, to measure velocity gradients across stenoses, and to quantify shunts (20–22). This technique is based on phase-contrast sequences. The MRI signal possesses both phase and amplitude. It is possible to encode velocity or acceleration in the phase of a signal by applying a gradient in the direction of flow. After reversing the gradient, the moving protons experience a phase shift proportional to the velocity, meanwhile the static spins are rephased.

The velocity is displayed using different gray levels to represent intensity and direction of flow. Velocity curves and instantaneous flow volume can be calculated. With this technique, CMR can reliably measure the aortic flow and the elastic properties of aorta. In the aorta, there is forward flow during systole and early diastole. In diastole, there is both forward as well as retrograde flow, the latter is mainly posterior in the ascending segment and anterior in the descending aorta. The normal flow is at rest 6 l/min in the ascending aorta and 3.9 l/min in the descending aorta; peak systolic flow may reach 40 and 30 ml/sec, respectively (23).

Flow into the carotid arteries and into the other aortic major branches is continuous and no retrograde flow is normally seen. The stroke volume and cardiac output obtained with the flow analysis method consistently agree with those obtained from LV volume measures.

AORTIC ANEURYSMS

Clinical Background

An aortic aneurysm is a permanent dilatation of the aortic lumen, exceeding the expected diameter 1.5 times or more (24), that interests all the three layers of the wall (intima, media, and adventitia). Aneurysmal disease often is multifocal or diffuse so that the evaluation of the entire aorta is mandatory (25).

The shape of aneurysms can be saccular (Fig. 1) or fusiform (Fig. 2). Fusiform aneurysms are spindle-shaped, the dilatation involving the whole circumference of long segments of the arterial wall. In saccular aneurysms, the dilatation is more localized appearing as an outpouching of the wall, usually with a narrow neck.

Atherosclerosis is the most common cause of aortic aneurysms. They may involve all the aortic segments and are often multiple (Figs. 3 and 4). Atherosclerotic aneurysms are usually fusiform but may be saccular (26) as a result of penetrating ulcers. In a patient with an aortic aneurysm, the whole aorta should be examined. Infrarenal abdominal aortic aneurysms are the most common (Fig. 5) (27,28); the suprarenal aorta is mainly involved by thoraco-abdominal aneurysms (Fig. 6). In the thoracic aorta, they are more commonly found in the proximal descending tract. The aortic sinus, ascending aorta, and the arch are rarely affected.

Ascending aorta aneurysms are mainly caused by cystic medial degeneration. They are fusiform and spare the arch. In annulo-aortic ectasia, the proximal ascending aorta, the sinuses of Valsalva, and the aortic annulus are dilated with resulting aortic insufficiency (29). The aneurismal dilatation is confined to the ascending aorta with sparing of the arch. Cystic medial degeneration is frequent in patients with Marfan's syndrome (Figs. 7 and 8), and may be associated with other connective tissue disorders. The dilatation of the ascending aorta may lead to dissection or rupture (30). Surgical

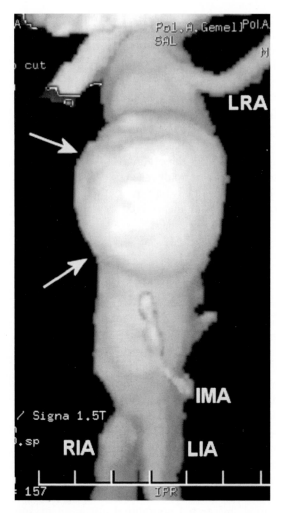

Figure 1 Descending aorta sacciform aneurysm. Contrast-enhanced-MRA 3D volume reconstruction. A sacciform atherosclerotic aneurysm (*arrows*) can be appreciated in the infrarenal descending aorta. *Abbreviations*: LRA, left renal artery; IMA, inferior mesenteric artery; RIA, right iliac artery; LIA, left iliac artery.

replacement must be considered when the diameter exceeds 55 mm. CMR allows an accurate follow-up of this condition. Aneurysmal ascending aorta dilatation can also be seen in severe aortic stenosis and aortic aneurysms can be associated with infectious or non-infectious aortitis.

Mycotic aneurysms originate from a primary infection of the aortic wall (31,32). It can be produced by septic embolization of the aortic vasa vasorum. The emboli may originate from infective endocarditis. Mycotic

(A) **(B)**

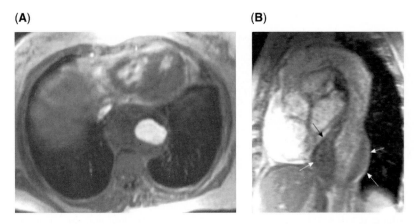

Figure 2 Thoracic fusiform aneurysm. (**A**) Fast gradient echo (GRE) axial image and (**B**) fast GRE oblique sagittal image. There is a fusiform aneurysm of the descending aorta. The aortic walls are lined with extensive thrombotic apposition.

aneurysms also result from trauma or super-infection of a pre-existing aneurysm. They are more often saccular, and more frequent in the ascending aorta. Unless resected, they tend to rupture.

Syphilitic aneurysms are nowadays rare, they are saccular, more often located in the ascending aorta, arch, or proximal descending tract (33–35).

(A) **(B)** **(C)**

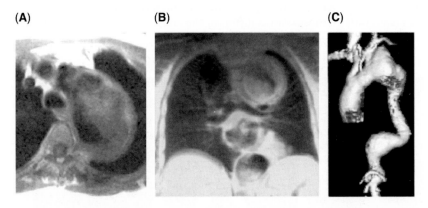

Figure 3 Aneurysm of the aortic isthmus and of the thoracic-abdominal descending aorta. (**A**) BBFSE axial image, (**B**) BBFSE coronal image, and (**C**) Contrast-enhanced-MRA 3D volume reconstruction. The aorta is dilated after the emergence of the left subclavian artery. The signal evident at this level in the aortic lumen is related to slow flow and mural thrombosis (**A,B**). The descending aorta is elongated and tortuous. A second aortic aneurysm can be seen at the thoracic-abdominal junction (**B,C**). *Abbreviations*: BBFSE, bromphenol blue, FICOLL®, SDS, EDTA loading dye; MRA, magnetic resonance angiography.

(A)   (B)   (C)

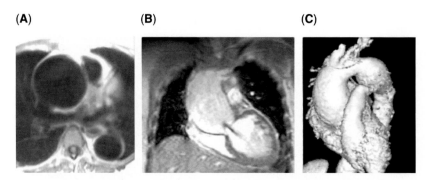

Figure 4 Aneurysms of the ascending aorta and of the proximal descending aorta.
(A) BBFSE axial image, (B) fast gradient echo (GRE) coronal image, and (C) Contrast-enhanced-MRA 3D volume reconstruction. The aortic root and the ascending
aorta are dilated. On the BBFSE image, there is no evidence of thrombosis. (A) A
turbulence jet of aortic regurgitation is evident on the fast GRE image. The 3D volume reconstruction shows a second aneurysm of the proximal descending aorta (C).
Abbreviations: BBFSE, bromphenol blue, FICOLL®, SDS, EDTA loading dye;
GRE, gradient echo; MRA, magnetic resonance angiography.

In Takayasu's arteritis, aneurysms are observed less commonly than
stenoses (Fig. 9) (36–39). In its early stage, the only morphologic change
may be subtle inflammatory wall thickening of the aorta and its branches
without significant stenosis. CMR displays concentric wall thickening, T2-
weighted hyperintensity, and post-contrast enhancement of the inflamed
vessel walls (40). Stenoses or occlusion of the arch vessels can be seen. Other

(A)   (B)   (C)

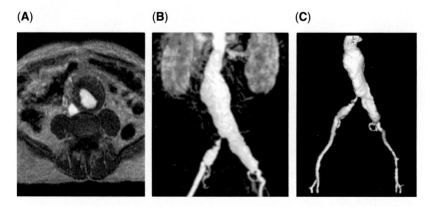

Figure 5 Abdominal aortic aneurysm. (A) Fast gradient echo (GRE) image,
(B) Contrast-enhanced-MRA MIP reconstruction, and (C) CE-MRA 3D volume
reconstruction. The infrarenal aorta is dilated. The aortic wall is lined with thrombotic apposition (A). The aneurysm extends into the iliac arteries. A stenosis of the
origin of the right iliac artery is appreciated (B,C). *Abbreviations*: CE-MRA, contrast-
enhanced MRA; MIP, maximum intensity projection.

(A) (B)

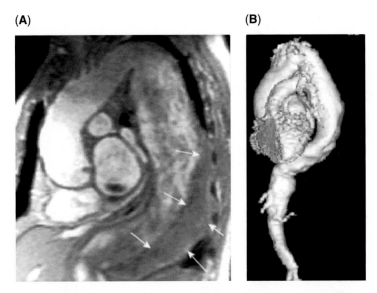

Figure 6 Thoraco-abdominal aneurysm. (A) Fast gradient echo (GRE) oblique sagittal image and (B) Contrast-enhanced-MRA 3D volume reconstruction. The thoracic aorta is aneurysmal and the dilatation extends to the upper abdominal aorta. There is extensive parietal thrombotic apposition at the thoraco-abdominal junction (*arrows*). *Abbreviations*: GRE, gradient echo; MRA, magnetic resonance angiography.

causes of aortitis include giant cell arteritis and HLA B27-associated spondyloarthropathies (41).

Abdominal inflammatory aneurysms demonstrate a thickened wall and a periaortic cuff of phlogistic tissue encasing the surrounding structures.

(A) (B) (C)

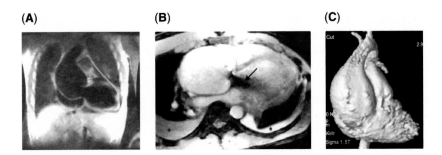

Figure 7 Marfan syndrome. (A) Coronal BBFSE, (B) left ventricular outflow tract (LVOT) fast GRE, and (C) Contrast-enhanced-MRA 3D volume reconstruction. The ascending aorta and the aortic root are markedly dilated. The aortic arch is spared and has normal diameter. A turbulence jet of aortic regurgitation can be appreciated (*arrow*). There is bilateral pleural effusion (*). *Abbreviations*: BBFSE, bromphenol blue, FICOLL®, SDS, EDTA loading dye; MRA, magnetic resonance angiography.

(A)   (B)

(C)   (D)

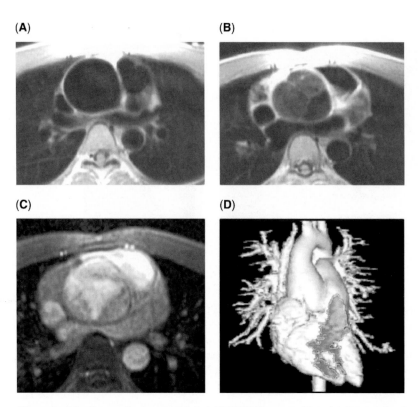

Figure 8 Marfan syndrome. (**A**, **B**) Axial BBFSE images, (**C**) axial fast gradiend echo, (**D**) Contrast-enhanced-MRA 3D volume reconstruction. Aneurysmal dilatation of the ascending aorta (**A**) and of the aortic root (**B**, **C**). The dilatation is confined to these segments while the aortic arch has normal diameter (**D**). *Abbreviations*: BBFSE, bromphenol blue, FICOLL®, SDS, EDTA loading dye; MRA, magnetic resonance angiography.

CMR demonstrates an intermediate signal, but with an intense enhancement after gadolinium injection.

Poststenotic aortic aneurysms can be found in or distal to a coarctation of the aorta. Pseudoaneurysms represent a contained perforation of the aorta; their wall is incomplete, does not contain intima, and is composed only by adventitia, portions of the media, and perivascular connective tissues. They communicate with the aortic lumen through a narrow neck (42).

Pseudoaneurysms can be acute or chronic and late presentation is not unusual. They can result from penetrating ulcers or infections. They may also developed as a complication after cardiac surgery (Fig. 10) arising from dehiscent aortic suture lines as in aortic valve replacement, bypass grafting, or from sites of aortic cannulation (43–45).

Posttraumatic pseudoaneurysms (Figs. 11 and 12) usually develop after a blunt trauma. They often arise near the ligamentum arteriosum

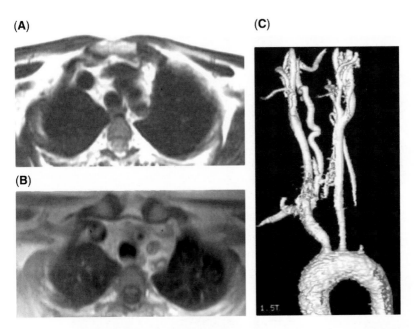

Figure 9 Takayasu's disease. (**A**) BBFSE T1-weighted axial image, (**B**) BBFSE T2-weighted axial image, and (**C**) Contrast-enhanced-MRA 3D volume reconstruction. The walls of the supraaortic vessels are thickened (**A,B**) and hyperintense on the T2-weighted image. The 3D volume reconstruction shows complete occlusion of the left subclavian artery and moderate stenosis of the origin of the brachiocephalic artery. Only the upper two-thirds of the left vertebral artery can be seen. *Abbreviations*: BBFSE, bromphenol blue, FICOLL®, SDS, EDTA loading dye; MRA, magnetic resonance angiography.

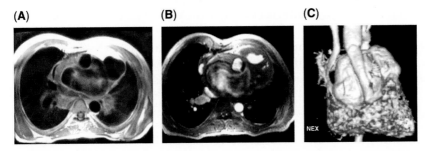

Figure 10 Postsurgical pseudoaneurysm of the ascending aorta. (**A**) BBFSE axial, (**B**) fast gradient echo axial, and (**C**) 3D volume reconstruction. The ascending aorta has been replaced by a tube graft (*arrow*). A large pseudoaneurysm can be seen posterior to the graft and posteromedial to the main pulmonary artery. The aneurysm is fed by a dehiscence of its proximal suture (**B**). The aneurysmal walls are lined with thrombosis (**A,B**).

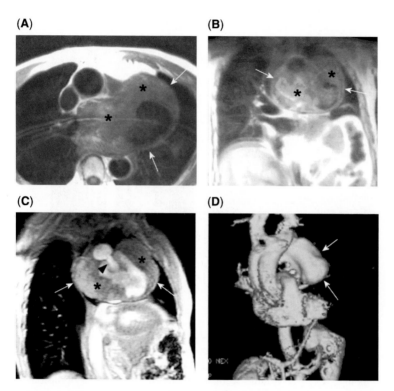

Figure 11 Pseudoaneurysm of the aortic arch. (**A**) BBFSE axial, (**B**) BBFSE coronal, (**C**) fast gradient echo (GRE) right anterior oblique images, and (**D**) 3D Contrast-enhanced-MRA volume reconstruction. A large pseudoaneurysm (*arrows*) is present inferiorly and on the left of the aortic arch. Its walls are extensively thrombosed (∗). Flow from the aortic arch to the pseudoaneurysm cavity can be appreciated as a high velocity laminar jet (*arrowhead*) on the fast GRE image. *Abbreviations*: BBFSE, bromphenol blue, FICOLL®, SDS, EDTA loading dye; GRE, gradient echo; GRA, magnetic resonance angiography.

because that is the less mobile portion of the aorta (70%) or in the ascending aorta just proximal to the innominate artery (30%). Pseudoaneurysms can rupture into nearby structures such as the mediastinum or pericardium.

Why CMR?

For most patients with aneurysmal disease, CMR is the most appropriate investigation (46,47). CMR can determine aortic dimensions and detect mural and intraluminal alterations with nearly 100% accuracy. Rapid breath-hold MRI and MRA techniques further strengthened the capability of CMR to evaluate the aorta. MRI is a safe, non-invasive investigation, allows a wide field of view and multiplanar imaging with ability to show complicated 3D relationships. Cine CMR provides all the functional information that can be obtained by echocardiography; it is not affected by acoustic shadowing

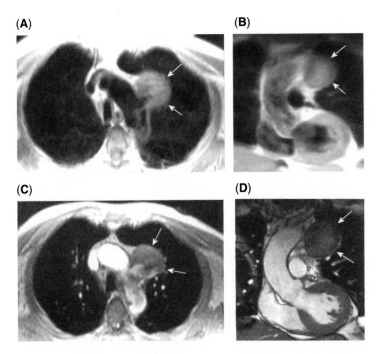

Figure 12 Pseudoaneurysm of the aortic arch. (**A**) BBFSE axial, (**B**) BBFSE coronal, (**C**) fast gradient echo (GRE) axial, and (**D**) fast GRE coronal. A pseudoaneurysm (*arrows*) is present on the left of the aortic arch. Its walls are extensively thrombosed. Flow from the aortic arch to the pseudoaneurysm cavity can be appreciated as a signal void on the axial BBFSE image (**A**) and as an high-intensity signal area on the axial fast GRE image (**B**). *Abbreviations*: BBFSE, bromphenol blue, FICOLL®, SDS, EDTA loading dye; GRE, gradient echo.

and beam hardening artifacts. In contrast, its major limitation is its inability to detect calcifications.

Image Analysis

It is important to define the shape of the aneurysm, its diameter and longitudinal extent, the extent of parietal thrombosis and of the residual flow within the lumen, the relationship with the emerging vessels, and surrounding structures (Table 2). The proposed imaging strategy can be applied to study the aorta in the suspect or presence of aneurysmal disease (Table 3). An aortic aneurysm has a diameter at least 1.5 times larger than that of the normal vessel; the normal luminal dimension varies with age, sex, physical constitution, and anatomical level; a threshold of 4 cm is often used. The ascending aorta is normally 1.5 times larger than that of the descending aorta. Aortic aneurysms are easily identified on SE images that allow a reliable measure of the vessel diameter (48). On axial images, it is more

Table 2 Relevant Information in Aortic Aneurysms

Localization
Shape
Length
Diameter and luminal dimensions
Wall assessment (thrombosis, aortitis, dissection, ulcers)
Relations to branch vessels
Effect on surrounding structures
Signs of rupture (paraaortic hematoma)
Involvement of aortic valve
Growth rate

accurate to measure the shorter aortic diameter, because measuring the longer diameter may lead to errors caused by the tortuosity of the vessel.

The longitudinal extension of the aneurysm is more easily measured on sagittal, left oblique sagittal, and coronal images. 3D CE-MRA accurately defines the aneurysm extension (49) but in the presence of parietal thrombosis it may underestimate the diameter (Figs. 5,6 and 13). Repeated studies are useful to document the expansion rate of the aneurysms. The mean growth rate is 0.12 cm/yr. Thoracic aneurysms grow more rapidly than the abdominal ones (0.42 vs. 0.28 cm/yr). High-resolution images provide a good definition of the aortic wall. Atherosclerotic lesions appear as areas of increased wall thickness, with irregular profile, of medium-to-high signal. Parietal thrombotic apposition may be crescentic or circumferential; the aneurysmatic lumen can be extensively thrombosed particularly in larger aneurysms (Figs. 5,6,13 and 14).

Organized thrombi are hypointense, whereas unorganized thrombi are hyperintense on both T1- and T2-weighted images; partially organized thrombi have inhomogeneous signal intensity with hyperintense areas on both T1- and T2-weighted images. Subacute thrombosis may appear bright on GRE images but its signal intensity remains constant throughout the cardiac cycle, whereas the signal intensity of flowing blood flow changes. MRI is unable to image calcifications. Organized thrombosis is hypointense on GRE images and is therefore easily distinguished from slow flow.

It is necessary to evaluate the relationship of the aneurysm with the aortic branches and assess their eventual involvement. The involvement of the arch vessels or of the celiac axis, mesenteric and renal arteries may change the surgical management. Aortic aneurysms can displace and compress the surrounding structures.

Thoracic aneurysms may displace/compress the superior vena cava, brachiocephalic veins, the pulmonary artery and its main branches, the trachea and main bronchi, the esophagus, the atria (more often the left atrium), and the pulmonary veins. Descending thoracic and abdominal aneurysms may cause erosion of the vertebral bodies and compress the inferior vena cava.

Table 3 Aneurysms: Imaging Strategy

Axial black blood FSE	FB or BH	From 1–2 cm above the arch to the diaphragm.
Axial fast GRE or SSFP	Single phase. Fast GRE BH SSFP BH o FB	Study of mural. luminal, parietal and extramural lesions Measure of ascending aortic dimensions. The examination is extended to the abdomen to assess the presence of pathology of the abdominal aorta
LAO SE	BH	Images the entire length of the thoracic aorta in a single plane. Obtained by setting the slice through the ascending and descending aorta and parallel to the arch
LAO Fast GRE or SSFP	multiphase BH	Longitudinal extension of the aneurysm Measure of aortic dimensions
CE-MRA sagittal	BH	3D sagittal slab planned to include both the ascending and descending aorta. Comprehensive evaluation of aortic anatomy and branches
Optional sequences Coronal oblique	BH	Ascending aorta aneurysms Planned on axial images or on an oblique coronal plan through the aortic root and the LVOT. Study of the ascending aorta and AV regurgitation
LVOT	BH	Ascending aorta aneurysms AV regurgitation
Axial T1W fat-sat GRE	BH	Inflammatory aneurysms Aortitis Suspect of ruptured aneurysm Suspect of graft leakage or endoleakage Evidence of periaortic enhancement
Axial T2W black blood FSE	BH	Inflammatory aneurysms Aortitis

Abbreviations: LVOT, left ventricular outflow tract; LAO, left anterior oblique; FB, free breathing; BH, breath-hold; AV, aortic valve.

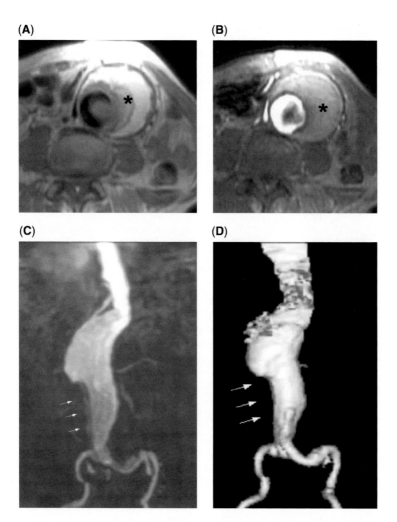

Figure 13 Abdominal aortic aneurysm. (**A**) BBFSE T1, (**B**) fast gradient echo (GRE) axial images, (**C**) Contrast-enhanced-MRA (CE-MRA) maximum intensity projection reconstruction, and (**D**) CE-MRA 3D volume reconstruction. Large abdominal aortic aneurysm. There is extensive mural thrombotic apposition (∗). The thrombus is inhomogeneously hyperintense on the T1 BBFSE and fast GRE images. The angiographic images demonstrate only the flow lumen so that the caudal part of the aneurysm appears to have a nearly normal diameter (*arrows*: **C,D**). *Abbreviations*: BBFSE, bromphenol blue, FICOLL®, SDS, EDTA loading dye; CE-MRA, contrast-enhanced magnetic resonance angiography.

The most serious complication of an aneurysm is its rupture (50–53). The mean dimension of aneurysm at the time of rupture is 6 cm for the ascending and 7.2 cm for the descending aorta. Most centers will repair a 5–5.5-cm ascending thoracic aneurysm or a 5.5–6.5-cm aneurysm of the descending aorta. A rapid increase in the aortic diameter, bleeding within the

(A)

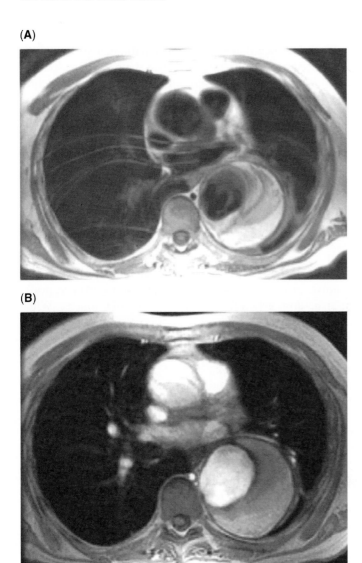

(B)

Figure 14 Thoracic aortic aneurysm. **(A)** BBFSE axial and **(B)** fast gradient echo (GRE) axial image. Fusiform aneurysm of the thoracic aorta. There is extensive parietal thrombus of high signal intensity both in the BBFSE and fast GRE sequences. The flow lumen is eccentric, anteromedial. *Abbreviations*: BBFSE, bromphenol blue, FICOLL®, SDS, EDTA loading dye; GRE, gradient echo.

parietal thrombus or a contained paraaortic leak may precede the rupture (54). Clefts of T1 high signal thrombus within the outer layers of a low signal thrombus may represent contained rupture. Contrast-enhanced SE images and CE-MRA may demonstrate extravasation. Thoracic aneurysms rupture into the left hemithorax or into the mediastinum, less commonly into the right lung. Mediastinal pericardial and pleural hemathomas strongly indicate rupture. The "draped aorta sign," present when the posterior aspect of the aneurysm is in close apposition to the spine and drapes around a vertebral body, also suggests impending rupture. Abdominal aneurysms may rupture into the retroperitoneum or into the peritoneal cavity (55). Fistulae with the esophagus, bronchi, inferior vena cava, and duodenum are also possible.

POSTOPERATIVE ASSESSMENT

CMR can be considered the method of choice for monitoring the aorta after surgery, and to depict cardiac surgery complications. An accurate postoperative imaging evaluation of the aorta requires precise knowledge of the surgical technique performed and its anatomic consequences.

Aneurysms of the ascending aorta are completely transected and replaced with a dacron graft sutured to the distal ascending aorta and then to the proximal aorta just above the aortic commissures. Aortic grafts appear as tubular structures, generally hypointense on GRE images. When replacement of the ascending aorta and aortic root is necessary, a combined graft-valve prosthesis is sutured to the aortic root. Sometimes the repair is performed wrapping the native aorta around the prosthetic graft.

The presence of perigraft thickening or fluid collection, flow or thrombus outside the graft but within the aortic wrap, and mass effect on the graft can be identified with CMR (56). A slight thickening around the graft is sign of fibrosis (57); a large or asymmetric thickening may represent a localized hematoma from anastomotic leakage. A strong periprosthetic T2 signal 6 month after surgery may correspond to infection.

When the coronary sinuses are involved in the disease, the coronary arteries with the aortic tissue surrounding their ostia are attached to openings in the graft (Bentall technique). If required, a segment of graft or a vein is interposed between the coronaries and the aortic graft. If aneurysmal disease extends distally, the concavity of the aortic arch or the entire arch and the arch vessels origin can be replaced with Dacron grafts.

In patients with extensive aneurysmal disease involving the ascending aorta, arch, and descending thoracic or thoraco-abdominal aorta, the "elephant trunk technique" (Fig. 15) can be employed. The ascending aorta and aortic arch are replaced first, and a segment of graft is left within the proximal descending thoracic aorta. It will be used later at the descending aorta repair so that it will not be necessary to dissect the distal aortic arch.

In descending aorta aneurysms, the aorta is transected and replaced with a graft. Intercostal arteries, visceral, and renal artery ostia are reattached to one or more openings in the graft.

Aortic aneurysms may be repaired using an aortic endograft that can also extend into the common iliac arteries. With this technique, a fabric

(A)   **(B)**   **(C)**

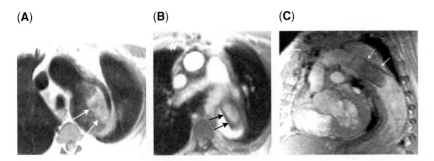

Figure 15 Ascending aorta prosthetic graft. **(A)** Axial BBFSE, **(B)** axial fast gradient echo (GRE), and **(C)** oblique sagittal fast GRE. The ascending aorta has been replaced by a prosthetic graft; a graft segment (*arrows*) is left within the proximal descending thoracic aorta. It will be used later during the descending aorta repair so that it will not be necessary to dissect the distal aortic arch. *Abbreviations*: BBFSE, bromphenol blue, FICOLL®, SDS, EDTA loading dye; GRE, gradient echo.

covered metallic stent or endograft is inserted into an abdominal aortic aneurysm to protect it from rupture through an incision in the femoral artery. Some endoprotheses are totally MRI-compatible allowing clear depiction of the vessel, some cause complete signal reduction from the lumen (and also of the adjacent structures) while other types are non-MRI safe (58). MRI/MRA demonstrates changes in aneurysm/endograft morphology, endoleakage, thrombus formation, and peri-aortic inflammation (59,60).

INTRAMURAL HEMATOMA

Intramural hematoma (IMH) is a contained hemorrhage within the external layers of the tunica media. The hemorrhage extends for a variable distance by dissecting along the outer media beneath the adventitia. The IMH may interest both the ascending and the descending aorta and as the dissecting aneurysm is classified in types A and B. The right anterolateral wall of the ascending aorta and the left postero-lateral wall of the proximal descending aorta are preferably involved. There are not intimal tears or direct communications between the media and the lumen but IMH is however considered a precursor of dissection. Images show localized concentric or eccentric increased wall thickness (Fig. 16), more than 7 mm and up to 30 mm (61–63). Intramural blood of the early-stage acute IMH (up to 48 hr) has "intermediate" signal intensity on both T1- and T2-weighted images, similar to that of the normal aortic wall (64). During this phase, aortic wall thickness may be overestimated on SE images because of the signal of slow moving blood. On day 3, the IMH contains sufficient quantities of methhemoglobin and becomes T1 hyperintense (65). As IMH does not communicate directly with the aortic lumen, the thickened aortic wall does not generally show enhancement after contrast administration (66).

(A)   **(B)**

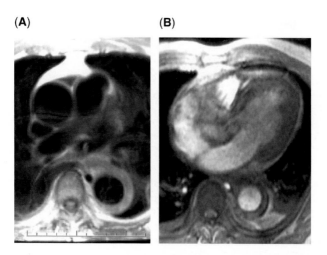

Figure 16 Intramural hematoma. (**A**) T1-weighted BBFSE axial and (**B**) fast gradient echo (GRE) axial images. The descending aorta wall is homogeneously thickened. It shows intermediate signal intensity on the T1-weighted BBFSE image while is hypointense on the fast GRE sequence. *Abbreviations*: BBFSE, bromphenol blue, FICOLL®, SDS, EDTA loading dye; GRE, gradient echo.

PENETRATING ULCER

Penetrating ulcers are a complication of the atherosclerotic plaque. The ulceration penetrates through the elastic lamina into the media (67) resulting in an IMH and a limited aortic dissection (68) that communicate with the lumen through a narrow neck. Penetrating ulcers are more common in the descending aorta, often in the wall of aneurysms; their length is limited, always shorter than 10 cm. Penetrating ulcers appear as a focal outpouching of the aortic lumen (69,70) with irregular edges, often in the presence of extensive aortic atheroma (Fig. 17). They can reach the adventitia and complicate with formation of false aneurysms, rupture, or form fistulas into adjacent organs.

AORTIC DISSECTION

Acute dissection of the aorta is the most common aortic emergency. It is 2–3 times more frequent than the acute rupture of an aneurysm, occurring more frequently in the sixth and seventh decades of life; its incidence is two times higher in men than in women (71). Predisposing causes are listed in Table 4. Most commonly the initial event is a tear of the intima. This exposes the media to the pressure of the intraluminal blood that cleaves the layer into two and dissects the aortic wall. An intimomedial flap separates the true from the false lumen that is the blood-filled space between the dissected layers of the aortic wall. The dissection extends along the aortic wall,

(A) **(B)**

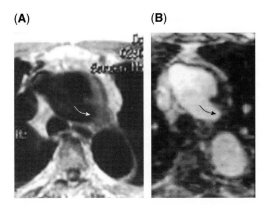

Figure 17 Penetrating atherosclerotic ulcer. **(A)** T1-weighted BBFSE axial and **(B)** fast gradient echo axial images. The ascending aorta presents an atherosclerotic plaque with irregular edges. It is evident a crater-like ulcer (*curved arrow*) that appears as focal outpouching of the aortic lumen.

typically antegrade but sometimes retrograde from the site of intimal tear. Further tears in the intimal flap produce exit sites or additional entry sites for blood flow in the false lumen. The false lumen may become distended with blood, causing the intimal flap to bow into the true lumen, thereby narrowing its caliber and distorting its shape.

In some cases, an intimal tear cannot be identifiable. A dissection present since less than 2 weeks is defined as "acute." The diagnosis of acute dissection is an emergency that cannot be delayed as the mortality rate is 1–2%/hr in the first 24–48 hr after onset. About two-thirds of aortic dissections are acute; "chronic" aortic dissections are present since 2 weeks or

Table 4 Aortic Dissection Predisposing Causes

Marfan syndrome
Hypertension
Bicuspid aortic valve
Coarctation of the aorta.
Turner syndromes
Aortitis
Cocaine abuse
Third trimester pregnancy
Early postpartum period
Direct trauma to the aorta
Intraarterial catheterization
Intraaortic balloon pumps
Aortic valve replacement

Table 5   Relevant Information in Aortic Dissection

Visualization of double lumen

Presence of dissection membrane
Involvement of the ascending aorta
Extent of dissection
Sites of entry or reentry
Intramural hematoma
Patent or thrombosed false lumen
Branch vessel involvement
Aortic valve regurgitation
Pericardial effusion

more; at this time, the mortality curve for untreated aortic dissections is
75–80%. Two major classification systems define the location and extent
of aortic involvement. De Bakey (72) classified dissections into three types
depending on the site of origin and extent of the dissection (72) (Table 5).
The Stanford classification (Table 6) is based on prognostic factors as the
involvement of the ascending aorta requires emergency surgery, whereas
descending aortic dissections are usually managed with medical therapy
alone (73). The vast majority of aortic dissections originate in the proximal
ascending aorta (65%) within several centimeters of the aortic root. The next
most common area is in the descending aorta, just distal to the origin of the
left subclavian artery at the site of the ligamentum arteriosum (20%). Only
10% originate in the aortic arch, and 5% in the abdominal aorta.

Why CMR?

CMR is highly sensitive, specific, and accurate for detection of all forms of
dissection (74,75). The International Registry of Acute Aortic Dissection
(IRAD) reports an CMR sensitivity of 100% for both type A and B dissections (76). CMR can be safely performed even on acute aortic dissection
patients (77–79). Most CMR facilities allow continuous ECG and blood
pressure monitoring and ventilatory assistance. The study may be time-
consuming, but the most important sequences can be performed in
15 min; the recently available rapid scanning techniques and real-time
sequences will further facilitate the diagnosis in unstable patients. In

Table 6   DeBakey Classification

Type I	Originates into the ascending aorta, extends at least to the arch
Type II	Originates and is limited to the ascending aorta
Type III	Originates and involves only the descending aorta. Type IIIa is confined to the thoracic aorta; Type IIIb extends to the abdomen

contrast, in the acute setting MRI could be less practical than other modalities as lacking the mobility of TEE requires the transportation of the patient; patient accessibility is limited during the study and his immobility is required. Some monitoring and support devices may not be allowed near the scanner.

CMR is considered the most accurate technique and the diagnostic gold standard for stable or chronic dissections and for the follow-up of dissections to monitor for extension of the disease or the formation of aneurysms (80–82). In patients with preexisting aortic disease, CMR can easily distinguish dissection from other pathology.

Image Analysis

Rapid detection and accurate diagnosis of relevant anatomic detail with CMR are critical for successful detection and management of dissecting aneurisms (Table 7). The proposed imaging protocol can be performed rapidly even in the acute or noncooperative patient (Fig. 18) (Table 8).

The primary sign of dissection is the identification of a true and a false lumen separated by the intimal flap (Figs. 19–21). The intimo-medial flap appears as a medium intensity linear structure in all sequences. Although, SE readily identifies the dissection flap GRE images offer high diagnostic yield. Multislice (single shot) SSFP images have demonstrated high accuracy in the detection of the dissection flap separating the true and false lumen. The SSFP sequence can be acquired without breath-hold in less than 2 minutes, even in acute non-cooperative patients. The true lumen tends to be semilunar and smaller (Fig. 19A and B), whereas the false lumen appears oval and larger. In the true lumen, early laminar systolic flow is usually detected, whereas in the false lumen diastolic, slow flow, late systolic or slow swirling flow can be documented. The false lumen more often demonstrates thrombosis. Cobweb or strands of dissected media are a pathognomonic for a false lumen (83).

In the SE images, the absence of signal in both lumens is expression of high velocity blood flow; the evidence of signal in the false lumen may be expression of slow flow (Fig. 21A) or thrombosis. The distinction between slow flow and thrombosis is more easily made on cine GRE images: laminar flowing blood is hyperintense (Fig. 21B) and its signal intensity varies throughout the cycle, whereas thrombosis demonstrates a constant medium/low signal. Flow velocity mapping will confirm the diagnosis showing different flow velocities in the true and false lumens (84,85). CE-MRA provides also valuable information detecting

Table 7 Stanford Classification

Type A	Involves the ascending aorta (include DeBakey types I and II)
Type B	Interests only the descending aorta (includes DeBakey types IIIa/b)

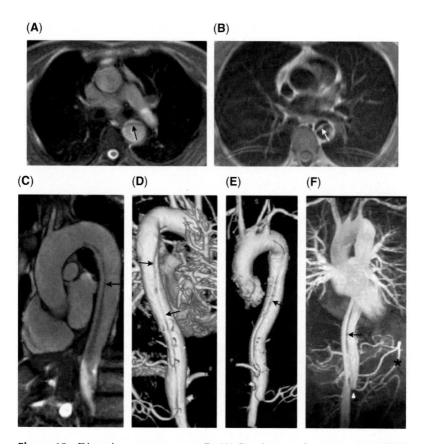

Figure 18 Dissecting aneurysm type B. (**A**) Steady–state free precession (SSFP) axial (free breathing); (**B**) BBFSE axial (free breathing); (**C**) Oblique sagittal SSFP; (**D, E**) Contrast-enhanced MRA (CE-MRA) 3D volume reconstructions, and (**F**) CE-MRA) maximum intensity projection reconstruction. The dissection flap (*arrow*) is evident on the axial and oblique sagittal images. True and false lumens are well evident on CE-MRA 3D volume reconstructions. False lumen is obstructed immediately below the left renal artery origin (**F**, *arrowhead*). Extensive collateral flow is provided through the colic vessels (**F**, ***). The whole examination has been acquired in less than 15 minutes. *Abbreviations*: BBFSE, bromphenol blue, FICOLL®, SDS, EDTA loading dye; CE-MRA, contrast-enhanced magnetic resonance angiography; SSFP, steady–state free precession.

the intimal flap, differentiating the true from the false lumen, and slow flow from thrombus (Figs. 19 and 21). Axial reformatted images better show the intimal flap than maximum intensity projecton (MIP) reconstructions.

A thickening of the aortic wall may represent an IMH that could progress into a typical dissection. T1 hyperintense areas within the thickened wall are consistent with subacute hemorrhage; a dissection where small intimal tears cannot be identified can also be postulated. Also it is difficult

Table 8 Acute Aortic Syndromes: Imaging Strategy

	Acute: FB	
Axial Black Blood FSE	Chronic: BH	From 1–2 cm above the arch to the diaphragm. Evidence of the dissecting membrane Evidence of true and false lumen Measures of ascending and descending aorta dimensions Pericardial effusion Extended to the abdomen to assess the presence of pathology of the abdominal aorta
Axial Fast GRE or SSFP	Acute: Single phase eventually multi-phase. Fast GRE BH SSFP FB Chronic: Single- or multiphase. Fast GRE BH SSFP FB or BH	
LAO SE	BH	Images the entire length of the thoracic aorta in a single plane. Obtained by setting the slice through the ascending and descending aorta and parallel to the arch
LAO Fast GRE or SSFP	Multiphase BH	Longitudinal extension of the dissection Evidence of entry and re-entry sites
CE-MRA sagittal	BH	3D sagittal slab planned to include both the ascending and descending aorta. Comprehensive evaluation of aortic anatomy and branches
Accessory sequences		

(Continued)

Table 8 Acute Aortic Syndromes: Imaging Strategy (*Continued*)

	Acute: FB	From 1–2 cm above the arch to the diaphragm.
Coronal Oblique GRE or SSFP	Multiphase BH	Planned on axial images or on an oblique coronal plan through the aortic root and the left ventricular outflow tract Study of the ascending aorta and aortic valve regurgitation Pericardial effusion
LVOT	Multiphase BH	Aortic valve regurgitation Pericardial effusion
Axial T1W fat-sat GRE pre- and postcontrast	BH	IMH: evidence of blood in the aortic wall Postcontrast: aortic wall and periaortic enhancement

Abbreviations: LVOT, left ventricular outflow tract; LAO, left anterior oblique; FB, free breathing; BH, breath-hold; GRE, gradient echo; SSFP, steady—state free precession; IMH, intramural hematoma.

(A)

(B)

(C)

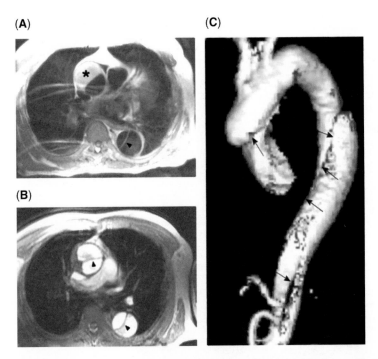

Figure 19 Dissecting aneurysm type A. (**A**) BBFSE axial, (**B**) fast gradient echo axial images, and (**C**) Contrast-enhanced–MRA 3D volume reconstruction. The dissecting aneurysm involves both the ascending and descending aorta. Slow flow in the false lumen in the ascending aorta demonstrates high signal in the BBFSE image (∗). The intimal flap (*arrowhead*) is well evident. The spiral course of the dissection can be seen in the 3D MRA volume reconstruction (*arrows*). *Abbreviations*: BBFSE, bromphenol blue, FICOLL®, SDS, EDTA loading dye; MRA, magnetic resonance angiography.

to differentiate a dissection with a completely thrombosed false lumen from an aneurysm with mural thrombosis.

It is crucial to determine if the dissection involves the ascending aorta (Fig. 19) or is limited to the descending aorta (Figs. 20 and 21). In general, acute dissections involving the ascending aorta require emergency surgery.

The ability of MRI to acquire high-quality images along multiple planes is helpful in determining the presence of entry/reentry sites. Entry sites are identified as discontinuities of the intimal flap (Fig. 21C). Flow across the membrane can be easily seen in GRE images: more often as turbulenct jets (flow void), and less often as areas of localized hyper-intensity directed from the true lumen toward the false lumen.

Rupture into the pericardial sac with cardiac tamponade is a frequent life-threatening complication of Type A aortic dissection. Pericardial effusions that demonstrate medium/high signal intensity on both T1- and

(A)

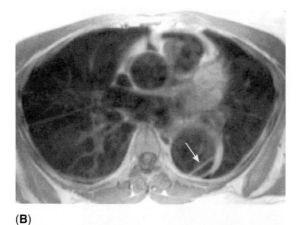

(B)

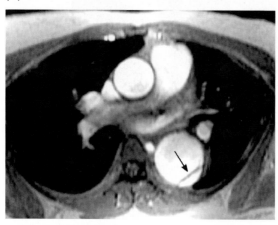

Figure 20 Dissecting aneurysm type B. **(A)** BBFSE axial, **(B)** fast gradient echo axial images. The descending aorta is dilated; a dissection flap is seen inside its lumen (*arrows*). Both true and false lumens are patent. There is no evidence of thrombosis. *Abbreviations*: BBFSE, bromphenol blue, FICOLL®, SDS, EDTA loading dye.

T2-weighed images indicate a bloody component and impending rupture of the dissecting aneurysm into the pericardium. Signs of tamponade include diastolic collapse of the right ventricle and indentation of the right atrium, dilatation of the inferior vena cava. Rarely a dissecting aneurysm may rupture into the heart cavities, the superior vena cava, esophagus, tracheo-bronchial tree, or into the pleural cavities (hemothorax).

The dissection flap may involve the ostium of a coronary artery (1–2% of the cases) and cause acute myocardial infarction (86). The dissection more often affects the right coronary artery than the left, explaining why these myocardial infarctions tend to be inferior in location.

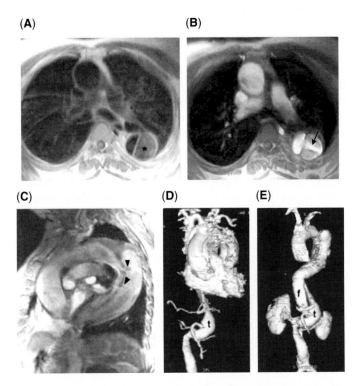

Figure 21 Dissecting aneurysm type B. (**A**) BBFSE axial; (**B**) fast gradient echo (GRE) axial; (**C**) Oblique sagittal fast-GRE; (**D,E**) CE-MRA 3D volume reconstructions. The axial images demonstrate the presence of an intimal flap in the descending aorta. On the BBFSE image there is signal void in the true lumen while the slower flow in the false lumen has low to intermediate signal (∗). An entry site is evident on the axial fast GRE image; blood passing from the true into the false lumen is evident as a hyperintense jet (*arrow*) against the darker signal of flow in the false lumen. On the oblique sagittal image the intimal flap, the true and false lumens can be appreciated in the descending aorta; jets of turbulent flow through the communication sites appear hypointense (*arrowheads*). At the abdominal level 3D MRA obtained early after contrast injection (**D**) only visualizes the true lumen (f); a later images (**E**) show both the true (t) and false (f) lumens. Celiac axis, mesenteric and renal arteries originate from the true lumen. BBFSE, bromphenol blue, FICOLL®, SDS, EDTA loading dye; GRE, gradient echo.

The dissection may also be the cause of aortic insufficiency: widening the aortic root and the annulus, depressing one leaflet, disrupting the annulus or the leaflets, or by prolapse of the intimal flap into the left ventricular outflow tract (LVOT). However, aortic regurgitation is generally antecedent to the dissection due to dilatation of the aortic root. Cine GRE images along the LVOT and left anterior oblique (LAO) are used to determine the presence and the severity of aortic regurgitation that can be quantified with velocity mapping.

CMR can assess the extension of the intimal flap into the branch vessels. Dissection of the aortic arch may extend into and eventually occlude the supraaortic vessels with neurological compromise. Accordingly, the abdominal aorta must be explored (87). Abdominal aortic dissections may extend into or occlude one or both renal arteries (5–8%) with resulting renal ischemia, or compromise the mesenteric vessels (3–5%) causing bowel ischemia and infarction. Caudally aortic dissection may extend into the iliac arteries and lead to lower extremity ischemia. Branch vessels may originate from the true or the false lumen. If the false lumen is widely communicating with the true lumen through entry and reentry sites, flow into the branch vessels may be preserved. Surgical treatment of proximal aortic dissection is intended to prevent ascending aortic rupture. A segment of the ascending aorta is resected and replaced by a Dacron graft. If necessary, the native aortic valve is replaced with a prosthetic valve. The distal false lumen may be left open so that it may give rise to vital arteries.

Close surveillance with CMR three months after surgery followed CMR exams at six and 12 months is recommended (83). CMR can be useful to detect a variety of postsurgical complications.

Dilatation and rupture of distal aorta is the most common cause of death after treatment, so rapid changes of dimension (that often precede rupture) must be accurately monitored (88–90). The usual expansion rate is 3.4 mm/yr with thrombosis of the false lumen and 5.6 mm/yr when the false lumen is patent (91). Residual dissection in the abdominal branches or supraaortic vessels may be observed. Thrombosis of the false lumen is a good prognostic factor. Formation of periprosthetic pseudoaneurysms caused by dehiscence of the sutures or re-dissection is also possible.

AORTIC COARCTATION

Coarctation is the most common congenital abnormality of the thoracic aorta; its incidence is 4.1/10,000 newborns and 7% in patients with congenital heart disease. Coarctation of the aorta is a congenital narrowing of the upper descending thoracic aorta adjacent to the site of attachment of the ductus arteriosus, which is sufficiently severe that there is pressure gradient across the area. Coarctation varies in severity, when it is localized, the lumen must be reduced in cross-sectional area by more than 50% before there is pressure gradient across it, but longer tubular coarctation may be hemodynamically significant with lesser narrowing.

The localized lesion of classic coarctation is a ridge or infolding of the aortic media protruding into the lumen, distal to the origin of the left subclavian artery, at or near the insertion of the ligamentum arteriosus. Coarctation with a patent ductus arteriosus distal to the narrowing called preductal coarctation, the aortic isthmus is invariable narrowed. This lesion

Table 9 Relevant Information in Aortic Coarctation

Position (pre or postductal)
Length
Severity of narrowing
Extent of turbulence (width, length, duration)
Flow velocity mapping quantization
Aortic isthmus hypoplasia
Poststenotic dilatation (smooth fusiform/asymmetric)
Collateral circulation
Bicuspid aortic valve
VSD
After surgery
Residual coarctation
Aneurysm formation

Abbreviation: VSD, ventricular septum defect.

nearly always present in infancy in association with a still patent ductus arteriosus and usually in combination with other congenital cardiac defects.

Some hearts with coarctation show a more diffuse narrowing due to hypoplasia of the aortic isthmus. This lesion is called tubular hypoplasia which may be present without coarctation.

Occasionally, the adult aorta may be redundant and severely kinked opposite to the ligamentum arteriosum without a significant pressure gradient, the so-called pseudocoarctation or nonobstructive coarctation (92).

In about half of the cases, the coarctation is associated with an aortic bicuspid valve (Fig. 23C) that is prone to stenosis. It can also be associated with the presence of a ventricular septal defect (Table 9).

Image Analysis

The coarctation may appear as a membrane partially or completely obstructing the lumen near the ductus arteriosus (Fig. 22B) or as a narrowed aortic segment. The most informative examination planes are the axial and the left sagittal oblique including the aortic root, the arch with the coarctation site, and the descending aorta (Figs. 22 and 23) (93). SE images are useful to assess morphology and length of the coarctation, the size of aortic isthmus, and of the aorta pre/post-coarctation. Cine GRE images contribute to assessment of severity by displaying flow across the coarctation site, the extent and duration of the turbulent jet beyond it (Fig. 23A). An oblique coronal GRE sequence across the aortic valve is useful to show aortic stenosis. Oblique axial SE and GRE images parallel to the aortic valve will show the number of valve leaflets.

(A)   **(B)**   **(C)**

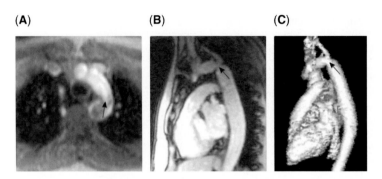

Figure 22 Aortic coarctation. (**A**) Axial fast gradient echo (GRE), (**B**) Oblique sagittal fast-GRE, (**C**) Contrast-enhanced-MRA 3D volume reconstruction. The aorta is narrowed immediately after the emergence of the left subclavian artery (*arrow*). The coarctation is more evident on its medial and inferior surface. The descending aorta is mildly dilated. *Abbreviations*: GRE-gradient echo; MRA, magnetic resonance angiography.

Flow velocity mapping can be used to measure the peak velocity across the site of coarctation, quantifying its severity. A flow velocity $> 3\,\text{m/sec}$ and diastolic prolongation of forward flow are signs of significant obstruction. A careful alignment of the scanning plane with the narrowing and the jet beyond is necessary to accurately measure the velocity of the jet. The pressure gradient across the stenosis can be calculated from peak velocity.

The obstruction to normal flow determines the formation of extensive collateral circulation with enlarged arch vessels, particularly from branches of the subclavian arteries through enlarged and tortuous intercostal arteries (that cause the well-known rib-notching evident on chest radiographs), where flow is reversed.

CE-MRA displays lumen geometry, severity of the narrowing, and the extent of collateral circulation providing important information for surgery (Fig. 22C). Collateral circulation develops through the intercostal arteries and subclavian branches. Collateral blood flow can be quantified with CMR velocity mapping (Table 10). Normally, flow volume in the proximal descending aorta is 7% higher than that in the distal thoracic aorta. In patients with a hemodynamically significant coarctation, collateral distal aortic flow may be greater than proximal flow due to retrograde collateral blood flow into the aorta from the intercostal arteries and other aortic branches (94).

Correction of the coarctation may be performed by subclavian flap aortoplasty, end-to-end anastomosis, synthetic patch flap aortoplasty, replacement with a tubular graft, simple bypass, or by balloon angioplasty. The best balloon angioplasty results are achieved in focal coarctation distal to the subclavian artery.

After surgery less than 10% of patients develop recoarctation (Fig. 23). Other post-surgical complications include the development of true or false

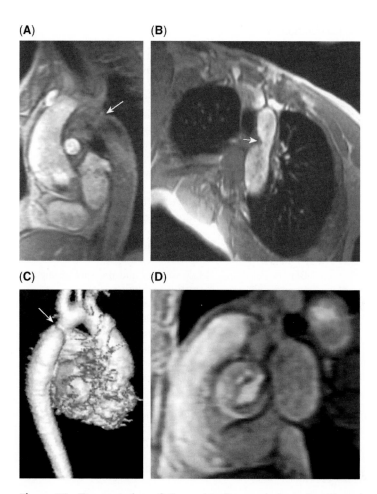

Figure 23 Recoarctation of the aorta after surgical repair with end-to-end anastomosis. (A) Left anterior oblique fast gradient echo (GRE), (B) axial oblique fast-GRE image at the level of the aortic arch, (C) CE-MRA 3D volume reconstruction, and (D) axial oblique fast-GRE image at the level of the aortic valve. The aortic isthmus is narrow at the recoarctation point (*arrows*). The postcoarctation segment is mildly dilated. Mild turbulence can be appreciated at this level (A). The aortic valve (D) is bicuspid, as demonstrated on the oblique axial cine fast-GRE images conducted on a plane parallel to the annulus. *Abbreviations*: GRE, gradient echo; CE-MRA; contrast-enhanced magnetic resonance angiography.

aneurysms adjacent to the site of repair (especially near a Dacron patch) or a dissecting aneurysm after balloon dilatation. Follow-up by CMR is recommended for monitoring for recurrence of coarctation or aneurysm formation.

A congenital defect in which there is complete discontinuity between two segments of the aortic arch is called interruption of the aortic arch (95).

Table 10 Aortic Coarctation: Imaging Strategy

Axial Black Blood FSE	BH	From 1 to 2 cm above the arch to the diaphragm
Axial fast GRE or SSFP	BH multi-slice	Measures of ascending and descending aorta dimensions The arch is imaged longitudinally and its morphology and orientation are easily appreciated
LAO black-blood FSE	BH	Images the entire length of the thoracic aorta in a single plane
LAO GRE	BH multi-phase	Coarctation dimension and length Turbulence jet conspicuity (GRE)
CE-MRA sagittal	BH	Comprehensive evaluation of aortic anatomy 3D coarctation display
Optional sequences		
Flow velocity mapping	BH	Flow velocity and pressure gradient at the coarctation site Collateral flow volume quantification (differential flow below the coarctation site and at the diaphragm level)
Coronal oblique Aortic valve plane Fast GRE or SSFP	BH multi-phase	Ascending aorta and aortic valve study to exclude bicuspidy

Abbreviations: BH, breath-hold; FB, free breathing; GRE, gradient echo; LAO, left anterior oblique; SSFP, steady–state free precession.

Morphologically, interruption of the aortic arch is divided into two categories:

1. Interruption of the left aortic arch and
2. Interruption of right aortic arch.

Only rarely the interruption occurs in right side of the aortic arch, where both right and left ducti may remain patent and give origin to the sub-clavian arteries.

Interruptions of both right and left aortic arches can be subdivided according to the location of the interruption:

1. Interruption beyond origin of the left subclavian artery (40% of the cases): in this case flow into the descending aorta is from ductus arteriosus.
2. The most common site of interruption (55%) is proximal to the origin of the left subclavian artery, between it, and the left common carotid artery.

3. In only 5% of the cases is the interruption proximal to the left common carotid artery, between it and the right innominate artery.

An aberrant right subclavian artery is not uncommon in interrupted aortic arch. The ascending aorta is half of normal diameter, it courses straight, dividing into two branches of about equal size (V sign), whereas the pulmonary artery is markedly dilated. The descending thoracic aorta is a direct continuation of the ductus arteriosus, and it is usually a little larger than the ascending aorta. Associated malformations include: ventricular septal defect (often perimembranous), stenosis of the left ventricular outlet due to abnormally left positioned infundibular septum, valvular aortic stenosis, transposition of the great arteries, and aorto-pulmonary window.

AORTIC ARCH ANOMALIES

CMR has high sensitivity in demonstrating aortic arch anomalies, allowing to image a large field of view along multiple planes, and providing high anatomical detail. CMR accurately shows the relationship of the vascular structures with esophagus and trachea, the eventual tracheo-bronchial compression, and the co-existence of cardiac malformations. The morphological evaluation is based principally on axial and coronal SE/FSE images. CE-MRA 3D volume and MIP reconstructions are helpful in understanding three-dimensionally the anomalous anatomy (Table 11) (96–98). Congenital anomalies of the thoracic aorta are classified according to the course of the aortic arch and of its branches.

Double Aortic Arch

Double aortic arch describes an anomaly characterized by the presence of two aortic arches. The ascending aorta arises anteriorly to the trachea and divides into two arches which pass to the right and to the left of the trachea and esophagus. The arches join each other posterior to form the thoracic aorta (99,100). The right common carotid and the right subclavian artery arise from the right arch. Similarly, the left common carotid and the left subclavian artery arise from the left aortic arch. More commonly, the descending thoracic aorta is on the right of the spine. The right aortic arch is usually the largest. Double aortic arch result in a constricting ring of vessels completely encircling the trachea and esophagus (vascular ring) producing various degrees of obstruction. When the compression by the vascular ring is severe, it results in respiratory difficulties dating from birth. Rarely, patients with this anomaly do not have symptoms and the anomaly is discovered incidentally. The left aortic arch may be in part atretic persisting as a fibrous cord without a lumen, whereas the other arch is patent.

Table 11 Acute Aortic Syndromes: Imaging Strategy

Axial black-blood FSE	Acute: FB Chronic: BH	From 1 to 2 cm above the arch to the diaphragm Evidence of the dissecting membrane Evidence of true and false lumen
Axial fast GRE or SSFP	Acute: single-phase eventually multi-phase Fast GRE BH SSFP FB Chronic: single-phase or multi-phase Fast GRE BH SSFP FB or BH	Measures of ascending and descending aorta dimensions Pericardial effusion Extended to the abdomen to assess the presence of pathology of the abdominal aorta
LAO SE LAO fast GRE or SSFP	BH Multi-phase BH	Images the entire length of the thoracic aorta in a single plane; obtained by setting the slice through the ascending and descending aorta and parallel to the arch Longitudinal extension of the dissection Evidence of entry and re-entry sites
CE-MRA sagittal	BH	3D sagittal slab planned to include both the ascending and descending aorta; comprehensive evaluation of aortic anatomy and branches
Accessory sequences Coronal oblique fast GRE or SSFP	Multi-phase BH	Dissection type A Planned on axial images or on an oblique coronal plan through the aortic root and the LVOT Study of the ascending aorta and aortic valve regurgitation Pericardial effusion
LVOT fast GRE or SSFP	Multi-phase BH	Dissection type A Aortic valve regurgitation Pericardial effusion

Abbreviations: BH, breath-hold; FB, free breathing; LAO, left anterior oblique; LVOT, left ventricular outflow tract; SSFP, steady-state free precession.

Anomalies of the Left Aortic Arch

Left Aortic Arch with Aberrant Right Subclavian Artery

Left aortic arch with aberrant right subclavian artery is the commonest malformation of the aortic arch (Figs. 24 and 25). Approximately one person in 200 has this anomaly. It usually does not produce symptoms and it is discovered accidentally with imaging (Table 12). The right subclavian artery arises as the fourth branch from the distal left arch; it is characteristically seen as a vascular structure crossing obliquely upward the mediastinum from right to left behind the esophagus and extending to the right arm (Fig. 24C). The descending aorta lies to the left of the spine.

Left Aortic Arch with Right Descending Thoracic Aorta

In this anomaly, the left aortic arch arises from the ascending aorta and passes backward to the left of the trachea and esophagus. The terminal portion of the aortic arch, crosses to the right side of the mediastinum behind the esophagus, turning abruptly downward, to continue as the right descending thoracic aorta.

Anomalies of the Right Aortic Arch

A right aortic arch courses the arch to the right of the esophagus and trachea, with the descending thoracic aorta to the right of the spine. The specific type of anomaly depends on the point where the left aortic arch is interrupted.

(A)   **(B)**

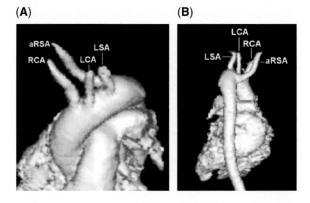

Figure 24 Aberrant RSA contrast enhanced MRA 3D volume reconstructions: (**A**) antero-superior view and (**B**) posterior view. The aortic arch gives rise to the RCA, LCA, LSA, and aRSA that courses towards right in the posterior mediastinum. *Abbreviations*: aRSA, aberrant right subclaviar artery; LCA, left carotid artery; LSA, left subclaviar artery; RCA, right carotid artery; RSA, right subclaviar artery.

(A)   (B)

(C)

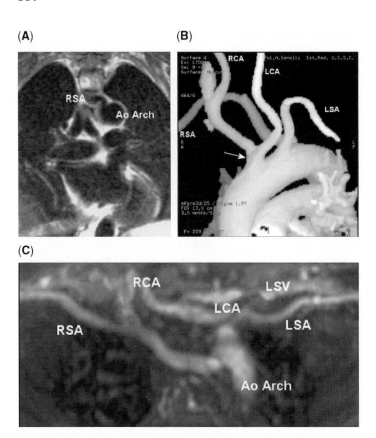

Figure 25 Aberrant right subclavian artery with common origin of the carotid arteries. (**A**) BBFSE coronal contrast-enhanced-MRA, (**B**) 3D volume reconstruction, (**C**) axial subvolume maximum intensity projection reconstruction. The aortic arch gives rise to a first branch (*arrow*) that divides into the RCA and LCA. Successively gives origin to the LSA and to the aberrant RSA that courses towards right in the posterior mediastinum. *Abbreviations*: LCA, left carotid artery; LSA, left subclavian artery; LSV, left subclavian vein; RCA, right carotid artery; RSA, right subclavian artery.

Right Aortic Arch with Mirror Image Branching

The first branch off this type of right aortic arch is the left brachiocephalic artery, followed by the right common carotid and right subclavian artery in that sequence (Fig. 26). It frequently associated with congenital heart disease.

Right Aortic Arch with Aberrant Left Subclavian Artery

In this anomaly, four branches originate from the aortic arch in the following sequence: left common carotid, right common carotid, right subclavian, and the aberrant left subclavian artery. The aorta may descend either to the

Table 12 Aortic Anomalies: Imaging Strategy

Axial black-blood FSE	FB or BH	From 1 to 2 cm above the arch to the diaphragm
Axial GRE/SSFP	Single-phase or multi-phase Fast GRE BH SSFP FB or BH	Measures of ascending and descending aorta dimensions The arch is imaged longitudinally and its morphology and orientation are easily appreciated Position of aortic arch with respect to trachea and esophagus
Coronal black-blood FSE	FB or BH	Position of aortic arch with respect to trachea
Sagittal black-blood FSE	FB or BH	Optional; relationship of supraaortic vessels with trachea and esophagus
CE-MRA coronal	BH	Comprehensive evaluation of aortic anatomy and of its branches Epi-aortic vessels origin and course

Abbreviations: BH, breath-hold; CE-MRA, contrast-enhanced MRA; FB, free breathing; GRE, gradient echo; SSFP, steady–state free precession.

right or left of the spine. It may be associated with aortic diverticulum. Right aortic arch with aberrant left subclavian artery is the most common anomaly in patients with right aortic arch (0.1%). If the ligamentum arteriusus is on the left side, it may form a vascular ring.

Right Aortic Arch with Aberrant Left Innominate Artery

In this type of right aortic arch, the left innominate artery arises as the third branch from the distal right arch, passing behind the esophagus to give off the left common carotid and left subclavian arteries (101). A vascular ring is present, formed by the right arch, as it runs posteriorly adjacent to the retroesophageal left innominate artery, and laterally to the left of the left ductus arteriosus.

Right Aortic Arch with Isolation of the Left Subclavian Artery

In this anomaly, the left common carotid, the right common carotid, and the right subclavian arteries arise independently from the aortic arch in that sequence. The left subclavian artery no longer has connection with the aorta, but it is connected to the left pulmonary artery by way of the left ductus arteriosus. The right arch is anterior to the trachea and esophagus. Right aortic arch with isolation of the left subclavian artery is an uncommon congenital anomaly. It is frequently associated with cyanotic congenital heart

(A)   (B)

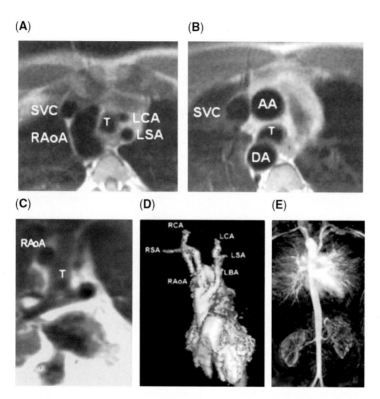

(C)   (D)   (E)

Figure 26   Right-sided aortic arch with mirror branching. (**A, B**) BBFSE axial images. (**C**) BBFSE coronal image contrast-enhanced-MRA. (**D**) 3D volume reconstruction. (**E**) maximum intensity projection reconstruction. The RAoA is on the right side of the T and the DA courses on the right side of the spine. The aortic arch gives rise to the LBA, RCA, and RSA. The LBA courses in front of the trachea and divides into the LCA and subclavian artery (LSA). *Abbreviations*: DA, descending aorta; LBA, left brachiocephalic artery; LCA, left carotid artery; LSA, left subclavian artery; RAoA, right aortic arch; RCA, right carotid artery; RSA, right subclavian artery; SVC: superior vena cava; T, trachea.

malformation, especially Tetralogy of Fallot. Some patients with this anomaly do not have other cardiac malformations. In these cases, the clinical symptoms have resulted from the associated subclavian steal syndrome, either in the form of cerebral symptoms or difference in blood pressure and pulse, between the two arms.

CONCLUSIONS

The aorta is subject to various pathologies including aneurysms, dissections, and congenital anomalies. As the main conduit of the bodies blood supply, it is vital to make a timely and accurate diagnosis of anatomy and flow dynamics. While Spin Echo technique is ideal to capture the anatomy of the aortic wall and slower moving blood, bright blood sequences such as gradient echo cine and SSFP techniques can be employed to taylor the imaging to the specific needs regarding timing, patient's clinical status, function, and highlighting specific features of the aortic pathologies. CMR imaging is the gold standard in diagnosis and monitoring of aortic disease both because of its accuracy and versatility offered in no other imaging modality.

REFERENCES

1. Hager A, Kaemmerer H, Rapp-Bernhardt U, et al. Diameters of the thoracic aorta throughout life as measured with helical computed tomography. J Thorac Cardiovasc Surg 2002; 123(6):1060–1066.
2. Mohiaddin RH, Kilner J, Pennell DJ. Aortic diseases. In: Pohost GM, O'Rourke RA, Berman DS, Pravin MS, eds. Imaging in Cardiovascular Disease. Philadelphia: Lippincott William & Wilkins, 821–842.
3. Blackwell GG, Cranney GB, Pohost GMP. Diseases of the aorta. In: Blackwell GG, Cranney GB, Pohost GMP, eds. MRI: Cardiovascular System. New York: Gower Medical Publishing, 1992:12.4–12.21.
4. Carr JC, Finn JP. MR imaging of the thoracic aorta. Magn Reson Clin N Am 2003; 11:135–148.
5. Reddy GP, Higgins CB. MR imaging of the thoracic aorta. Magn Reson Imaging Clin N Am 2000; 8(1):1–15.
6. White RD, Higgins CB. Magnetic resonance imaging of thoracic vascular disease. J Thorac Imaging 1989; 4:34–50.
7. Nienaber CA, Spielmann RP, von Kodolitsch Y. Diagnosis of thoracic aortic dissection: magnetic resonance imaging versus transesophageal echocardiography. Circulation 1992; 85:434–447.
8. Stemerman DH, Krinsky GA, Lee VS, Johnson G, Yang BM, Rofsky NM. Thoracic aorta: rapid black-blood MR imaging with half-Fourier rapid acquisition with relaxation enhancement with or without electrocardiographic triggering. Radiology 1999; 213(1):185–191.
9. Campos S, Martinez Sanjuan V, Garcia Nieto JJ, et al. New black blood pulse sequence for studies of the heart. Int J Card Imaging 1999; 15(2):175–183.
10. Scott Pereless F, McCarthy RM, Baskaran V, et al. Thoracic aortic dissection and aneurysm: evaluation with nonenhanced true FISP MR Angiography in less than 4 minutes. Radiology 2002; 223: 270–274.
11. Ho VB, Prince MR. Thoracic MR aortography: imaging techniques and strategies. Radiographics 1998; 18(2):287–309.
12. Ko SF, Wan YL, Ng SH, et al. MRI of thoracic vascular lesions with emphasis on two-dimensional time-of-flight MR angiography. Br J Radiol 1999; 72(858): 613–620.
13. Krinsky G, Rofsky N, De Corato DR, et al. Thoracic aorta: comparison of gadolinium-enhanced three-dimensional MR angiography with conventional MR imaging. Radiology 1997; 202:183–193.

14. Krinsky G, Rofsky N, Flyer M, et al. Gadolinium-enhanced three-dimensional MR angiography of acquired arch vessels disease. Am J Roentgenol 1996; 167:981–987.

15. Prince MR, Narasimham DL, Jacoby WT, et al. Three dimensional gadolinium-enhanced MR angiography of the thoracic aorta. Am J Roentgenol 1996; 166:1387–1397.

16. Shetty AN, Bis KG. Dynamic contrast-enhanced 3D breath hold MRA using a multiple variable orientation slab acquisition. Magn Reson Imaging 1999; 17(6):837–841.

17. Prince MR, Grist TM, Debatin JF. 3D contrast MR angiography. Berlin: Springer, 1997.

18. Prince MR. Gadolinium-enhanced MR aortography. Radiology 1994; 191: 155–164.

19. Hany TF, McKinnon GC, Pfammatter T. Optimisation of contrast timing for breathhold 3D MR-angiography. J Magn Reson Imaging 1997; 7:551–556.

20. Higgins CB, Caputo G, Wendland MF, et al. Measurement of blood flow and perfusion in the cardiovascular system. Invest Radiol 1992; 27:S66–S71.

21. Hopkins KD, Leheman ED, Gosling RG. Aortic compliance measurements: a noninvasive indicator of atherosclerosis. Lancet 1994; 334:1447.

22. Niezen RA, Doornbos J, van der Wall EE, et al. Measurement of aortic and pulmonary flow with MRI at rest and during physical exercise. J Comput Assist Tomogr 1998; 22:194–201.

23. Mohiaddin RH, Kilner PJ, Rees RSO. Magnetic resonance volume flow and jet velocity mapping in aortic coarctation. J Am Coll Cardiol 1993; 22:1515–1521.

24. Johnston KW, Rutherford RB, Tilson MD. Suggested standards for reporting on arterial aneurysms. J Vasc Surg 1991; 13:444.

25. Schoenberg SO, Wunsch C, Knopp MV, et al. Abdominal aortic aneurysm: detection of multilevel vascular pathology by time-resolved multiphase 3D gadolinium MR angiography: initial report. Invest Radiol 1999; 34(10):648–659.

26. Devereux RB, Roman MJ. Aortic disease in Marfan's syndrome. N Engl J Med 1999; 340:1358.

27. Bickerstaff LK, Hollier LH, Van Peenan HJ. Abdominal aortic aneurysms: the changing natural history. J Vasc Surg 1984; 1:6.

28. Anidjar S, Kieffer E. Pathogenesis of acquired aneurysms of the abdominal aorta. Ann Vasc Surg 1992; 6:298.

29. Kersting-Sommerhoff BA, Sechtem UP, Schiller NB. MR imaging of the thoracic aorta in Marfan patients. J Comput Assist Tomogr 1987; 11:633.

30. Strotzer M, Aebert H, Lenhart M. Morphology and hemodynamics in dissection of the descending aorta: assessment with MR imaging. Acta Radiol 2000; 41(6):594–600.

31. Walsh DW, Ho VB, Haggerty MF. Mycotic aneurysm of the aorta: MRI and MRA features. J Magn Reson Imaging 1997; 7(2):312–315.

32. McCuskey WH, Loehr SP, Smidebush GC. Detection of mycotic pseudoaneurysm of the ascending aorta using MRI. Magn Reson Imaging 1993; 11:1223–1226.

33. Bickerstaff LK, Pairolero PC, Hollier LH. Thoracic aortic aneurysms: a population based study. Surgery 1982; 92:1103.

34. Dapunt OE, Galla JD, Sadeghi AM. The natural history of thoracic aortic aneurysms. J Thorac Cardiovasc Surg 1994; 107:1323.

35. Itazawa T, Noguchi K, Ichida F, Miyawaki T. Magnetic resonance imaging for early detection of Takayasu arteritis. Pediatr Cardiol 2001; 22(2):163–164.

36. Matsunaga N, Hayashi K, Sakamoto I. Takayasu arteritis: MR manifestations and diagnosis of acute and chronic phase. J Magn Reson Imaging 1998; 8(2):406–414.

37. Choe YH, Han BK, Koh EM, et al. Takayasu's arteritis: assessment of disease activity with contrast-enhanced MR imaging. Am J Roentgenol 2000; 175(2): 505–511.

38. Yamada I, Nakagawa T, Himeno Y. Takayasu arteritis: diagnosis with breath-hold contrast-enhanced three-dimensional MR angiography. J Magn Reson Imaging 2000; 11(5):481–487.

39. Choe YH, Kim DK, Koh EM. Takayasu arteritis: diagnosis with MR imaging and MR angiography in acute and chronic active stages. J Magn Reson Imaging 1999; 10(5):751–757.

40. Flamm SD, White RD, Hoffman GS. The clinical application of 'edema-weighted' magnetic resonance imaging in the assessment of Takayasu's arteritis. Int J Cardiol 1998; 66(suppl 1):S151–S159.

41. Berkmen T. MR angiography of aneurysms in Behcet disease: a report of four cases. J Comput Assist Tomogr 1998; 22(2):202–206.

42. Goarin JP, Le Bret F, Riou B. Early diagnosis of traumatic thoracic aortic rupture by transeosphageal echocardiography. Chest 1993; 103:618–620.

43. Mesana TG, Caus T, Gaubert J, et al. Late complications after prosthetic replacement of the ascending aorta: what did we learn from routine magnetic resonance imaging follow-up? Eur J Cardiothorac Surg 2000; 18(3):313–320.

44. Fattori R, Nienaber CA. MRI of acute and chronic aortic pathology: pre-operative and post-operative evaluation. J Magn Reson Imaging 1999; 10(5):741–750.

45. Fattori R, Descovich B, Bertaccini P. Composite graft replacement of the ascending aorta: leakage detection with gadolinium-enhanced MR imaging. Radiology 1999; 212(2):573–577.

46. Hartnell GG. Imaging of aortic aneurysms and dissection: CT and MRI. J Thorac Imaging 2001; 16(1):35–46.

47. Schmidta M, Theissen P, Klempt G, et al. Long-term follow-up of 82 patients with chronic disease of the thoracic aorta using spin echo and cine gradient magnetic resonance imaging. Magn Reson Imaging 2000; 18(7):795–806.

48. Kawamoto S, Bluemke DA, Traill TA, et al. Thoracoabdominal aorta in Marfan syndrome: MR imaging findings of progression of vasculopathy after surgical repair. Radiology 1997; 203:727–732.

49. Krinsky G, Rofsky N, Flyer M, et al. Gadolinium-enhanced three-dimensional MR angiography of acquired arch vessels disease. Am J Roentgenol 1996; 167:981–987.

50. Lederle FA, Wilson SE, Johnson GR. Variability in measurement of abdominal aortic aneurysms. J Vasc Surg 1995; 21:945.

51. Katz DJ, Stanley JC, Zelenock GB. Operative mortality rates for intact and ruptured abdominal aortic aneurysms in Michigan: an eleven-year statewide experience. J Vasc Surg 1994; 19:804.

52. Gott VL, Greene PS, Alejo DE, et al. Replacement of the aortic root in patients with Marfan's syndrome. N Engl J Med 1999; 340:1307.

53. Coselli JS, Buket S, Djukanovic B. Aortic arch operation: current treatment and results. Ann Thorac Surg 1995; 59:19.

54. Blum U, Voshage G, Lammer J. Endoluminal stent-grafts for infrarenal abdominal aortic aneurysms. N Engl J Med 1997; 336:13.

55. Muluk SC, Gertler JP, Brewster DC. Presentation and patterns of aortic aneurysms in young patients. J Vasc Surg 1994; 20:880.

56. Rofsky NM, Weinreb JC, Grossi EA, et al. Aortic aneurysm and dissection: normal MR imaging and CT findings after surgical repair with the continuous-suture graft-inclusion technique. Radiology 1993; 186:195–201.

57. Gaubert J, Moulin G, Mesana T, et al. Type A dissection of the thoracic aorta: use of MR imaging for long term follow-up. Radiology 1995; 201: 363–369.

58. Merkle EM, Klein S, Kramer SC. MR angiographic findings in patients with aortic endoprostheses. Am J Roentgenol 2002; 178(3):641–648.

59. Weigel S, Tombach B, Maintz D, et al. Thoracic aortic stent graft: comparison of contrast-enhanced MR angiography and CT angiography in the follow-up: initial results. Eur Radiol 2003; 13(7):1628–1634.

60. Whitaker SC. Imaging of abdominal aortic aneurysm before and after endoluminal stent-graft repair. Eur J Radiol 2001; 39:3–15.

61. Mohr-Kahaly S, Erbel R, Kearney P, et al. Aortic intramural hemorrhage visualized by transoesophageal echocardiography: findings and prognostic implications. J Am Coll Cardiol 1994; 23:658–664.

62. Price R, Johnson K, Delany D. Magnetic resonance imaging of intramural haematoma of the ascending aorta in Marfan's syndrome. Clin Radiol 2000; 55(11):885–887.

63. Murray JG, Manisali M, Flamm SD. Intramural hematoma of the thoracic aorta: MR image findings and their prognostic implications. Radiology 1997; 204(2):349–355.

64. Casolo F, Dore R, Cardinale L. Acute spontaneous aortic pathologies associated with intramural hematoma: can a differential diagnosis be made by imaging techniques? Radiol Med 2002; 103(1–2):20–33.

65. Wolff KA, Herold CJ, Tempany cm, et al. Aortic dissection: atypical patterns seen at MR imaging. Radiology 1991; 181:489–495.

66. Vilacosta I, Roman JA. Acute aortic syndrome. Heart 2001; 85(4):365–368.

67. Hayashi H, Matsuoka Y, Sakamoto I. Penetrating atherosclerotic ulcer of the aorta: imaging features and disease concept. Radiographics 2000; 20(4): 995–1005.

68. Troxler M, Mavor AID, Homer Vaiassikam H. Penetrating aortic ulcers of the aorta. Br J Surg 2001; 88:1168–1177.

69. Yucel EK, Steinberg FL, Egglin TK, et al. Penetrating atherosclerotic ulcers: diagnosis with MR imaging. Radiology 1990; 177:779–781.

70. Mohiaddin RH, McCrohon J, Francis JM, Barbir M, Pennell DJ. Contrast-enhanced magnetic resonance angiogram of penetrating aortic ulcer. Circulation 2001; 30;103(4):E18–E19.

71. Hagan PG, Nienaber CA, Isselbacher EM, et al. International Registry of Acute Aortic Dissection (IRAD)—new insights into an old disease. J Am Med Assoc 2000; 283:897.

72. DeBakey ME, Henley WS, Cooley DA. Surgical management of dissecting aneurysms of the aorta. J Thorac Cardiovasc Surg 1965; 49:130.

73. Dailey PO, Trueblood HW, Stinson EB. Management of acute dissection. Am J Thorac Surg 1970; 10:237.

74. Danias PG, Edelmann RR, Manning WJ. Magnetic resonance angiography of the great vessels and the coronary arteries. In: Pohost GM, O'Rourke RA, Berman DS, Pravin MS, eds. Imaging in Cardiovascular Disease. Philadelphia: Lippincott William & Wilkins, 449–462.

75. Erbel R, Alfonso F, Boileau C, et al. Diagnosis and management of aortic dissection. Recommendations of the Task Force on Aortic Dissection, European Society of Cardiology. Eur Heart J 2001; 22(18):1642–1681.

76. Moore G, Eagle KA, Bruckman D, et al. Choice of computed tomography, transesophageal echocardiography, magnetic resonance imaging, and aortography in acute aortic dissection: International Registry of Acute Aortic Dissection (IRAD). AJC 2002; 89:1235–1238.

77. Panting JR, Norell MS, Baker C. Feasibility, accuracy and safety of magnetic resonance imaging in acute aortic dissection. Clin Radiol 1995; 50:455–458.

78. Cigarroa JE, Isselbacher EM, De Sanctis RW, et al. Diagnostic imaging in the evaluation of suspected aortic dissection. N Engl J Med 1993; 328:35–43.

79. Nienaber CA, Fattori R. Aortic diseases—do we need MR techniques? Herz 2000; 25(4):331–341.

80. Nienaber CA, von Kodolitsch Y, Nicolas V. The diagnosis of thoracic aortic dissection by noninvasive imaging procedures. N Engl J Med 1993; 328:1–9.

81. Gaubert JY, Caus T, Dahan M, et al. MRI for follow-up after surgery for thoracic aorta dissection. MAGMA 2000; 11(1–2):78–79.

82. Di Cesare E, Giordano AV, Cerone G, De Remigis F, Deusanio G, Masciocchi C. Comparative evaluation of TEE, conventional MRI and contrast-enhanced 3D breath-hold MRA in the post-operative follow-up of dissecting aneurysms. Int J Card Imaging 2000; 16(3):135–147.

83. Williams DM, Joshi A, Dake MD, et al. Aortic cowebs: an anatomic marker identifying the false lumen in aortic dissection. Imaging and pathological correlation. Radiology 1994; 190:167–174.

84. Bogren HG, Underwood SR, Firmin DN. Magnetic resonance velocity mapping in aortic dissection. Br J Radiol 1988; 61:456–462.

85. Chang JM, Friese K, Caputo GR. MR measurement of blood flow in the true and false channel in chronic aortic dissection. J Comput Assist Tomogr 1991; 15:418–423.

86. Holland AE, Barentsz JO, Heijstraten FM, et al. Images in cardiovascular medicine: aortic dissection at the coronary artery sinus: magnetic resonance angiography findings. Circulation 2000; 102(5):597.

87. Bogaert J, Meyns B, Rademakers FE, et al. Follow-up of aortic dissection: contribution of MR angiography for evaluation of the abdominal aorta and its branches. Eur Radiol 1997; 7(5):695–702.

88. Fann JL, Smith JA, Miller CD, et al. Surgical management of aortic dissection during a 30 year period. Circulation 1995; 92:110–121.

89. Moore NR, Parry AJ, Trottman-Dickenson B, et al. Fate of the native aorta after repair of acute type A dissection: a magnetic resonance imaging study. Heart 1996; 75:62–66.

90. Kawamoto S, Bluemke DA, Traill TA, et al. Thoraco-abdominal aorta in Marfan syndrome: MR imaging findings of progression of vasculopathy after surgical repair. Radiology 1997; 203:727–732.

91. Fattori R. MRI and MRA of the thoracic aorta. In: Higgins CB, De Roos A, eds. Cardiovascular MRI and MRA. Philadelphia: Lippincott Williams & Wilkins, 2003:371–392.

92. Munjal AK, Rose WS, Williams G. Magnetic resonance imaging of pseudo-coarctation of the aorta: a case report. J Thorac Imaging 1994; 9(2):88–91.

93. Greenberg SB, Marks LA, Eshaghpour EE. Evaluation of magnetic resonance imaging in coarctation of the aorta: the importance of multiple imaging planes. Pediatr Cardiol 1997; 18(5):345–349.

94. Varaprasathan GA, Araoz PA, Higgins CB, Reddy GP. Quantification of flow dynamics in congenital heart disease: applications of velocity-encoded cine MR imaging. RadioGraphics 2002; 22(4):895–906.

95. Roche KJ, Krinsky G, Lee VS, et al. Interrupted aortic arch: diagnosis with gadolinium-enhanced 3D MRA. J Comput Assist Tomogr 1999; 23(2):197–202.

96. Soler R, Rodriguez E, Requejo I, et al. Magnetic resonance imaging of congenital abnormalities of the thoracic aorta. Eur Radiol 1998; 8(4):540–546.

97. Beekman RP, Hazekamp MG, Sobotka MA. A new diagnostic approach to vascular rings and pulmonary slings: the role of MRI. Magn Reson Imaging 1998; 16(2):137–145.

98. Thoracic Aorta. In: Didier D, Ratib O, eds. Dynamic Cardiovascular MRI. Stuttgard: Georg Thieme Verlag, 2003:75–98.

99. Kastler B, Livolsi A, Germain P. Diagnosis of double aortic arch in the neonatal period: contribution of magnetic resonance imaging. Apropos of a Case. J Radiol 1988; 69(10):625–628.

100. Bernard C, Galloy MA, Marcon F, et al. Contribution of MRI to the diagnosis of double aortic arch. Arch Mal Coeur Vaiss 1988; 81(10):1277–1280.

101. Midiri M, Finazzo M, Pilato M, et al. Right aortic arch with aberrant left innominate artery: MR imaging findings. Eur Radiol 1999; 9(2):311–315.

18

MRI and MRA Techniques for the Evaluation of the Systemic Arterial Vasculature

Mark A. Lawson

*Division of Cardiovascular Medicine, Vanderbilt University Medical Center,
Nashville, Tennessee, U.S.A.*

INTRODUCTION

Magnetic resonance imaging (MRI) and angiography (MRA) are recognized as useful tool for the noninvasive evaluation of arteries by providing clinicians with high-quality diagnostic images, in any imaging plane, without interference from surrounding soft tissues or bones, using only a peripheral intravenous (IV) catheter, and administration of MRI contrast agents characterized by an excellent safety profile. MRI can depict often complex and intertwined vascular anatomy due to the free choice of imaging planes by the scan operator and acquisition of 3D data sets that overcome many limitations of projection techniques.

PRIOR TO BEGINNING MRI/MRA

Appropriate patient selection, preparation, and education are essential to a successful study. Usual contraindications for MRI apply. A thorough history is necessary to prescribe the MRI/MRA examination to obtain useful images and provide a useful report.[a] Details of prior surgeries, especially locations of stents, sternal wires, and surgical clips, should be known. Stents are generally safe to image, but will obscure the repaired region. Fasting for four to six hour prior to the exam may minimize peristalsis that can lead to bowel motion artifacts during abdominal imaging.

To obtain optimal image quality, the patient needs to remain perfectly still, be capable of suspending breathing for brief periods of time, and cooperate with breath-hold commands. The patient should be educated regarding breath-hold techniques, and breath-holding should be rehearsed prior to going into the scanner. Placement of a respiratory bellow around the patient's chest can help monitor the patient's respiratory cycle. Although most patients can hold their breaths for 20 sec, some find this easier using supplemental oxygen. If the patients are unable to suspend respirations for the entire time to complete the scan, they should be instructed to breathe in gently (rather than starting with a gasp) to minimize motion artifacts. In ill or uncooperative patients, shallow breathing may still work well enough to obtain useful, albeit not high quality, images. As most arterial CMR examinations will use MRI contrast agents, peripheral venous access via a 20G (but no less than a 22G) IV catheter in an antecubital vein should be established. The right antecubital vein is preferred due to (i) the shorter, more direct route to the heart, (ii) the larger venous luminal caliber able to accept larger bore catheters, and (iii) a lower vessel wall fragility to power injection. Syringes or tubing with twist or leur-lock fittings are used to ensure a secure seal during rapid injection. Depending on the type of pulse sequences desired, a surface phased-array coil should be considered to improve signal-to-noise ratio (SNR). Phased-array coil placement adds to setup time, and care must be taken to ensure proper centering on the patient or vessel of interest. In most patients, it is often best to extend the arms over the head to reduce wrap artifact on chest and sometimes abdominal MRA. Care should be taken that the IV lines do not become occluded as the patient goes into the scanner. Placement of ECG electrodes (necessary for certain pulse sequences) and drawing up contrast and saline flush in advance while the patient is in the prep area will diminish the demands on scanner time.

---

[a] Given the high mortality of ascending aortic dissection, in a patient with a high index of suspicion for aortic dissection, the most rapid and readily available imaging study should be performed. Although several papers in the literature have documented equal diagnostic utility between CMR, computed tomography (CT), and transesophageal echocardiography (TEE), the choice of the initial diagnostic imaging modality will depend chiefly on availability. Limitations of CMR in this setting are the lack of immediate availability with subsequent delay from bedside to scanner, the relatively longer CMR examination time compared to that of CT and TEE, and the limited access to and restricted monitoring of potentially critically ill patients.

COMMONLY USED MRI AND MRA TECHNIQUES

Factors that determine the appearance of blood on MRI are flow velocity, flow patterns, flow direction, and the T1 relaxation properties of blood (which can be markedly shortened by MRI contrast agents) (1). Inherent in every type of MRI/MRA acquisition are the important interrelationships between acquisition time, spatial resolution, anatomic coverage, SNR, bolus timing, acquisition strategy (2D or 3D), and pulse sequence parameter manipulation of the repetition time (TR), echo time (TE), flip angle, k-space ordering, slice thickness, use of flow compensation or saturation prepulses, and slice location. Knowledge of these parameter interrelationships, the clinical question, and the ability of the patient to cooperate with breath-holding is critical when prescribing an CMR examination.

Black-Blood Techniques

Following scout images, most arterial CMR examinations include some form of black-blood imaging to evaluate the arterial wall and to provide a survey of intra-thoracic or intra-abdominal organs and structures. The blood appears black due to the washout of blood prior to the refocusing pulse and sampling of the echo. Typical black-blood pulse sequences include T1- and T2-weighted spin echo [or fast spin echo (FSE)] and single-shot FSE. The double-inversion recovery FSE acquisition has found increased utility over conventional FSE because it uses two magnetization preparation inversion pulses to suppress the signal within the vascular lumen. First, a nonselective inversion pulse is applied followed by a slice-selective inversion pulse that restores the signal in the imaged section. The time delay between the second inversion pulse and image acquisition is chosen to null the signal from blood. The saturated blood from outside the imaged section will replace blood within the imaged section that receives the second restorative pulse. Selecting an imaging plane perpendicular to the vessel of interest maximizes black-blood appearance. Accordingly, axial imaging is ideal for evaluating most of the aorta, coronal imaging is useful for the arch and abdominal organs, and sagittal imaging depict long segments of the descending thoracic and abdominal aorta. Ideally, axial imaging should be carried out from the level of the aortic arch to the bifurcation. Increasing slice thickness and adding an interslice gap will help complete imaging in a reasonable period of time. These images should be performed with cardiac gating and breath-holding to minimize artifacts that could mimic intimal flaps. Subsequent oblique cine CMR imaging planes (Fig. 1) are planned from the black-blood images.

White-Blood or Cine Techniques

One of the strengths of the CMR is the ability to obtain dynamic information regarding blood flow and heart function. Conventional gradient

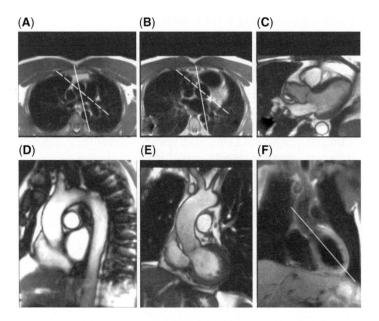

Figure 1 Axial T2-weighted HASTE images at the (**A**) pulmonary artery bifurcation and (**B**) aortic root. Cine MRI images in the (**C**) left ventricular outflow tract (LVOT), (**D**) left anterior oblique (LAO) aorta, and (**E**) ascending aorta orientations. (**F**) Coronal T2-weighted HASTE through the artic root. The solid line defines the cine LAO aorta imaging plane (**D**). The dashed line defines the cine ascending aorta imaging plane (**E**). The cine LVOT imaging plane (**C**) is planned from a coronal HASTE (**F**).

echo (GRE) and steady-state free precession (SSFP) techniques have been discussed previously (Chapter 5). They can be performed as breath-hold sequences on most current scanners. Similar imaging parameters are used as described in previous chapters to acquire these images. Turbulent blood flow may be less apparent on SSFP imaging due to the ultrashort TE used. When examining the aorta, special oblique views are often helpful. First, the left anterior oblique (LAO) view of the aorta is planned from the axial black-blood images. This plane intersects the ascending and descending aorta (Fig. 1D). This plane usually, but not always, includes the aortic arch and may need to be repeated as a parallel plane moved slightly to the left to image the arch. This plane emulates the LAO aortogram from the catheterization laboratory. Another imaging plane also planned from the axial black-blood images is an angulated coronal view that isolates the ascending aorta and aortic valve. This plane intersects the ascending aorta and aortic valve (Fig. 1E). Finally, a view through the left ventricular outflow tract (LVOT) provides information regarding LV size and function as well as the aortic valve competency. This plane is planned from the coronal images and intersects the aortic valve and the LV apex (Fig. 1C).

Phase Contrast Techniques

Phase contrast (PC) methods create contrast between stationary and moving spins as a result of velocity-induced phase shifts of moving spins acquired along a magnetic gradient. In its basic form, PC is a gradient echo-based technique that utilizes bipolar gradients. Stationary tissues will experience no net phase shift by the combination of positively and negatively applied gradients while flowing blood accumulates a phase shift that is directly proportional to the velocity of blood. PC methods are used to measure volumes and velocities of flowing blood and to form PC angiograms (PCAs).

The 2D PC ECG-gated technique can be used in the same way as it is used for valvular regurgitation (Chapter 6) to calculate blood flow velocity, volume, and to depict blood flow profiles though arteries in graphic form across the cardiac cycle. A single imaging plane perpendicular to the long axis of vessel is selected to display the cross-sectional blood flow. The information from a 2D PC acquisition is processed into two data sets: magnitude and phase velocity images. In the phase images, the gray value of each pixel represents velocity information in that pixel, with higher flow velocities represented by higher signal intensities. Blood flow volume can be calculated by circumscribing a region of interest encompassing the target vessel. The operator must carefully select the velocity-encoding factor (VENC) that should be close to the anticipated maximal velocity of the flowing blood in the target vessel. In normal patients, an appropriate VENC for ascending aortic flow is 200–220 cm/sec, 60–12 cm/sec for carotids and 60–80 cm/sec for renal arterial flow. In the presence of stenosis, blood flow velocities can be much higher (up to 400–500 cm/sec). The renal arterial VENC should be set lower (30–40 cm/sec) for patients with congestive heart failure or large aortic aneurysms.

3D phase contrast MRA (PCA) is a noncontrasted flow-dependent MRA technique that acquires three PC data sets, each in the three orthogonal directions, to generate a complete map of flow regardless of direction. Although this technique is less susceptible to signal fallout at vessel tortuosities, it has not found widespread acceptance due to signal loss in areas of turbulence from stenosis. Flow accelerating through a tight stenosis becomes disorganized, separated, swirling, and turbulent. This chaotic flow destroys the MRI phase coherence causing dephasing of the MRI signal. This is especially problematic with 3D PCA due to the relatively long TE resulting in overestimation of vessel stenosis during interpretation. Although this is a disadvantage for estimating percent luminal stenosis, many CMR practitioners recommend PCA to complement contrast-enhanced renal MRA. With PC imaging, if a flow void is seen distal to the site of stenosis demonstrated on contrasted MRA, then a significant stenosis is present such that it has caused a disruption of poststenotic laminar flow sufficient to result in intravoxel phase dispersion and a drop of signal. When performing PCA, select the VENC about 10% to 20% greater than the anticipated blood flow velocity. If the VENC is set too high, SNR is low due to small differences between velocity signals. Meanwhile, VENC values set too low will result in aliasing, a condition where velocities faster than the VENC are incorrectly reconstructed or displayed as low velocities. 3D PCA has also been found to be useful as a scout scan to identify the location of the carotid bifurcation.

Time-of-Flight MRA

Time-of-flight (TOF) is a gradient echo-based imaging technique that takes advantage of the intrinsic contrast created between flowing blood and static tissue. 2D TOF techniques depend on the inflow of unsaturated blood outside the imaging plane. Stationary tissues within the imaging plane become saturated by application of repeated radiofrequency (RF) pulses at a very short TR and high flip angle. The short TR saturates stationary tissues by driving its CMR signal down. Meanwhile blood flowing from outside the imaging plane has not been exposed to these repetitive RF pulses and the unsaturated blood (spins) is capable of generating signal when it washes into the imaging plane. This phenomenon has been referred to as "flow-related enhancement" or "inflow refreshment." As this technique relies on "inflow" of blood for the intravascular signal, the axial plane is selected to maintain signal due to the cranial–caudal orientation of the aorta, carotid, or lower extremity arteries. Maximal signal is achieved when a totally new column of blood enters the slice every TR period. Therefore, TR and slice thickness must be adjusted depending on the velocity of the flowing blood. The sections should be thin enough to allow for sufficient inflow between RF pulse repetitions, but thick enough to ensure adequate SNR and anatomic coverage. A slice thickness of 3–4 mm is adequate for larger vessels and 1.5–2 mm for smaller vessels. Thicker slices (also called partitions by some vendors) used to shorten acquisition time have the untoward effect of increased saturation effects and decreased spatial resolution. The typical TR for TOF is about 20–50 msec. The short TR keeps background tissue saturated but should not be too short to allow for satisfactory inflow of unsaturated blood between successive repetitions. The flip angle is usually maintained between 30° to 60°. High flip angles are effective in suppressing background tissues but may begin to saturate blood and reduce the separation between blood and stationary tissues. In addition, pulsatile artifact is greater at higher flip angles.

For 3D TOF, data are collected as a 3D volume set rather than individual slices as done in a 2D TOF acquisition. Thinner slices are possible on 3D acquisitions, and therefore results in less dephasing because of a smaller voxel size and shorter TE. Compared with 2D TOF, 3D TOF acquisition time is shorter and SNR is higher. In contrast, 3D TOF is more susceptible to saturation effects because unsaturated spins from outside the volume may have to travel a few centimeters into the imaging volume to produce flow enhancement. Saturation effects can be minimized in 3D TOF by using the thinnest volume to encompass the target vessel, low flip angle, and longer TR. 3D TOF can be acquired as a single slab or as a series of multiple overlapping slabs that are combined to cover the entire course of the vessel of interest.

As TOF relies in part on the direction of flowing blood, a "presaturation" pulse can be applied prior to image acquisition to suppress signal from veins. For example, to perform TOF of the carotid arteries, a spatial presaturation slab can be positioned superior to the imaging slice and programmed to move together with each section that is being acquired (the so-called "traveling sat band"). This will eliminate venous flow from the jugular veins by "presaturating" the caudally flowing venous blood. If venous flow is slow, more space between acquired sections and the saturation band is required.

TOF methods have limited use for imaging the aorta and renal arteries due to longer acquisition times, sensitivity to flow direction, saturation of slow spins, and intravoxel dephasing from turbulent blood flow that overestimate stenosis severity.

Contrast-Enhanced MRA

With images resembling conventional X-ray angiography, contrast-enhanced MRA (CE-MRA) is the preferred, currently available (2,3) MRA technique used today. This technique does not rely on the flow characteristic of blood but rather on T1-shortening effects of a circulating MRI contrast agent making it less prone to flow-related artifacts. CE-MRA requires the coordination of an intravenously administered MRI contrast agent bolus with image acquisition during the arterial phase. Although CE-MRA can be performed on any MRI system, implementation on systems equipped with high-performance gradients reduces imaging times so that the entire 3D data set covering the target vessel can be sampled within a breath-hold. With such a short acquisition time, respiratory artifacts are reduced, and the scan can be completed before venous enhancement occurs.

Injectable MRI Contrast Agents

In the United States, no agent is approved for MRA by the Food and Drug Administration at the time of the writing of this chapter. Any use constitutes off-label use of an approved drug. Nevertheless, gadolinium chelates have revolutionized MRA by eliminating in-plane saturation effects and flow voids related to the turbulence that were often encountered with TOF imaging. Gadolinium has a favorable side effect profile with no adverse hemodynamic or pharmacological effects. Gadolinium is not nephrotoxic and has a low incidence of anaphalactoid reactions. They are safe in patients with renal insufficiency and in patients with a history of allergic reactions to iodinated contrast. Although gadolinium is being used as a blood pool agent as it passes through a vessel of interest, it is not the gadolinium that is visible on the images; rather gadolinium alters the relaxation properties of surrounding blood (spins) and drastically shortens the T1 relaxation time of blood. For practical purposes, however, it is sufficient to conceptualize gadolinium as being imaged with a behavior similar to what is experienced with iodinated contrast during X-ray angiography. Currently available gadolinium-based contrast agents do not remain in the vascular space but diffuse into the extracellular space. Thus for MRA to be successful, a sufficient concentration of contrast material should be maintained in the target artery during the entire acquisition time.

Contrast Agent Injection

Contrast volume, delivery rate, delay time from injection to image acquisition, and saline flush are important parameters to select for high image quality. To make blood appear bright compared to the background tissues, it is necessary to inject a sufficient volume of gadolinium at a sufficient rate. The arterial phase of the gadolinium infusion is the optimal time to acquire image data of the target vessel to take advantage of the higher arterial SNR and to eliminate overlapping venous enhancement. An extremely fast acquisition is essential to capture the gadolinium bolus during the brief moment that the agent is present in the arteries but not yet in the veins. To accomplish this goal, use of an MRI-compatible power injector has been advocated. Only a small volume of gadolinium is needed due to the marked relaxation properties of gadolinium. A typical contrast dosage of 0.1–0.2 mmol/kg (20–40 ml) is sufficient to shorten the T1 of blood below that of fat for the duration of the acquisition. Gadolinium has a viscosity lower than iodinated contrast and can be injected at 2–4 mL/sec using the power injector. The gadolinium injection is chased by 20 ml of normal saline injected at the same rate to ensure that the gadolinium bolus is flushed out of the tubing set into peripheral venous system and well into the central circulation. The right arm is preferred site because it has the most direct path to the heart.

Triggering MRA Acquisition

Once the gadolinium is injected, the first-pass arterial phase of the bolus is brief. There is only one shot at capturing the arterial phase of the injection. Circulation times can vary from patient to patient due to the differences in cardiac output, blood flow profiles, and plasma volume. Coordination of image acquisition and the arrival of the gadolinium bolus at the target vessel is crucial to achieve high image quality. Imaging prematurely can result in incomplete vascular depiction (Fig. 2). Imaging too late can result in

(A)   (B)

(C)   (D)

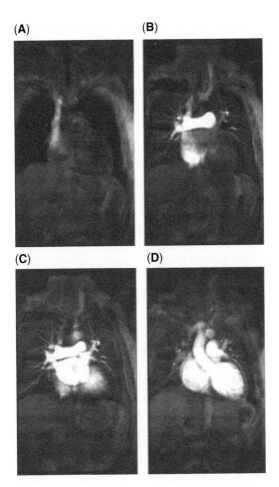

Figure 2   Time-resolved MRA: (A) contrast initially arrives in superior vena cava, (B) contrast transit through pulmonary artery, (C) contrast transit through left atrium, and (D) contrast arrives finally into left ventricle and aorta.

insufficient signal within the target vessel due to washout of the gadolinium and diffusion into the tissues. Images acquired too long after arterial arrival are frequently obscured by enhancement of the veins and soft tissues. Different triggering strategies have been developed to optimize the proper timing to synchronize the beginning of image acquisition with arterial enhancement to avoid the enhancement of unwanted structures.

Empiric or Fixed Triggering: Following the bolus injection of gadolinium, the peak signal intensity in the ascending aorta occurs 15 ± 1.6 sec and 20 ± 6 sec in the abdominal aorta in the average patient. However, one must anticipate longer transit times in patients with slow flow from aortic aneurysms or decreased cardiac output. Because timing mismatch is more often encountered with empiric triggering, a longer and larger gadolinium infusion should be considered. Delay times of 15–25 sec for the thoracic aorta and 20–30 sec for the abdominal aorta are generally reliable for most cases.

Bolus Timing Scan or Test Injection: The purpose of the bolus timing scan is to calculate the time required for peak enhancement of the targeted vessel. This method is performed using a 1–5 ml test bolus of contrast followed by saline flush injected at the same rate as the planned CE-MRA. For MRA of the aorta, axial imaging at the targeted aortic level is performed using a fast 2D GRE sequence with a temporal resolution of about one image per second. A time–intensity curve is constructed of the aorta and the arrival time of the test bolus is determined, to which is added 5–10 sec for the actual imaging delay. If an axial imaging plane is used for the timing scan (i.e., perpendicular to the aorta), some MRI practitioners advocate that addition of superior and inferior saturation pulses minimizes the signal from the inflowing blood and ensure that the vascular signal is attributable only to the gadolinium bolus.

Automated Bolus Detection: With automated bolus detection technique, the operator positions a small tracker volume in the aorta at the desired level. The signal intensity of the tracker volume is repeatedly sampled during gadolinium injection, and image acquisition is started automatically when the signal level rises above a predetermined threshold. A delay of 5–10 sec between bolus detection and the start of the acquisition is added to allow the contrast concentration to achieve a plateau and initiate a breath-hold. The patient should breathe quietly and remain still during bolus detection to avoid false triggering. A "fail-safe" triggering time using the empirical method described above should be programmed to begin MRA acquisition if no bolus is detected.

MRI Fluoroscopy with Manual Triggering: Another real-time method of timing the bolus arrival is MRI fluoroscopy. In this technique, time-resolved 2D GRE images are obtained and displayed on the operator's monitor at near real-time rates. The operator manually triggers the start of CE-MRA acquisition when enhancement of the target vessel is visualized.

k-space Ordering

Different regions of k-space have varying importance for CE-MRA. As image contrast depends mainly on the central region of k-space, collection of the central lines of k-space during the plateau phase of arterial enhancement would therefore be optimal for CE-MRA. The periphery of k-space contributes primarily to image detail, but its acquisition is less time-sensitive. Arterial phase images are achieved by preferentially timing the acquisition of central k-space during arterial transit of gadolinium resulting in selective arterial enhancement.

For most CMR pulse sequences, *sequential* ordering of k-space is employed whereby the center of k-space is acquired during the middle or center of the imaging period. Sequential ordering is a linear method of filling k-space from top to bottom (or bottom to top) of k-space, so filling of the central lines must fall in the middle of the acquisition time. If sequential ordering is used for CE-MRA, the scan should start when the bolus arrives one-quarter of the total scan time. An improved method for k-space filling for CE-MRA applications is *centric* ordering where crucial image contrast data are acquired first. k-space filling starts with the center lines and progresses out towards the periphery. Centric ordering is beneficial for imaging patients with limited breath-holding capability, ensuring that the critical central k-space data are acquired earlier during the breath-hold. Incomplete breath-holding would thus corrupt peripheral filling of k-space and result in less significant degradation of the final image. Centric ordering is optimized for only one of the two phase-encoding directions. *Elliptic centric* k-space ordering is performed in both phase-encoding directions and progresses from the center out to the next most radial point in k-space. This results in a compact acquisition of the center of k-space and is also less sensitive to motion artifact caused by loss of breath-hold. A partial Fourier acquisition scheme can also decrease total acquisition time by acquiring only a little more than half of k-space and extrapolating the unsampled data by exploiting the symmetry of signals in k-space.

If the central portion of k-space is filled prior to or during the upslope of gadolinium bolus arrival, severe ringing artifacts limit the diagnostic usefulness of the images. This artifact is recognized by alternating bright and dark bands that parallel vascular structures. In contrast, images acquired too long after peak arterial gadolinium arrival are frequently obscured by enhanced veins and soft tissues.

The "Dry Run"

It is recommended that before injecting gadolinium, a noncontrasted MRA sequence be executed. This "dry run" serves multiple purposes. First, it verifies that the sequence parameters selected (including the FOV and imaging slab position) are correct to ensure adequate anatomical coverage and assess for excessive wrap artifact that may obscure the target vessel. Second, it tests the patient's ability to breathe hold and follow the appropriate commands. Third, this acquisition can serve as a mask for subtracting residual background signal (mostly fat) from the arterial phase images. If the subtraction processing method will be used, both the mask (noncontrasted MRA) and CE-MRA images should be obtained with breath-holding and the patient should not move between the "dry run" and actual CE-MRA ("wet run").

The "Wet Run"

Following the injection of gadolinium and acquisition of the first arterial phase CE-MRA, routine use of a second and even a third MRA acquisition (the so-called "equilibrium-phases") is useful. Although the equilibrium phases are less than ideal than the arterial phase because of the increased background signal and venous contamination, equilibrium-phase MRA can detect late enhancing vessels and recover diagnostic information when the arterial-phase data were acquired too early following injection. Equilibrium-phase MRA can provide additional information regarding slow flow (e.g., flow in aneurysms or false channels) and parenchymal enhancement.

Multistation MRA

To cover larger vascular territories, CE-MRA can be performed using several overlapping contiguous CE-MRA acquisitions, the so-called multistation MRA. This technique is frequently employed when abdominal MRA is combined with peripheral MRA of the legs to evaluate the adequacy of lower extremity arterial inflow. Typically, the initial station is centered on the abdomen, and the first scan is initiated with arrival of gadolinium in the abdominal aorta. Each subsequent MRA station is acquired in rapid succession moving more distal than the first to capture the arterial transit of gadolinium down the lower extremity. A stepping table is essential to perform this "bolus chase" and consists of the progressive movement of the imaging field of view to coincide with gadolinium run-off. Each station requires an optimized spatial resolution (FOV and matrix) and imaging volume (slab and slice thickness) to minimize the total acquisition time at each station.

The main challenge of multistation MRA is to avoid enhancement in the infrapopliteal veins which contaminates the infrapopliteal arterial images. MRA of the infrapopliteal station occurs only after the scans of the proximal stations (plus time for table movement) are completed. As bolus arrival time varies widely, venous enhancement may occur when the combined time of proximal multistation MRAs exceeds the aorta-to-infrapopliteal vein circulation time. To improve distal arterial visualization, several approaches have been proposed. One technique uses a 2D TOF MRA of the infrapopliteal arteries prior to CE-MRA. Time-resolved MRA or a separate single-station CE-MRA of just the infrapopliteal arteries using a low-dose gadolinium injection has also shown merit. However, with these approaches, it is recommended that a mask image of the proximal stations be acquired before running the CE-MRA bolus chase. The mask images will subsequently be used during image subtraction to eliminate the effects of gadolinium tissue accumulation from the initial injection. Finally, with the availability of parallel imaging techniques, substantial time savings can be achieved from increased acquisition speeds. When employing parallel imaging, time savings can be invested in the proximal stations to maintain synchronization of the bolus with image acquisition but use higher spatial resolution parameters for the infrapopliteal arteries. All these approaches have certain attractive features, and no single technique has yet emerged as the clear method of choice in every case.

CE-MRA PARAMETER SELECTION

For thoracic and abdominal imaging, CE-MRA is performed during a breath-hold to minimize artifacts (image blurring) related to respiratory motion. For this reason, the fastest possible T1-weighted 3D imaging sequence should be selected, typically a fast gradient echo-based sequence. The imaging parameters should be tailored to achieve the highest spatial resolution for the allotted time period for image acquisition. The total acquisition time for CE-MRA is equal to the product of the number of phase-encoding steps, NEX, and TR. Some of the imaging parameters that can be adjusted for optimal results using CE-MRA are discussed in Table 1.

Time-Resolved MRA

Time-resolved MRA is a method of obtaining high temporally resolved images. The imaging technique enables rapid updating of 3D data sets in several seconds, eliminating the need for timing acquisitions or triggering methods. Two techniques have been used. TRICKS (time-resolved imaging with contrast kinetics) samples low-spatial frequency data more often than high-spatial frequency data, as they are shared among adjacent frames to fill k-space for each frame. The so-called "subsecond angiography" is based on a 3D MRA acquisition made ultrafast by using markedly short TRs of < 2 msec and TEs of < 1 msec along with partial Fourier and fractional FOV k-space schemes. The transit of gadolinium through the target vessel can be displayed using these techniques as a continuous loop of contrast wash-in during the arterial phase and wash-out during the venous phase (Fig. 2). The high temporal resolution can be achieved only at the price of compromising spatial resolution. With the use of consecutive rapid acquisitions, at least one data set will be obtained during peak arterial enhancement producing a sufficient arterial angiogram without venous overlap. Subtraction is less problematic by acquiring precontrast data together with postcontrast data during a single breath-hold.

Postcontrast Black-Blood Techniques

Black-blood imaging may also be repeated following CE-MRA. Postcontrast fat-suppressed T1 spin echo may reveal inflammatory changes in and around the aorta. Postcontrast T1- and T2-weighted FSE images can aid in better delineating a mural thrombus lining the aortic aneurysm, the fibrous cap of the atherosclerotic plaque, and an increased inflammatory component (4).

Table 1 Parameters for Contrast Enhanced-MRA

Parameter	Value	Comments
Shortest TR	Typically 4–6 msec	Short TR leads to better background suppression, enhances CNR, reduces scan time, and increases sensitivity to the short T1 of contrast-enhanced blood.
Shortest TE	Typically 1–3 msec	Short TE eliminates dephasing (signal loss from regions of chaotic or nonlaminar flow), minimizes $T2^*$ decay, maximizes differences between fat and water artifact, and minimizes pulsatile ghosting artifact.
Matrix	Typically 256×192 (frequency × phase-encoding steps)	Higher matrix results in higher resolution at a penalty of diminished SNR and increased scan time; to decrease scan time, phase-encoding steps can be reduced using a rectangular FOV (also called phase FOV by some vendors) usually set to a value of 0.75–0.9.
Flip angle	Typically 20–45°	By increasing the flip angle, background suppression and SNR increase but so does imaging time; for slower injections, lower contrast dose, or a very short TR (<5 msec), flip angles near the low end of this range are more appropriate; in patients with stents, a higher flip angle may improve visualization of flow in the stent; some advocate using "variable" flip angle whereby the flip angle is automatically varied as a function of position along the slice-select direction; mitigating the loss of signal from flowing blood that is deeper in the imaging slab where a larger flip angle is used.
Bandwidth	Typically 32–64 kHz	Bandwidth is a compromise setting balance between SNR and acquisition time (or in practical terms, the time the patient can hold their breath); as bandwidth decreases, the SNR and imaging time increase.
Imaging volume (or "slab")	Customized for each patient	The number of slices (also called partitions by some vendors) and slice thickness, together with the FOV, determine the imaging volume; the dimensions are prescribed to achieve the smallest possible voxel size (ideally 2 mm or less), include sufficient spatial anatomical coverage of the target vessel, and yet, still be acquired within a breath-hold; the FOV is usually about 30–40 cm depending on patient's body habitus; a volume of 36–40 slices each 2–4 mm thick provides adequate coverage of the aorta; if too small of a volume is prescribed, critical anatomical structures will be excluded;

the volume is oriented along the coronal plane and extends from the anterior to the posterior aspects of the target vessel; the critical technical issue for achieving diagnostic CE-MRA of aortic branch vessels is spatial resolution; the thinner the imaging volume, the thinner the effective slices (or partitions) can be made, increasing the through-plane spatial resolution for improved multiplanar reformatted 3D reconstructions.

NEX	Typically 0.5–1	Lower values result in faster scanning but lead to a reduction in SNR related to diminished signal averaging; this reduction, however, is overcome by the increase in signal intensity associated with the shorter T1 of contrast-enhanced blood.
Spoiling	Yes	Spoiling destroys the residual magnetization after each echo thereby suppressing background signal and enhancing the signal from gadolinium in the vasculature.
Coil selection	Surface	The body coil can provide adequate signal for aortic MRA; however, SNR can be significantly improved using a surface phased-array coil at the expense of a somewhat restricted FOV; it is acceptable and easiest to use the body coil because it provides a larger FOV and homogeneous signal; phased-array surface coils are less sensitive to motion outside the FOV that can lead to artifacts and improve SNR, but can cause bright, near-field artifact from tissue closer to the coil (unless a normalization or depth correction algorithm is used to even the displayed signal).
Fat saturation	Yes	Additional background signal suppression can be achieved by fat saturation pulses, but this incurs additional time.
Zero-filling	Yes	This data manipulation scheme has gained popularity by visually improving MIP images at no additional cost to imaging time; although zero-filling generates better reformations and MIPs, it does not improve the true spatial resolution of the images; this scheme involves filling peripheral lines of k-space data with zeroes before performing the Fourier transform; this helps eliminate volume averaging and creates a smoother visualization of small vessels on the reformatted image.
ECG-gating	No	CE-MRA is independent of ECG triggering.

Abbreviations: TR, repetition time; TE, echo time; CE-MRA, contrast-enhanced MRA; MIP, maximal intensity projection; SNR, signal-to-noise ratio; FOV, field of view.

PROCESSING IMAGE DATA

Dexterity and understanding of the postprocessing workstation utilities are critical for accurate interpretations of imaging data. Some vendors offer filtering algorithms to improve image quality. A variety of processing tools are available to display the results of MRA. These include maximal intensity projections (MIPs), multiplanar reformatting (MPR), volume rendering (VR) display, and virtual arterial endoscopy. Care must be taken when viewing MIPs or MPRs created by another person because an apparent occlusion or stenosis may be an artifact related to an incorrectly oriented display plane that excluded a portion of the target vessel. When reviewing the MIP images, it is strongly encouraged to simultaneously review the source data to detect possible artifacts and nonvascular abnormalities. Some MRI practitioners believe that volume-rendered MRA data facilitate more accurate detection of artery stenosis over MIP images by displaying the sometimes complex geometry of the target vessel in a more appealing and intuitive 3D representation. This is because the MIP algorithm selects only the voxel with the highest signal intensity along a ray projected through the data set so that volume-averaged voxels may be erroneously excluded from the final image. This would result in overestimation of stenosis severity. However, the VR algorithm allows volume-averaged voxels to be included in the final image because it calculates a weighted sum of data from all voxels along a ray projected through the data sets. Because of the limited spatial resolution of MRA, even minimal misclassification of marginal voxels between vascular and perivascular tissues may lead to an anatomical miscategorization of the voxel and worsen the degree of stenosis. MIP and VR images are often performed on the subtraction data sets to improve SNR and remove unwanted high background signal that may persist. However, if the patient held their breath inconsistently between the dry and wet runs, the subtraction sets may produce worse results than the unsubtracted image data set. Most vendors offer workstations which can automatically display all the three orthogonal MPR views along with an interactive oblique view selected by the operator. This allows the operator to aid in judging whether abnormalities of arterial segments noted on MIP or VR images are pathological or artifactual.

INTERPRETATION OF MRI/MRA OF THE ARTERIAL VASCULATURE

Black-Blood Images

Vascular pathology often first becomes evident on review of the black-blood images. When scrolling through the image set, the reader should initially observe the relationship of the great arterial vessels to the heart and organ viscera as the initial clue for congenital heart and vascular disease (5–8). In

Table 2 Aortic and Pulmonic Valve Relationship using the Van Praagh Convention

Label	Description	Relationship	Condition
S	Normal sidedness and concordant connection	The aortic valve is posterior and to the right of the pulmonary valve.	Describes the normal heart
I	Inverted sidedness and normal connection	The aortic valve is posterior and to the left of the pulmonary valve.	
D	Rightward malposition and discordant connection	The aortic valve is anterior and to the right of the pulmonary valve.	The most common arrangement is complete transposition of the aorta, designated S, D, D.
L	Leftward malposition and discordant connection	The aortic valve is anterior and to the left of the pulmonary valve.	The most common arrangement is congenitally corrected transposition of the great arteries, designated S, L, L.

congenital heart disease, some pediatric cardiologists have adopted the Van Praagh classification (Table 2) to describe the anatomic relationship of the venoatrial, atrioventricular, and ventriculoarterial connections viewed on axial sections. Aortae that crossover the left pulmonary artery and pass left of the trachea are termed left-sided; they are right-sided when they crossover the right pulmonary artery and to the right of the trachea. For the most part, adult patients will have normal ventriculoarterial concordance and left-sided aortae.

Next, each maximum transverse arterial segment dimension should be measured perpendicular to the longitudinal course of the vessel to quantify the degree of ectasia or aneurismal dilatation. Attention should then be directed towards examination of the arterial wall to detect possible atherosclerosis, inflammation, dissection, or hematoma. Systemic arterial atherosclerosis is a systemic disease common in the United States and throughout the world. Atherosclerotic lesions can be quite heterogeneous even within the same patient and all subtypes of lesions likely coexist together but in unpredictable proportions. The proportional distribution of different plaque types is inherently variable within individual patients because of the continuous, evolutionary nature of atheroma formation. Plaque structure and composition importantly impact the clinical expression of atherosclerosis. Fortunately, MRI has a unique ability to differentiate plaque components based on water and chemical composition and concentration, along with other properties of molecular motion, diffusion, and magnetization transfer. Thus, T1- and T2-weighted images for the same anatomy can appear quite different (9,10). Accordingly, fibrous plaque tissues (mainly composed of extracellular matrix elaborated by smooth muscle cells) have a short T1. Plaque lipids (mainly composed of unesterified cholesterol and cholesteryl esters) have a short T2. Perivascular fat (mainly composed of triglycerides) has even a shorter T1 than atherosclerotic plaque lipid. Calcific regions have low signal intensities due to low proton density and susceptibility artifacts. On the basis of these differing relaxation times, it is possible to predict plaque components based on signal intensity on T1- and T2-weighted images (Table 3).

In addition to atherosclerosis, the arterial wall should be examined for a mural thrombus lining an aortic aneurysm or for a thrombus-filled false lumen of an aortic dissection because neither of these may be apparent on the arterial phase of CE-MRA alone. In these instances, intraluminal or intraaortic signal may be high from thrombus, slow flow, or a combination of the two. In patients presenting with pain, the aortic wall should also be inspected for a penetrating aortic ulcer (PAU) and intramural hematoma (IMH). PAU is characterized by an atherosclerotic plaque ulcer that penetrates through the intima into the media of the aortic wall (11). Progressive penetration deep into the aortic wall may result in hematoma and a weakening of the aortic wall, which in turn may result in aortic enlargement and aneurysm formation. PAU is typically seen as an outpouching or "crater" extending beyond the contour of the aortic lumen usually located in the descending aorta surrounded by extensive atherosclerosis and can be associated with a variable degree of aortic wall thickening and adjacent subintimal hematoma within the aortic wall. There may be an area of aortic dissection, but unlike classic aortic dissection, the length of dissection is

Table 3 Appearance of Atherosclerotic Plaque and Hemorrhagic Components on Magnetic Resonance Imaging

Component	T1-weighted appearance	T2-weighted appearance
Lipid	Hyperintense	Hypointense
Fibrocellular	Iso-/hyperintense	Iso-/hyperintense
Calcium	Hypointense	Hypointense
Fibrous cap	Hyperintense (especially on postcontrast images)	Hypointense
Acute thrombosis	Hypo-/isointense	Hyperintense
Subacute thrombosis	Hyperintense	Hyperintense
Chronic thrombosis	Isointense	Isointense

limited and the intimal flap is thick, irregular, and does not usually encroach on the aortic lumen. A prominent feature of advanced atherosclerosis is *superficial* ulcerations limited just to the intima. These shallow atheromatous ulcers sometimes radiographically appear similar to PAU. Therefore, care should be taken in making a diagnosis of PAU, particularly if discovered incidentally. IMH is characterized by the absence of an intimal tear with no direct flow communication between true and "false" lumens. Diagnostic CMR features of IMH are increased wall thickness (>5–7 mm) and the presence of multiple layers of aortic wall with splitting due to hemorrhage (12). Crescentic sequestration of blood between the intima and adventitia is a characteristic finding. Thrombus signal characteristics on T2-weighted images depend on thrombosis age, with a higher signal seen in thrombus up to 1 week of age and declining thereafter. It may be difficult to distinguish IMH from limited aortic dissection with a thrombosed false lumen, a laminated thrombus of an aortic aneurysm, or severe atherosclerotic changes. MRI contrast agents rarely fill the intramural space. Fat-suppressed images can differentiate IMH from surrounding periaortic or mediastinal fat. In patients presenting with a prodrome of systemic inflammatory symptoms, the edema and inflammation of vasculitis can be demonstrated by arterial wall thickening and signal enhancement of the wall and adjacent vascular soft tissues on T2-weighted and on both precontrast and postcontrast T1-weighted sequences. These findings are especially apparent during the acute and active phases of the disease.

Finally, the images for nonvascular anatomy and pathology are inspected. Comment on any anatomy that is seen that may impact on surgical planning (such as horseshoe kidney or accessory renal arteries in the presence of an abdominal aortic aneurysm). In dissection cases, extravasation of fluid or blood into the pericardial, pleural, mediastinal, or periaortic space often signals a high likelihood for rupture into these spaces and requires urgent surgical consultation. Arterial dilatation may compress and erode into adjacent structures such as vertebrae, the tracheobronchial tree, esophagus, duodenum, pulmonary vessels, and vena cavae.

Vascular Cine CMR

Cine CMR is invaluable for depicting flowing blood. Stagnant or slow flowing blood may appear bright on black-blood sequences and subsequently misinterpreted as thrombosis without the aid of cine CMR. The sine qua non of aortic dissection is the documentation of an intimal flap and systolic expansion of the true lumen. Cine CMR can demonstrate the location of entry and reentry sites as well as the extent of the tear. Measurements of the true and false lumen dimensions should be recorded from the various parts of the affected aorta. On cine CMR, thrombus in the false lumen is hypointense compared with the faster flowing bright blood of the true lumen. Although often larger in diameter than the true lumen, the false lumen demonstrates little circumferential change during the cardiac cycle because pulsatile motion is diminished. Atherosclerotic plaques of the aorta that are at high risk for atherothrombotic embolization are those >4 mm in diameter, ulcerations >2 mm deep, or protruding mobile lesions. However, freely mobile aortic debris may be better visualized by TEE.

Cardiac Cine MRI

A cardiac cine MRI study (whether complete or abbreviated) should be performed before CE-MRA to examine the left ventricle for clues of comorbid conditions. The MRI reader should record ventricular cavity size and mass, and assess the global and segmental function as well as for the presence of aortic value insufficiency in cases of aortic dissection or aneurysm. Left ventricular hypertrophy may be an indication of uncontrolled hypertension. Segmental wall motion abnormalities provide a clue of previously undiagnosed coronary artery disease, but could also indicate ongoing myocardial ischemia due to extension of aortic dissection down the coronary artery or coronary compression by an external hematoma. Myocardial ischemia sufficient to cause global left ventricular systolic dysfunction contributes to hypotension and shock in patients with aortic dissection. Aortic valve morphology (such as bicuspid or calcific) and the mechanism of aortic regurgitation, especially in cases of aortic dissection, should be discussed. Dilatation of the aortic root and annulus, tearing of the annulus or valve cusps, downward displacement of one cusp below the line of valve closure, loss of support of the cusp, and physical interference in the closure of the aortic valve by an intimal flap are possibilities. 2D PC methods through the aortic root can calculate the regurgitant fraction or estimate aortic stenosis severity by measuring peak aortic valve velocity (Chapter 6).

Vascular PC MRI

For cases where the morphological findings of dissection are ambiguous, 2D PC MRI can differentiate true and false lumens on the basis of blood flow profile pattern. Thrombosed channels exhibit absent flow. Patent false lumens exhibit delayed or even reversed flow and diminished mean flow velocity and volume. The amount of flow volume in a patent false lumen correlates positively with the prediction of aneurysm formation and aneurysm growth rate.

3D PCA is sensitive to turbulent flow due to intravoxel dephasing and can confirm the presence of a hemodynamically significant stenosis. A disadvantage with this approach is that patients often have poor arterial blood flow as a result of a critical stenosis, thus minimizing the added value of this sequence. However, if a stenosis is apparent on CE-MRA but appears minimal on PCA, then the stenosis can be graded moderately.

2D PC MRI can also be used to determine hemodynamic significance for a stenotic lesion, usually in cases of renal artery stenosis. For 2D PC flow measurements, a scan plane is selected perpendicular to the renal artery approximately 1 cm distal to the ostium or 1–2 cm distal to the stenosis in diseased vessels. Normally, an early systolic maximal velocity ("early systolic peak") and a lower second midsystolic velocity peak should be present. Changes in vascular resistance and loss of autoregulation alter the slope and shape of the flow curve in a characteristic way that correlates with the degree of stenosis. A moderate stenosis is present when there is near-complete or complete loss of the early systolic peak or a decrease of the midsystolic peak. A featureless, flattened flow profile with no systolic velocity components represents severe high-grade stenosis.

In cases of aortic coarctation, transverse 2D PC imaging should be carried out just distal to the coarctation and at the level of the diaphragm. If the aortic flow measured at the level of the diaphragm is more than the flow that is immediately distal to the stenosis, then collateral flow, mostly through intercostals arteries, is present. Peak instantaneous pressure gradient across the aortic narrowing using the modified Bernoulli's equation can be calculated from the peak flow velocity measurement obtained just distal to the coarctation on 2D PC.

Contrast-Enhanced MRA

CE-MRA has emerged as a technique of choice for vascular imaging (2,3). Due to their three-dimensional appearance, the tendency of the reader to rely solely on the MIP or VR image reconstruction is only natural. However, the careful CMR practitioner will develop a disciplined approach that includes review the coronal raw data set and even a series of stacked axial MPRs. If the CE-MRA is acquired in multiple phases, examining each equilibrium phase is important because flow within a patent false channel or large aneurysm may be slow and not adequately filled with gadolinium during the earlier arterial phase. Remember that laminated thrombus often lines the aneurysm, so that gadolinium opacification of the lumen does not completely delineate the size and extent of the aneurysm.

First, the practitioner should comment on the quality of the images (Table 4). Importantly, the reader should review old studies and compare with prior study measurements, e.g., to determine the expansion rate of aortic aneurysm. Given the adverse outcomes of patients with aortic dissection, in the appropriate clinical setting, special attention should be given to examining the images for dissection by looking for evidence of an intimal flap, describing the location of entry and reentry sites, assessing the extent of the tear, and measuring the true and false lumen dimensions in the various parts of the affected aorta (Fig. 3). As discussed earlier, these entry sites may be more easily identified using cine techniques. Arterial size and

Table 4 Potential Artifacts Affecting Image Quality

Source of artifact	Effect on image
Chemical shift artifact	If both water and lipid protons coexist in a voxel, the signal emitted by the lipid protons will have a lower frequency than that of the water protons; consequently, when the scanner is tuned to water, the signal from the lipid protons will appear to have arisen from water protons from another voxel in a lower part of the field; this spatial mismapping of MRI signal is based on frequency and will be observed in the frequency-encoding direction within a section; chemical shift artifact will appear as a light crescent or halo aside the aorta, one to several pixels in width; one simple way to work around the chemical shift artifact is to swap the frequency and phase-encoding directions; if the "halo" moves, the finding is artifact; alternatively, the bandwidth or FOV can be expanded to minimize the artifact.
Off-resonance artifact	If the scanner is not tuned to water frequency, artifactual flow disturbances may be seen in the aorta.
Susceptibility artifact	Susceptibility artifacts occur at interfaces between substances with different magnetic susceptibilities that cause local distortion of the magnetic field; susceptibility artifact appears as a black outline that follows the anatomical boundary between two different tissues; metallic materials typically have large susceptibility and distort the magnetic field sufficiently to cause signal dropout over a larger area adjacent to the metal.
Dephasing artifact	This artifact is common in regions with complex geometry or stenosis that unfortunately are typically the regions of clinical interest; all MRA sequences suffer signal loss due to intravoxel-phase dispersion or phase incoherence, commonly referred to as dephasing; signal loss from dephasing can be minimized using the smallest voxel size, minimum TE, and first-order flow compensation; TOF MRA becomes unreliable when blood flow is slow, turbulent, or complex resulting in signal loss that can overestimate stenosis severity, or even simulate vascular occlusion; 3D PC angiography commonly demonstrates artifactual dephasing at the renal artery origins; it is more of a problem with 2D methods due to larger voxel size and longer minimum TE.
Saturation artifact	Slow flow may cause this artifact within the lumen of the aorta; incomplete washout of saturated blood results in persistence of signal within the vessel lumen; this may mask of underlying luminal pathology such as an intimal tear or

(Continued)

Table 4 Potential Artifacts Affecting Image Quality (*Continued*)

Source of artifact	Effect on image
	may erroneously simulate vascular occlusion or thrombus; flow stasis and recirculation of flow (e.g., large aneurysms) result in intravascular signal due to saturation effects.
Flow artifact	There are many types of flow patterns that can lead to artifacts; retrograde flow during diastole can cause image distortion; artifactual stenosis can occur in the vessels that run parallel with the plane of acquisition; pulsatile flow in vessels with relatively brisk inflow can produce external ghost artifacts that extend across the image in the phase-encoding direction; turbulent, nonlaminar flow with complex vortex and eddy current result in intravoxel-phase dispersion and loss of signal as mentioned above.
Artifacts from hemorrhage and thrombosis	Methhemoglobin in hemorrhage or acutely thrombosed vessels produces bright signal that may simulate flowing blood; in partially thrombosed aneurysms, signal loss from the susceptibility effects of deoxyhemoglobin, hemosiderin, and ferritin may be encountered obscuring the margins of the residual lumen; on spin echo images, chronic mural thrombus has intermediate signal intensity within the lumen of the aorta and may be difficult to differentiate this from slow flow in patients with aneurysm; PC angiography is not affected by methhemoglobin and can be used to distinguish thrombus from flow
Artifacts from gadolinium injection	Ringing artifacts (seen as alternating black and white lines about the edges of arteries) are the result of acquiring the central lines of k-space too early, when gadolinium arriving in the imaging volume is still increasing to its peak arterial blood concentration; when using centric k-space ordering, delaying the onset of scanning an additional 3–4 sec beyond the actual bolus arrival time avoids acquiring the center of k-space during the rapid rise of arterial gadolinium concentration; ringing may mimic intimal flap or periaortic fluid; if a suspected flap is found on the first data set, but not on the equilibrium-phase MRAs, then dissection can be excluded; another artifact from gadolinium injection occurs when $T2^*$ is transiently decreased due to the high concentration of gadolinium in the subclavian or brachiocephalic veins and may cause signal dropout in adjacent arteries or structures; poor bolus timing will affect image quality in many ways, including venous overlap, ringing artifacts, and insufficient signal within the target vessel.

(*Continued*)

Table 4 Potential Artifacts Affecting Image Quality (*Continued*)

Source of artifact	Effect on image
Motion artifacts	Respiratory, cardiac, patient movement, bowel peristalsis, and arterial pulsation during image acquisition all produce spatial blurring and ghost artifacts; these artifacts are more prominent in the direction of the motion; due to the long acquisition times of TOF techniques, patient motion causes a characteristic stair-step or "Venetian blind" appearance to the images that may simulate luminal disease.
Metallic artifact	Stents, sternal wires, prosthetic aortic valves, vein graft markers, and clips result in signal loss that may interferes with the visualization of the target vessel.
Normal anatomical structures	The azygous vein and the thoracic duct lie just to the right of the descending aorta; the hemiazygous vein and the accessory hemiazygous vein travels to the left of the aorta where they meet, cross the midline, and join the azygous vein; these vessels should not be confused with aortic dissection or ulcers; the transverse sinus of the pericardium surrounds the aortic root and proximal ascending aorta; fluid in this pericardial space may mimic dissection.
Irregular heart rhythm or poor ECG gating	Can blur images making dissection difficult to assess
Incorrect TE	Selecting a long TE on MRA that may exaggerate stenosis due to dephasing effects
Vessel truncation	Positioning the imaging volume so that part of the target vessel lies outside the imaging volume resulting in apparent occlusion; truncation can also occur when processing the MRA data, the operator may not include a portion of the target vessel into the reconstructed image
Wrap artifact	Wrap occurs whenever the dimensions of the object exceed the defined FOV; this results in the lateral parts of the FOV being "wrapped around" or "folded over" (i.e., spatially mismapped due to phase shifts) into the image.

Abbreviations: MR, magnetic resonance; TE, echo time; TOF, time of flight; PC, phase contrast; FOV, field of view; MRA, magnetic resonance angiography.

morphology should be noted. In cases of aneurysm (Fig. 4), its location, course, and size should be reported along with the maximal cross-sectional (i.e., perpendicular to course of the vessel) dimension. Aneurysm morphology can be fusiform (uniform, symmetric, circumferential shape) or saccular (eccentric, focal outpouching shape). It may be helpful to reference the location to another anatomical landmark. The pattern of aneurysm appearance may give a clue to its underlying etiology. In Marfan's syndrome, an ascending aortic aneurysm characteristically begins proximally at the sinuses and extends distally to just short of the innominate artery giving the classic "onion bulb" appearance on MRA and often is associated with significant aortic insufficiency. In traumatic aortic injury, up to 80% will have a circumferential aortic tear, but partial transaction can lead to saccular aneurismal formation occurring at the aortic isthmus where the mobile aorta is fixed by the *ligamentum arteriosum* just distal to the origin of the left subclavian artery. Traumatic tears may appear as a small intimal flap, blood clot localized to the intima or media, pseudoaneurysm, mediastinal hemorrhage, or as simply an abnormal contour of the aortic lumen. Cases of sinus of Valsalva aneurysm involve dilatation of only the aortic root. Most sinus of Valsalva aneurysms that rupture originate from either the right coronary sinus or the noncoronary sinus. Aneurysms arising from right sinus tend to rupture into the right ventricle (occasionally the right atrium), whereas noncoronary sinus aneurysms rupture into the right atrium. Left sinus of Valsalva aneurysms are much less common. Aneurysms that are eccentric or saccular in shape or that appear in atypical locations are keys to mycotic aneurysms usually secondary to infection and are confined to patients with predisposing causes such as intravenous drug users, valvular or congenital disorders of the heart, pericardiac infections, or compromised immunity. In cases of pseudoaneurysm, the aortic wall is penetrated completely and surrounding tissues form the wall of the pseudoaneurysm. As long as the aortic wall remains intact, dilatation represents a true aneurysm. Pseudoaneurysms are most commonly a consequence of surgery, trauma, or inflammation. Pseudoaneurysms are often focal and saccular in appearance. As discussed previously, PAU is seen as an outpouching or "crater" extending beyond the contour of the aortic lumen.

Next, the MRA should be examined for the presence of stenoses and the pattern in which these stenoses appear. Scattered stenoses from atherosclerotic lesions may be evident in many older patients. Leriche originally described complete obliteration of the aortic bifurcation, but "Leriche Syndrome" is commonly used to describe obstruction at any level of the infrarenal aorta. This aggressive form of the atherosclerotic process is often chronic allowing time for the development of periaortic collateral circulation. MRA is an ideal image modality for this condition because gadolinium contrast remains visible in very low concentrations in the collateral vessels secondary to the vast differences in T1 between tissues and contrast-enhanced blood.

Certain common developmental abnormalities of the aorta are readily apparent on MRA, especially in young adults. Two of these are coarctation of the aorta and supraortic stenosis. Coarctation of the aorta is classically described as a congenital narrowing of the proximal descending aorta adjacent to the site of the *ligamentum arteriosum*. Although the arch may have a steep angulated configuration (often found with arch hypoplasia),

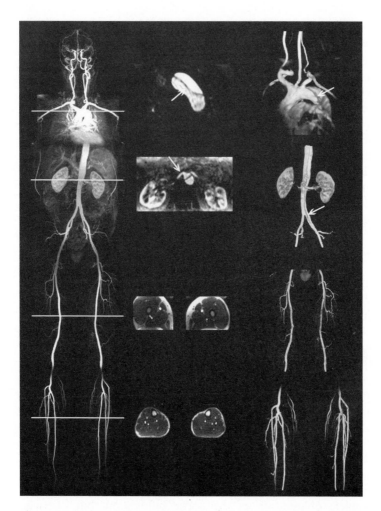

Figure 3 Patient with repaired type I aortic dissection. Whole body MRA was acquired in four stations during bolus administration of contrast. Axial multiplanar reformatting (MPR) and volume rendering (VR) of first station demonstrate residual dissection (*arrow*) and origin of the arch vessels from the true lumen. Axial MPR and VR of second station demonstrate origin of right renal artery from true lumen (*arrow*) and dissection extending down left iliac artery (*arrow*). Axial MPR and VR of third and fourth stations demonstrate normal iliofemoral segments with patent infrapopliteal trifurcation. *Abbreviation*: MRA, magnetic resonance angiography.

coarctation occurring proximally in the aortic arch between the left common carotid and left subclavian arteries is uncommon. The aorta may occasionally be redundant and severely kinked opposite the *ligamentum arteriosum*; but without a pressure gradient, this should be called pseudocoarctation.

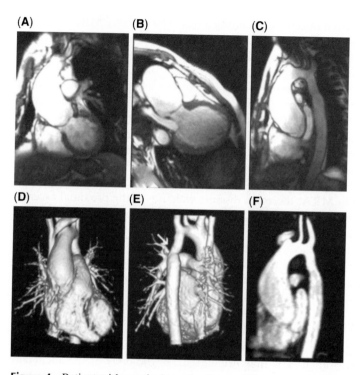

(A) **(B)** **(C)**

(D) **(E)** **(F)**

Figure 4 Patient with surgical repair of coarctation of the aorta and interval development of ascending aortic aneurysm. End-diastolic steady-state free precession images in the **(A)** ascending aorta, **(B)** left ventricular outflow tract, and **(C)** left anterior oblique (LAO) aorta imaging planes demonstrating dilatation of the ascending aorta. 3D volume-rendered MRA images in the **(D)** anterior and **(E)** posterior projections demonstrating ascending aortic aneurysm and coarctation repair (*arrow*). **(F)** maximal intensity projection in LAO aorta imaging plane. *Abbreviation*: MRA, magnetic resonance angiography.

Percent luminal stenosis of the coarctation does not always predict hemodynamic significance because a 50% reduction in cross-sectional area of a localized coarctation may be equally as obstructive as a longer tubular coarctation of lesser narrowing. As coarctations can vary in severity, they are considered hemodynamically significant when (1) a pressure gradient of more than 20 mmHg across the coarctation is present or (2) collateral flow development is present. Collateral circulation develops between the aorta proximal and distal to the coarctation. Collateral circulation inflow pathways rely on the subclavian arterial branches: vertebral artery (to anterior spinal artery), internal mammary artery, lateral thoracic artery, costocervical trunk (to the supreme intercostal artery), and thyrocervical trunk (to the transverse cervical and transverse scapular arteries). These inflow channels anastamose with the intercostal arteries, which in turn reverse flow to drain into the descending aorta. The primary MRI feature of classic untreated coarctation is a localized shelf or projection of aortic media into the lumen of the aorta which occurs along the posterior and leftward wall of the aorta just opposite the *ligamentum arteriosum*. On MRA, it may appear as an indentation or waisting of the left proximal descending thoracic aortic wall. When describing the coarctation, it is important to include measurements of the aorta, the anatomic relationship between the aortic narrowing and the origin of the major arch vessels, and visualization of collateral vessels bypassing the coarctation. Supravalvular aortic stenosis is characterized by a localized narrowing of the aortic lumen just distal to the aortic valve beginning immediately above the attachments of the valve commissures. On MRA, there is a discrete waisting of the proximal ascending aorta associated with some degree of dilatation of the aortic root. If poststenotic dilatation occurs, the ascending aorta may take on an hourglass shape. Patients may have thickening and redundancy of the aortic valve, but stenosis from leaflet fusion or bicuspid aortic stenosis is rare. The MRA should also be examined for peripheral pulmonary stenosis that can be severe enough to produce right ventricular hypertrophy.

Branch Vessels

In all forms of aortic disease, it is important to identify the origins of the branch vessels. Branch ostia may originate from the body of the aneurysm or from the false lumen in cases of dissection. It is important to identify and describe the branch vessel origins in these cases because a complete surgical repair will be determined in part by this information. In aortic dissection, branch vessels should also be examined independently for dissection or obstruction. Branch vessels may become obstructed from (a) the intimal flap extending into the branch artery, separating the branch vessel into two lumens, one which is supplied by the true lumen and the other by the false lumen, (b) thrombosis of the false lumen and compression of the true lumen, (c) compression of the branch artery by external hematoma, (d) prolapsing dissected intimal flap across the origin of the branch artery, covering it like a curtain overlying the orifice, or (e) reduced flow in the true branch vessel lumen due to collapse of the aortic true lumen.

Arch Vessels: The most common indication for extracranial carotid MRA is for atherosclerosis detection with its severity expressed as the percentage of stenosis of the common and internal carotid arteries (Fig. 5). 2D TOF MRA can overestimate the degree of stenosis and is generally not used. Many MRI practitioners recommend that 3D TOF MRA be acquired prior to CE-MRA because jugular venous contamination frequently occurs on CE-MRA. When reviewing TOF images, be aware that signal may decrease in areas of eddy currents that naturally form in the proximal internal carotid artery just cranial to the carotid bifurcation. These eddy currents contribute

(A)

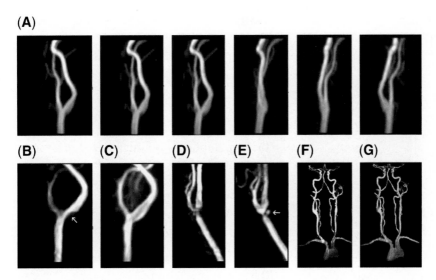

(B) **(C)** **(D)** **(E)** **(F)** **(G)**

Figure 5 (A) Series of 3D time of flight (TOF) MRA of the carotid artery rotated 180° about its longitudinal axis. (B) 3D TOF MRA and (C) contrast-enhanced MRA (CE-MRA) of the carotid bifurcation with pseudostenosis of the internal carotid artery (*arrow*). (D) 3D TOF MRA and (E) CE-MRA of the carotid artery bifurcation with ulcerated plaque (*arrow*) apparent only on contrasted study. (F) maximal intensity projection and (G) volume rendering of aortic arch and branch vessels. *Abbreviation*: MRA, magnetic resonance angiography.

to the loss of phase coherence and result in pseudostenosis at this location. In the arch vessels, arterial dissection can occur from trauma, extension of aortic dissection, or spontaneously from congenital abnormalities of the vessel wall. When subclavian stenosis is present, it is often helpful to acquire an axial 2D PC MRI throughout the neck to document subclavian steal phenomenon where systolic reversal of flow down the ipsilateral vertebral artery is present (Fig. 6). In the appropriate clinical setting, Takayasu's or Giant Cell arteritis should be considered when inflammatory changes of the aorta along with branch occlusions or stenosis (occasionally with dilatation) of the arch vessels are apparent.

Celiac and Mesenteric Arteries: Atherosclerosis of the splanchnic arteries is considered to be the main pathophysiological mechanism for chronic mesenteric ischemia (postprandial abdominal pain, food aversion, and weight loss). Acute onset of symptoms suggests a thromboembolic or vasculitic etiology. Extrinsic compression of the celiac axis by the median arcuate ligament can simulate celiac stenosis ("pseuodostenosis"). Often, this has the appearance of the celiac trunk as being "pulled" inferiorly.

Renal Arteries: Renal artery stenosis (RAS) is implicated as the underlying cause of elevated blood pressure in 1–5% of patients, so-called

(A)   (B)

(C)   (D)

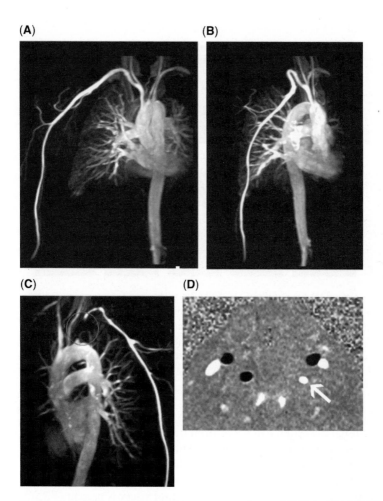

Figure 6 Right upper extremity contrast-enhanced MRA (CE-MRA) in the (**A**) anterior and (**B**) RAO projections. (**C**) CE-MRA of the left upper extremity with occlusion of the proximal left subclavian artery. (**D**) Mid-systolic axial 2D phase contrast MRI through the neck demonstrating reversal of flow (*arrow*) in the left vertebral artery. (Key: Blood flowing in the cranial direction coded black and in the caudal direction coded white). *Abbreviations*: MRA, magnetic resonance angiography; RAO, right anterior oblique; MRI, magnetic resonance imaging.

renovascular hypertension (13,14). The most common etiologies of renovascular hypertension are atherosclerosis and fibromuscluar dysplasia (FMD). Atherosclerotic RAS is a manifestation of generalized atherosclerosis being present in 39–45% of patients with peripheral arterial disease and 22% of patients with coronary artery disease (but can be as high as 40% in patients with left main coronary artery stenosis). However, 15–20% of cases of atherosclerotic RAS are not associated with identifiable disease elsewhere.

Atherosclerosis is usually present in the aorta and typically involves the ostium or the proximal 1–2 cm of one or both renal arteries. In rare cases, atherosclerosis may be isolated to the distal renal artery or renal artery branches. Bilateral disease is reported to occur in 32–78% of cases. Atherosclerotic lesions are responsible for 60–90% of all renovascular disease and are found more often in the older age group. FMD is the second most common cause of RAS but a less frequent cause of renovascular hypertension. It is seen more frequently seen in women of younger age (typically <40 yr old). It manifests as a nonatheromatous vascular lesion in medium sized and small arteries. Medial fibroplasia is the most common type of FMD having an angiographic appearance of a "string-of-beads" with web-like stenoses alternating with small fusiform or saccular aneurysms. The distal two-thirds of the main renal artery are involved, sometimes with extension into segmental vessels. Medial fibroplasia is bilateral in the majority of cases, and rarely advances to complete occlusion. In contrast, perimedial fibroplasia is considered a more progressive lesion that also affects the distal main renal arteries and may advance to occlusion. The remaining two forms of FMD, medial hyperplasia and intimal fibroplasias, affect children and teenagers and appear angiographically as smooth linear stenosis in the proximal and distal main renal arteries. As FMD affects the distal renal arteries, its angiographic findings can be subtle, and MRA may not always demonstrate delicate irregularities because of low spatial resolution, small caliber distal vessels, lower SNR and contrast to noise ratio, and motion artifact.

When reviewing a renal MRA (Fig. 7), the practitioner should account for the number and origin of the renal arteries (30% of kidneys are supplied by more than one renal artery). Accessory renal arteries usually arise from the abdominal aorta and rarely from the common iliac arteries. Although segmental and smaller renal artery branches usually are visualized on these studies, identification of pathology is less reliable because of their small size and limited spatial resolution of MRA. Stenotic regions are localized and characterized by describing the grade of severity, morphology, and length of lesions. The typical angiographic feature of atherosclerotic renovascular disease is eccentric plaque lesions involving the ostial and proximal portions of the renal arteries. Distal lesions occur less common, and when present, usually occur at branch points. Concomitant aortoiliac disease is common. The distal renal arteries for the "string of pearls" angiographic sign of FMD are examined; however, this angiographic feature may be subtle. Poststenotic dilatation from an accelerated jet that impacts the artery wall just distal to the stenosis is observed. An increase in renal artery diameter of more than 20% distal to a stenosis is common in severely stenotic renal arteries.

Finally, the anatomy and structure of the kidney are inspected. The normal kidney measures 11–13 mm in cranial–caudal length with a tendency for the right kidney to be slightly smaller (up to 1 cm). Long-term ischemia results in nephron loss and renal atrophy, further reducing parenchymal volume. Typical cortical thickness is 1.7 ± 0.3 cm, and the cortex appears brighter on T1-weighted images than the medulla. Loss of corticomedullary differentiation on unenhanced T1-weighted images is a nonspecific marker of renal dysfunction. After gadolinium, loss of corticomedullary differentiation

(A)   **(B)**

(C)   **(D)**

(E)   **(F)**

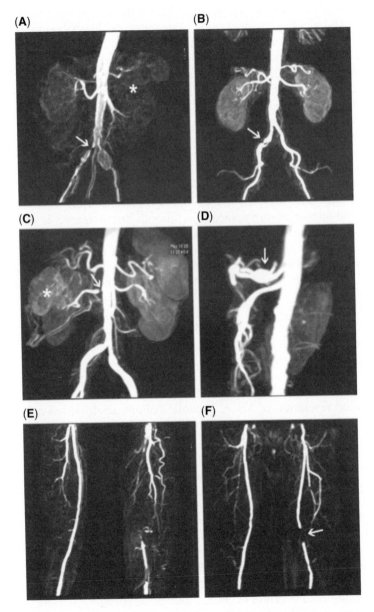

Figure 7 (*Caption on facing page*)

results from decreased blood flow that is more pronounced in the cortex than the medulla. Renal cysts are common. CE-MRA can differentiate simple cysts from complex cysts containing malignancy. Mural irregularity and intense mural enhancement are indicators of malignancy, whereas simple cysts are completely avascular. Kidney perfusion on multiphase CE-MRA is observed. Gadolinium arrival time to the cortex following bolus injection can be delayed in ischemic kidneys. A reduction in the cortical-aortic signal intensity ratio and the cortical–aortic time delay (typically an additional 10 sec) is greatest in patients with severe RAS. Lack of enhancement or asymmetric enhancement of the kidneys on equilibrium-phase MRA suggests organ hypoperfusion. A delayed T1-weighted scan 10 min after gadolinium injection can assess renal excretory function. Asymmetric signal intensity in the collecting system is a reliable indicator of unilateral renal dysfunction. As many renal MRAs are performed to assess uncontrolled hypertension, adrenal mass enhancement is also observed.

Aortoiliac and Distal Runoff Vessels: Atherosclerosis commonly involves the arteries of the lower extremities making CE-MRA ideal for evaluating ischemic syndromes but also for evaluating the patency of peripheral vascular bypass grafts. TOF methods have largely been replaced by CE-MRA because TOF images were prone to motion artifact due to long acquisition times, to overestimation of stenosis due to intravoxel dephasing, and to overestimation of segment lengths of occlusions due to elimination of the retrograde component of cranially flowing blood.

COMMON ARTIFACTS ENCOUNTERED WITH VASCULAR MRI/ MRA TECHNIQUES

Recognition of artifacts is important when interpreting MRI and MRA findings and distinguishes the accomplished MRI practitioner, especially when called upon to interpret poorer quality studies. Artifacts can be introduced into the final image at the time of image acquisition due to

---

Figure 7 (*Figure on facing page*) MRA of the abdomen and lower extremities. (**A**) Abdominal MRA in the anterior projection demonstrating right common iliac stenosis (*arrow*) and aneurysm of the left common iliac artery. The left kidney (∗) is absent. (**B**) Abdominal MRA in the anterior projection again with stenosis of right common iliac arterial stenosis but normal bilateral renal arteries and nephrograms. (**C**) Abdominal MRA in the anterior projection demonstrating right renal artery stenosis (*arrow*). Tumor blush (*) is noted of the right kidney. (**D**) Abdominal MRA in the lateral projection demonstrating celiac trunk aneurysm and scattered atherosclerotic disease of the aorta. (**E**) Femoral MRA in the anterior projection demonstrating occlusion of the left proximal superficial artery and reconstitution distally. (**F**) Femoral MRA in the anterior projection with stent (*arrow*) in the left superficial femoral artery. *Abbreviation*: MRA, magnetic resonance angiography.

proton spin behavior, the CMR sequence, the patient, or errors by the operator (Table 4).

COMMON POSTOPERATIVE FINDINGS

A detailed knowledge of the surgical technique and its anatomic consequences is required to accurately evaluate postoperative images. In some patients, variations seen after surgery may suggest complications, whereas in others may be the result of routine postoperative findings. In cases of aortic repair, the two most widely used surgical techniques involve placement of an interposition graft (with excision of the diseased segment) or an inclusion graft (with closure of the diseased aorta around the graft, creating a potential space between the graft and the aortic wall). This perigraft space may contain thrombus, flowing blood, or both. Reconstruction of the aortic root can involve aortic valve replacement and reimplantation of the coronary arteries. The length of graft does not always match the extent of the aneurysm and residual dilatation of the remaining native abdominal aorta is often encountered. Usually, the ascending aorta is repaired by insertion of a short segment of graft material between the sinuses and the proximal arch. The segment of graft is seen between two small areas of aortic constriction of the vessel wall at the site of proximal and distal anastomoses. To ensure perfusion of branches arising from the patent false lumen, the proximal end of the dissection flap is tacked down to the aortic wall and a fenestration is created in the flap distal to this site. Total arch replacement involves reimplantation of the head and neck vessels, usually as a single patch incorporated into the graft. Meanwhile, hemi-arch replacement involves beveling the graft and anastomosing this to an appropriately beveled distal native arch that incorporates the head and neck vessels and the left subclavian artery. There may be small diverticuli at the anastomotic site where reapposition of the true and false lumina has been attempted. In type A dissection, a persistent intimal flap may be seen distal to the graft in up to 75% of cases. Patients with communicating dissections are at risk for secondary aneurysm formation involving the false lumen. A risk of anastomotic pseudoaneurysm formation results from partial dehiscence of the proximal or distal suture line or at the coronary reimplantation. The "elephant trunk" technique involves graft replacement of the ascending aorta and aortic arch and a free segment of graft is left projecting into the proximal end of an invariably diseased descending aorta. The "elephant trunk" should not be confused with new dissection. Repair of the descending aorta may involve anastomosis of the visceral arteries as a patch, incorporating part of the native wall and reattachment of lower intercostal and upper lumbar branches to preserve spinal cord supply. For aortic coarctation, an interposition graft, Dacron patch, or bypass graft can be used. Abnormal soft tissue is occasionally demonstrated outside a graft or anastomosis, especially when soft tissues have been wrapped around the anastomoses to aid in hemostasis or where the inclusion graft technique has been used. The post operative images are examined for complications of surgical repair including hemorrhage, pseudoaneurysm formation, infection, graft occlusion, clamp damage, and arterial–venous or arterial–enteric fistula. Endovascular stents for aneurysm exclusion or for treatment of coarctation are currently being investigated by MRA techniques with mixed success reported thus far.

RECOMMENDED PROTOCOLS

Vascular anatomy may be complex, and vessels may appear differently depending on the imaging plane, CMR pulse sequence, and CMR parameter selection. Rigid imaging protocols should probably be avoided. Rather, a well-devised patient imaging session that is customized and tailored to answer the clinically relevant information necessary for diagnosis and to accommodate individual patient variations that either appear normally or as the result of disease. An experienced CMR practitioner should ideally be present during the examination to manage unexpected adaptations of the imaging protocol. This approach to scanning will minimize the number of "call back" patients that may have to return for additional imaging.

The versatility and flexibility of CMR permit any number of variations of imaging protocols. CMR practitioners must be facile with imaging solutions and options offered by the vendor of their scanner and remain alert to introduction of new imaging solutions. The following protocols are suggested and tabulated by vascular beds (Table 5).

Carotid MRA

Most carotid MRAs are preformed to detect the severity of occlusive arterial disease. Scout imaging typically includes a sagittal, in-plane, PC-based sequence to identify the carotid bifurcation. As the timing of contrasted carotid MRA can be delicate given early jugular venous enhancement due to short circulation distance, a 3D TOF MRA prior to contrast MRA is usually performed as a series of multiple overlapping slabs centered on the carotid bifurcation. Then, contrast-enhanced 3D MRA is performed. If atherosclerosis imaging is requested, a form of black-blood imaging, such as double inversion recovery FSE imaging, can be performed before CE-MRA. Some investigators have repeated spin echo imaging after contrast to observe plaque components. If subclavian steal syndrome is suspected, axial 2D PC imaging through the neck can illustrate vertebral arterial flow patterns. Finally, some investigators continue to report success using time-resolved 3D CE-MRA as the sole imaging protocol to examine the extracranial circulation.

Table 5 MRA Protocols

Vascular bed	Protocol	Optional scans
Carotid artery	Scout imaging	Pre and post Gd axial spin echo imaging
	3D TOF MRA	Axial 2D PC MRI
	Contrast-enhanced 3D MRA	
Aorta	Scout imaging	Time-resolved contrast-enhanced 3D MRA
	Axial (and sagittal) black blood	Aortic valve cine MRI
	Ascending aorta cine MRI	Targeted axial cine MRI through aorta
	LAO aorta cine MRI	Post Gd spin echo imaging
	Contrast-enhanced 3D MRA	
Renal artery	Scout	Renal arterial cross-sectional 2D PC MRI
	Axial and coronal single-shot FSE	3D PCA
	Axial and coronal single-shot gradient echo	Post Gd spin echo
	Contrast-enhanced 3D MRA	
Lower extremity	Scout	Time-resolved contrast-enhanced 3D MRA of last station
	2D TOF MRA of last station	
	Contrast-enhanced 3D MRA	

Abbreviations: TOF, time of flight; PC, phase contrast; MRI, magnetic resonance imaging; LAO, left anterior oblique; FSE, fast spin echo; PCA, phase contrast angiogram; Gd, gradient; MRA, magnetic resonance angiography.

Aortic MRA

CE-MRA acquired as a coronal 3D spoiled gradient echo slab is the principal MRA technique to image the aorta. Depending on the acquisition speed of the MRI scanner, some practitioners advocate time-resolved CE-MRA either as a coronal slab or with an LAO angulation. This can be done either as a low-dose (6–10 ml) study before a full-dose conventional contrast-enhanced 3D MRA or as a standalone full-dose-contrasted MRA. Depending on the clinical question, additional imaging of the aorta including cine MRI and black-blood spin echo imaging should also be considered prior to CE-MRA. When acquiring black-blood images,

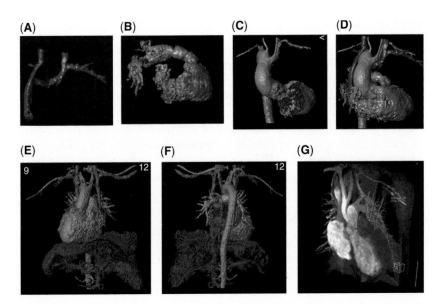

Figure 8 (*See color insert*) Congenital heart disease. Volume renderings in the anterior projection of (**A**) superior vena cava and brachiocephalic vein, (**B**) right ventricle, proximal right pulmonary artery stenosis and atretic left pulmonary artery, (**C**) right-sided aorta with mirror-order branching, and (**D**) composite image demonstrating retro aortic course of the venous drainage. (**E**) Anterior and (**F**) posterior projections of a patient with situs inversus, dextrocardia, bilateral vena cava, anterior systemic ventricle and aorta, and posterior pulmonic ventricle and pulmonary artery. (**G**) RAO sliced volume rendering of truncus arteriosus with interrupted aorta.

the double-inversion recovery technique can minimize blood signal and delineate the aortic wall.

Renal MRA

Although both contrast-enhanced and PC techniques have been used to image the renal arteries, CE-MRA is generally preferred. Prior to MRA, a series of axial and coronal single-shot spin echo (and gradient echo) images through the abdomen are helpful to measure kidney size and observe for renal pathology. Contrast-enhanced 3D MRA is typically performed next as a coronal slab. The slab should be planned from a sagittal scout view in order to include the most anterior part of the aorta and the most posterior extent of the renal pelvis. Depending on the speed of the scanner and the patient's ability to breath-hold, some MRI practitioners will add a slight cranial tilt to the slab to decrease slab thickness and acquisition time. PC imaging following CE-MRA may provide functional data regarding observed stenoses, if desired.

Lower Extremity MRA

When devising a protocol to evaluate ischemic disease of the lower extremity, the protocol should be adapted to accommodate the arteries distal to the popliteal trifurcation based, in part, on image acquisition speed of the scanner in order to minimize venous contamination of this most distal run-off station. Either a 2D TOF MRA or a low-dose time-resolved CE-MRA of the distal station should be considered prior to performing multistation full-dose conventional contrast-enhanced 3D MRA. By employing this strategy, the MRI practitioner can use image data from both studies to aid in the interpretation of distal arterial disease.

CURRENT EFFECTIVENESS OF CMR

MRA techniques have become widely accepted as noninvasive diagnostic tools. Image data are good when bolus timing in CE-MRA is accurate and patient cooperation is optimal. When reviewing the literature reporting diagnostic accuracy of MRA, it is important to critically review the imaging technique, chosen imaging parameters, coil selection, and scanner performance because older MRA studies may appear less promising than conventional X-ray angiography. This has been the experience for renal MRA where low sensitivities have been reported, especially for the detection of FMD. However, because of a high negative predictive value and the safety profile of gadolinium, renal MRA is often particularly attractive as an initial test to avoid unwanted nephrotoxic contrast agents in patients already with compromised renal function. Carotid MRA has proved to be highly sensitive and specific although subtotal occlusions ("string sign" on conventional X-ray angiography) can appear as total occlusions on MRA. Lower extremity MRA also performs favorably compared to conventional X-ray angiography with high sensitivity for arterial segments that are at least moderately stenosed. With percutaneous peripheral interventions being performed with increasing frequency, identification of arterial calcification will impact therapeutic options. It is important for the MRI practitioners to convey to the interventionalist that MRA is weaker than CTA for detecting calcium.

CONCLUSIONS

The material presented in this chapter describes the state-of-the-art imaging techniques present at the time of its printing. The interested reader is encouraged to stay abreast of the rapid technological changes that are likely to occur before the next revision. MRA scan time may be reduced in the future with even faster gradients that will reduce TR, but the resulting RF absorption may potentially cause tissue heating. There is limited experience with high-field (3T) MRA applications. It is believed that higher field strengths will increase spatial resolution, especially useful for lower extremity MRA applications. Contrast injection protocols will have to be optimized for 3T because T1 and susceptibility increase with high field strengths. New contrast agents may further revolutionize CMR angiographic techniques. These include agents with higher relaxivity or agents that can be given in higher concentrations. Blood pool agents that maintain stable blood pool signal for greater lengths of time may yield images that are more detailed with higher spatial resolution. However, as arteries and veins are equally enhanced during the blood pool equilibrium phase, more advanced projection techniques will be necessary to display the arteries separately from the veins. Targeted contrast agents are being developed to improve detection of disease, such as lipohilic agents that can accumulate in atherosclerotic plaque, ultrasmall particles of iron oxide that are phagocytozed by macrophages residing in early plaque, or fibrin-targeted agents that bind to thrombus.

REFERENCES

1. Schneider G, Price MR, Meaney JFM, Ho VB, eds. Magnetic Resonance Angiography. Milan: Springer, 2005.
2. Neimatallah NA, et al. Gadolinium-enhanced 3D magnetic resonance angiography of the thoracic vessels. JMRI 1999; 10:758–770.
3. Prince MR, Grist TM, Debatin JF, eds. 3D Contrast Angiography. 3rd ed. Milan, Italy: Springer, 2003.
4. Kramer CM, et al. Magnetic resonance imaging identifies the fibrous cap in atherosclerotic abdominal aortic aneurysm. Circulation 2004; 109:1016–1021.
5. Ho VB, et al. MR angiography of the abdominal aorta and peripheral vessels. Radiol Clin N Am 2003; 41(1):115–144.
6. Vogt FM, et al. MR angiography of the chest. Radiol Clin N Am 2003; 41(1):29–41.
7. Rajagopalan S, et al. Magnetic resonance angiographic techniques for the diagnosis of arterial disease. Cardiol Clin 2002; 20(4):501–512.
8. Tatli S, et al. MR imaging of aortic and peripheral vascular disease. RadioGraphics 2003; 23:S59–S78.
9. Toussaint JF, et al. Magnetic resonance images: lipid, fibrous, calcified, hemorrhagic, and thrombotic components of human atherosclerosis in vivo. Circulation 1996; 94:932–938.
10. Fayad ZA, et al. In vivo magnetic resonance evaluation of atherosclerotic plaques in the human thoracic aorta: a comparison with transesophageal echocardiography. Circulation 2000; 101:2503–2509.
11. Evangelista A, et al. Long-term follow-up of aortic intramural hematoma. Circulation 2003; 108:583–589.
12. Hideyuki H, et al. Penetrating atherosclerotic ulcer of the aorta: imaging features and disease concept. RadioGraphics 2000; 20:995–1005.
13. Dong Q, et al. Diagnosis of renal vascular disease with MR angiography. RadioGraphics 1999; 19:1535–1554.
14. Leung DA, et al. MR angiography of the renal arteries. Radiol Clin N Am 2002; 40(4):847–865.

19

Risks and Safety

Mark Doyle and Robert W. W. Biederman

Division of Cardiology, Cardiovascular MRI Laboratory, Allegheny General Hospital, Pittsburgh, Pennsylvania, U.S.A.

CARDIOVASCULAR MAGNETIC RESONANCE RISKS

Cardiovascular magnetic resonance (CMR) is widely reported as a safe modality, with no exposure limits, and thus is suitable for longitudinal studies. However, there are several conditions under which it would be unadvisable to scan a patient due to issues of safety. When evaluating safety issues associated with CMR studies of the heart, there are several approaches that can be taken to assess risk to the patient, including:

- comparing the ratio of the number of scans without adverse events to the number of scans with adverse events,
- sighting cases of patients who were scanned event-free with or without various implants, ranging from metallic eye liner to implantable cardiac devices (ICDs),
- determining the risk on an individual basis.

The first approach (i.e., sighting event rates) only gives us information regarding the event rate for the scanned population (which could be refined for certain sub-populations, for example, those with ICDs). While this approach is generally unsatisfactory, it is nevertheless the criterion that is routinely used to assess the risk to patients undergoing procedures such as cardiac catheterization (where mortality is 1/1100). Use of the second approach (i.e., sighting anecdotal cases) can be countered as being noninclusive, further it can be argued that even if some patients with ICDs were scanned event-free there may be known case of patients with such devices who have suffered adverse events. However, this method of assessing risk is commonly used to justify submitting patients to ionizing radiation. The third approach of assessing risk (i.e., on an individual basis) is commonly used in clinical practice to assess risk in complex cases. A question posed is "is the risk of using CMR to obtain a diagnosis substantially lower than the risk of not obtaining the diagnosis?" This approach is imperfect, since it relies on physician judgment and is often made from a standpoint of limited knowledge. Nevertheless, this is the approach that is routinely used and can be enhanced by educational programs and access to research data. To give physicians access to the latest information on contraindications for devices, a knowledge database is required. However, as knowledge increases, the list of devices and conditions that require consideration continues to grow. Thus, the process will always be imperfect because CMR technology and implantable devices are always changing. However, the number of resources available to physicians is increasing, including better patient records (searchable by computerized means) where the CMR compatibility of devices may be indicated and Internet web sites that provide up-to-date and searchable information on specific devices.

It is an encouraging sign that many manufacturers of implantable devices are generally aware of the issues involved with CMR and are increasingly accommodating of the requirements for compatibility. The best possible solution is for the devices to be made in a CMR-compatible manner, not only for current scanner systems but also for foreseeable future systems. The only way to ensure future compatibility is for the devices to be made of materials that do not interact with any of the components of a magnetic resonance (MR) scanner. This is important since there are trends for the components of CMR systems to increase in power, including the static magnetic field, the slew rates of the magnetic gradients, and the use of sequences that deposit higher levels of radio frequency (RF) power. All these developments potentially contribute to increasing risk to the patient. Thus, if a small interaction is noted on present day instrumentation, there is the possibility that the interaction could become larger on future systems. If no interaction is noted, then none would be expected in future systems. Given this rapidly changing technologic environment, it is unlikely that for any given situation that the exact combination of conditions encountered will match those reported in the knowledge databases or safety literature. Thus, to allow informed decisions to be made, certain fundamentals of the interaction of CMR technology and the patient must be understood and applied. Also, once the decision has been made to subject a patient to a CMR examination, there are certain precautions that can be taken to limit the potential for an adverse event (1). Following is a discussion of the major interactions between CMR and patients, with and without adornments and devices.

There is no reproducible evidence that exposure to strong magnetic fields is inherently dangerous to humans (2). Thus, the most obvious interaction of the main (static) magnetic field with humans exists through the attractive forces exerted on metallic devices placed in on or around the patient. This is arguably the easiest interaction to test for, since a number of standard examinations exist to quantifiably determine the strength of the attractive force that the static magnetic field exerts on a device (for example, a prosthetic heart valve). All metals exhibit an interaction with magnetic fields to some degree, but the attraction levels are almost negligible with certain alloys. While the degree of attraction between a device and a static magnetic field can be measured, it is possible that the device may experience stronger forces as it enters or exits the magnet. This phenomenon is due to the higher density of flux lines near the openings of the magnet, which results on higher forces for a given device. Thus, even this relatively straightforward measurement requires judicious interpretation to adapt it to clinical conditions. Since CMR scanners are available in a range of field strengths (with higher field strengths becoming more common), it is possible that documented data only exists for lower field strengths than the scanner under consideration (for example, 1.5 vs. 3 Tesla (T). For the example of comparing 1.5 to 3 Tesla (T), a good approximation would be to double the forces known to be present at 1.5 T. Many commonly encountered devices have been tested for their degree of attraction at 0.5 and 1.5 T and these data are presented in a book and Internet formats (3–5). A nonexhaustive list of such devices and substances includes: tattoo ink, aneurysm clips, stents, biopsy needles, catheters, dental implants, electrocardiograms (ECG) electrodes, heart valves, and cochlear implants. The degree of magnetic attraction displayed by these devices and their mode of implantation play a role in assessing risk. For devices that are firmly fixed in the body, such as bone fixation screws, higher thresholds of interactive forces can be tolerated. For devices such as aneurysm clips that are loosely constrained, displacement could result in severe morbidity and these require a higher threshold of justification prior to scanning.

Thus far, the main consideration has been the degree of deflection exhibited by a given device, assuming that its performance will not be impeded on entering or leaving the high magnetic field environment. For devices such as pacemakers, their function in the magnetic environment is an important issue (6). For patients who are not pacemaker-dependent, it may be possible to "safely" switch off the device or place it in fixed rate mode. The patient's ability to tolerate lack of pacing or fixed rate pacing should be tested outside of the magnet. Patients with pacemakers have been imaged without adverse events (7). However, one must consider the potential of electrode heating, disruption of pacer electronics, the effect of the magnet on the pacemaker reed switch, and the possibility of affecting the pacing rate by the scanning sequence. Now, pacing devices, once thought to be strictly contraindicated for CMR, are being manufactured to be safe for CMR.

Other devices that must be considered are those that accompany patients, such as ventilators, wheelchairs, infusion pumps, intravenous (IV) poles, oxygen cylinders, and sandbags (8). Since the forces exerted by the scanner's magnetic field are beyond that of every day experience, it is of paramount importance that all personnel (especially the patient) be screened prior to entering the scanner region. In one incident known to us, a patient entered the magnet with a "sandbag" that was pressurizing a wound. The "sandbag" proceeded to rapidly move upward and pin the patient's clothing to the inner wall of the magnet. It was later learned that the "sandbag" contained iron shot! Sadly, there have been reports of patient death associated with devices such as oxygen cylinders being attracted into the scanner and impacting the patient with tremendous force. Naturally, safety precautions should be taken to secure the CMR scan room from unauthorized (untrained) personnel. Reliance on any single barrier mechanism should be avoided. Instead, a combination of warnings and physical restraints is widely recommended. The logistics of each site are different, with some scanners protected by two or three doors while others may be protected by only one secure door in an otherwise unrestricted area (such a hallway lined with offices). Effective warning devices should be positioned at appropriate distances from the scanning room, including warning signs, walk-through metal detectors, and alarms. Further, access to the scanning area should be restricted to trained personnel (with formal certification preferred). Access, even for trained personnel should be granted via a keyed entryway (for example, by swipe card, combination lock, or key). Ideally, the scanning technician should have a direct line of site to the scan room door (9). While a direct line of site is potentially important to possibly prevent unauthorized entry into the scan room, it is unlikely that the technician could respond rapidly enough to prevent such a person from coming dangerously close to the magnet. For this reason, an alarm system, possibly linked to a metal detector, can give the technician additional warning time to respond. Additionally, the alarm may trigger the person to stop from proceeding. In the event that an unauthorized person is seen to approach the magnet, the technician, or some other knowledgeable person, should quench the magnet. Thus, one quench button should be located in the scan console area. Any hesitation in such a situation could result in serious injury or death, and training should emphasis this. In part, the knowledge that the authorities are willing to facilitate someone pressing a $50,000 quench button sends an important message regarding the importance of safety.

In addition to the static magnetic field, patients and their devices are subjected to time varying (i.e., oscillating) magnetic fields during a CMR scan. Time varying fields can induce voltages across conductors, causing a current to flow. Further, many body tissues are inherently susceptible to the generation of such currents. The impedance of body tissues to these currents is dependent on the oscillation frequency and the rate of change of field strength.

Thus, the body should be regarded as a conductive media in which there are many possible conductive pathways, each of which having the potential to sustain a voltage and a current. The rate of change of field strength generated by the oscillating gradients is characterized by the slew rate parameter. About 10 years ago, typical gradient systems had slew rates of about 10 mT/m/sec, whereas, presently, slew rates of 150 to 200 mT/m/sec are typical in cardiovascular systems. The slew rate is expected to increase further as higher scan resolution and reduced imaging times are sought. In gradients with field of view (FOV) as small as 32 cm, when the slew rate reaches about 150 mT/m/sec they are large enough to induce voltages that can stimulate neuromuscular interactions. Such interactions can result in sensations of involuntary muscular twitching. While such involuntary muscle twitching does not present a known danger to patients, it can be very uncomfortable (10,11).

However, induction of voltage/current loops can present an immediate danger when low impedance circuits are encountered in the form of wire loops (such as pacemaker leads). Such circuits may have voltages induced that could affect cardiac rhythm directly. Since the gradient strength increases with distance from the center of the scanner, the slew rate similarly increases with the distance from the center of the magnet. Thus, patients with residual pacemaker leads may possibly tolerate a cardiac scan without an event since the heart is positioned centrally in the scanner. However, the same patient, when repositioned to scan the abdominal aorta, may experience an adverse event since the heart and leads may now be in a higher slew rate environment (due to the offset along the Z gradient). While there is a trend for magnetic gradient slew rates to increase, there are several approaches that can limit such increases: (i) use of gradients designed to produce a large gradient only over the central region (i.e., cardiac-specific gradients) with the outer body regions experiencing lower slew rates, (ii) software that limits the maximum slew rate for individuals at risk, and (iii) use of imaging sequences that limit induced voltages (12).

The third distinct source of danger associated with cardiac imaging systems is associated with the RF transmitter of the system. All CMR sequences require delivery of RF power to the body, which has the potential to locally increase the body temperature. For individuals with a regularly functioning circulatory system and in whom there are no additional devices, the maximum allowable specific absorption rate (SAR) of the system/sequence is set low enough to protect against localized heating $>2°C$ (13). The typical mechanism by which heat is dissipated from the body is by directing blood from the body core to the periphery where heat is exchanged with the external environment. Thus, the patient should be appropriately dressed and the scanner bore sufficiently ventilated to allow such an exchange of heat to take place.

However, for individuals with implanted devices, especially if they form conducting loops (either in their own right or in combination with body tissue), there is the potential for extreme localized heating as resonant current loops may be induced by the RF pulses. Such current loops can develop enough localized heating to melt metallic devices such as catheters and electrodes and cause severe tissue damage related to burning. Recently, transdermal patches have been reported to result in patient burns. In particular, it is thought that it is the aluminum backing of the patches that was responsible for heating. Until further clarification is available, it is recommended that patients remove patches prior to receiving the CMR examination. It is even possible that certain configurations of patient tissue can form conduction loops, e.g., a hand touching the leg may form a loop involving the arm, torso, and thigh, and may lead to skin burns (14). However, the presence of loops is not necessary for excessive heat production to occur. In one in vitro test, a linear guidewire used for interventional MRI experienced a temperature rise from 26°C to 74°C after only 30 seconds of conventional scanning (15). The precipitous rise in temperature was attributed to a resonance phenomenon associated with the RF pulse frequency. Resonance phenomena are particularly important for conductors which are comparable in length to the wavelength of the RF waveforms. At the field strength of 1.5 T, the resonance frequency of water protons is 64 MHz, which corresponds to a wavelength of 4.6 m. For a conductor approximating to a length one-fourth of a wavelength (1.1 m) a high heating rate is expected. This length is comparable to the length of a typical catheter and in general, heating is maximal at the tip of a linear conductor (16). It can be appreciated that the exact interaction of the conductor and the MRI system is dependent on resonance effects and is therefore field strength-and orientation-dependent (17). To use catheters or guidewires in the CMR system, specialized circuitry is required to decouple the conductor during application of RF energy to the system. Unless a catheter is specifically designed for an MRI system and all the safeguards are working and in place, patients should not be scanned with a catheter inserted. When in use in the body, an MRI-compatible catheter will typically be surrounded by blood, which may rapidly conduct heat away from the catheter. However, this phenomenon should not be relied upon to safeguard the patient, since the catheter could easily come in contact with tissue, such as the arterial wall, and result in burning if the catheter was susceptible to heating. Reports that claim that a patient did not complain of any heating effects may be misleading, since the body generally cannot detect heat internally. Thus, safety of a device should be based on suitable ex vivo experiments that demonstrate an acceptably low heating effect, rather than on anecdotal patient-reported experiences.

Even if a device has been proven safe for use in an MRI scanner, it is important to establish that the device is in full working order. For example a device with a broken lead may form a configuration that can result in excessive heat generation (18). To establish that each device is intact may require a demonstration of its function and may also require that an X-ray be taken.

Attempts to monitor patients during a CMR examination may in itself lead to risk of serious burns; when for example a pulse oximeters is attached it may complete a circuit that results in high levels of RF heating (19). A general rule is that the patient should have the least number of devices, inserts, and attachments in place that is consistent with safety of monitoring and scanning.

Over the recent past, RF power in CMR systems has not increased to the same degree that the gradient power has. Nevertheless, there has been a trend for CMR imaging sequences to produce higher SAR levels. This is a result of being able to switch gradients faster, which has resulted in application of more RF pulses per unit time. Further, the recent development of steady state imaging methods has resulted in dramatically increased SAR levels, since high RF flip angles are required to be applied at short intervals. RF heating, amplified by conductive loops, is the most difficult danger to assess. For CMR to be considered in patients with implanted devices, especially for the newer generation of scanners, more basic testing of these devices is required. This is potentially an enormous undertaking, requiring multiple tests to be performed, under a variety of conditions including field strength, magnetic gradient slew rates, and RF power. For completeness and uniformity of presentation of results, standardization of testing is required. Further, such standardization will aid in presentation of test results in a uniform and impartial manner. This presents an opportunity for a consortium of research and industry partners to collaborate to determine solutions for this growing issue (20).

In the event that a patient with an implanted device is at substantial risk and that CMR scanning is sought, if the decision is made to scan the patient, it is advisable to proceed with caution. If RF heating is perceived to be the limiting problem, then scans that require low SAR levels may be applied. Additionally, delays between individual scans can be prolonged to allow for heat dissipation.

Given the very serious sources of morbidity and mortality associated with CMR examination, the question is raised of "how should the daily practice of CMR be conducted?" The answer can be formulated in a stepped manner involving (i) education, (ii) screening, and (iii) testing.

EDUCATION

Referring physicians require training to be able to perform patient screening at a high level. Since cardiac CMR is outside the experience of the majority of referring physicians, it generally behooves a CMR center to involve the physicians in an educational program. With adequate instruction, the referring physicians can be alerted to the risks and benefits of CMR, and possibly disabusing them of erroneous preconceptions (for example, CMR is absolutely contraindicated for patients with aneurysm clips). In many instances, physicians may be unaware of the level of information provided by CMR, particularly for vascular imaging and functional cardiac imaging, which may result in increased referral of suitable patients. Conversely, reducing the number of patients who are referred with contraindications for receiving a CMR examination may reduce frustration on behalf of the referring physician.

SCREENING

When the patient presents at the CMR site, a screening form should be used to explain the risks to the patient. The form should not assume that the patient is aware of all the issues and terms involved and some tangential questions should be included, e.g., to assess the likelihood of the patient having metal splinters in their eyes, a question such as "have you ever worked in a metal shop?" could be included. If no implantable devices, shrapnel, or other objects are flagged, and if the procedure is indicated, the physician–CMR imager should further evaluate the patient prior to scanning. If there remains a suspicion that the patient may not have revealed all relevant data, then the patient should be questioned further by the physician or chief technologist. A review of the patient's chart should be conducted to corroborate the information provided by the patient. When implanted devices are detected, their configuration and condition should be ascertained (through chart review and/or performance of a planar X-ray).

In general, the presence of coronary artery stents should not pose a danger to patients. Patients with ICDs should be assessed by a cardiologist prior to scanning. Patients with wire conductors, e.g., residual pacemaker leads, can be at significant risk, since in vitro studies have demonstrated significant heating in such leads. If the indications for scanning the patient are great, with such leads in position, several factors should be considered; the heat may be dissipated more efficiently if the leads are intravascular and less heat may be generated if they are short. If possible, image patients with low duty cycles and low SAR value sequences. For patients with catheters in place, evaluation should be conducted to determine if the catheter contains metal (for example, a guide wire) and especially if it contains a coil. In such cases, imaging may be very hazardous, and the catheter and associated wires should be removed prior to imaging or an alternative imaging modality sought. The flow chart in Figure 1 summarizes the approach.

TESTING

Whenever possible, some elementary testing should be conducted prior to scanning a patient. For instance, a strong hand-held magnet should be

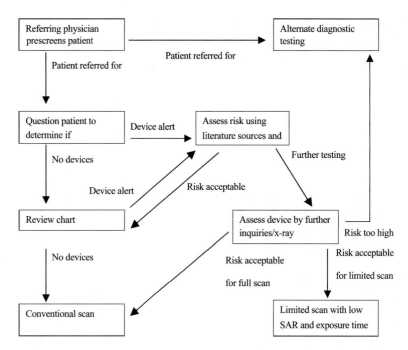

Figure 1 Flow chart for determining whether to scan a patient using cardiovascular magnetic resonance. *Abbreviation*: SAR, specific absorption rate.

available outside of the scan room for testing external devices for magnetic attraction, e.g., to test "sand bags," arm bracelets, metal plates, etc. To avoid the possibility of metallic objects imbedded in patient's clothing resulting in injury, patients should change into loose-fitting clothing (for example, scrub suits or similar covering without any pockets) and remove all footwear prior to scanning. In particular, all removable devices and adornments should be removed, including dentures and hairpins. If they cannot be removed, consider performing an appropriate test to assess them for safety.

    CMR has a good safety record, but this can be attributed to conservatism at scanning sites, in that suspicious cases are not generally scanned. This approach has proven generally effective in serving the patient and physician communities, in that patient safety is maintained and relevant information is obtained on the majority of patients scanned. However, an increasing number of patients, treated for both cardiac and noncardiac diseases, are having devices permanently installed. Fortunately, manufacturers of a wide variety of devices are attempting to make them CMR-compatible. Nevertheless, there exists a challenge to the CMR community to assess the risk associated with each device and publish this information. As the capabilities of CMR continue to grow, it is important to ensure that patients who may potentially benefit from the accuracy and comprehensiveness of an MR examination are not excluded due to devices or lack of knowledge concerning these devices.

CONCLUSIONS

Everyone using CMR must be intimately aware of its inherent risks. These include projectiles related to objects that have ferromagnetic properties, devices such as AICDs that are incompatible with CMR, the heating of tissue that can occur in association with RF, and the fact that the gradients are limited since they can lead to stimulation of neuromuscular tissue. It is important to follow the screening and testing guidelines described in this chapter, and maintain an awareness of the risks and safety issues of CMR. With appropriate education and knowledge in CMR laboratories, the safety of CMR remains high.

REFERENCES

1. Sawyer-Glover AM, Shellock FG. Pre-CMR procedure screening: recommendations and safety considerations for biomedical implants and devices. J Magn Reson Imaging 2000; 12(1):92–106.
2. Schenck JF. Safety of strong, static magnetic fields. J Magn Reson Imaging 2000; 12(1):2–19.
3. http://www.CMRsafety.com/.
4. Shellock FG, Shellock VJ. Cardiovascular catheters and accessories: ex vivo testing of ferromagnetism, heating, and artifacts associated with CMR. J Magn Reson Imaging 1998; 8(6):1338–1342.
5. http://kanal.arad.upmc.edu/MR_Safety/.
6. Sommer T, Lauck G, Schimpf R, et al. CMR in patients with cardiac pacemakers: in vitro and in vivo evaluation at 0.5 tesla. Rofo. Fortschritte auf dem Gebiete der Rontgenstrahlen nd der Neuen Bildgebenden Verfahren 1998; 168(1):36–43.
7. Gimbel JR, Johnson D, Levine PA, Wilkoff BL. Safe performance of magnetic resonance imaging on five patients with permanent cardiac pacemakers. Pacing Clin Electrophys 1996; 19(6):913–919.
8. Williams EJ, Jones NS, Carpenter TA, Bunch CS, Menon DK. Testing of adult and paediatric ventilators for use in a magnetic resonance imaging unit. Anaesthesia 1999; 54(10):969–974.
9. Kanal E, Borgstede JP, Barkovich AJ, et al. American College of Radiology white paper on MR safety. Am J Roentgenol 2002; 178(6):1335–1347.
10. Chronik BA, Rutt BK. A comparison between human magnetostimulation thresholds in whole-body and head/neck gradient coils. Magn Reson Med 2001; 46(2):386–394.
11. Irnich W, Schmitt F. Magnetostimulation in CMR. Magn Reson Med 1995; 33(5):619–623.

12. Jokela K. Restricting exposure to pulsed and broadband magnetic fields. Health Phys 2000; 79(4):373–388.
13. Strilka RJ, Li S, Martin JT, Collins CM, Smith MB. A numerical study of radio-frequency deposition in a spherical phantom using surface coils. Magn Reson Imaging 1998; 16(7):787–798.
14. Knopp MV, Metzner R, Brix G, van Kaick G. Safety considerations to avoid current-induced skin burns in CMR procedures. Radiology 1998; 38(9):759–763.
15. Konings MK, Bartels LW, Smits HF, Bakker CJ. Heating around intravascular guidewires by resonating RF waves. J Magn Reson Imaging 2000; 12(1):79–85.
16. Buechler DN, Durney CH, Christensen DA. Calculation of electric fields induced near metal implants by magnetic resonance imaging switched-gradient magnetic fields. Magn Reson Imaging 1997; 15(10):1157–1166.
17. Liu CY, Farahani K, Lu DS, Duckwiler G, Oppelt A. Safety of CMR-guided endovascular guidewire applications. J Magn Reson Imaging 2000; 12(1):75–78.
18. Chou CK, McDougall JA, Chan KW. RF heating of implanted spinal fusion stimulator during magnetic resonance imaging. IEEE Trans Biomed Eng 1997; 44(5):367–373.
19. Brown TR, Goldstein B, Little J. Severe burns resulting from magnetic resonance imaging with cardiopulmonary monitoring. Risks and relevant safety precautions. Am J Phys Med Rehab 1993; 72(3):166–167.
20. Young IR. Notes on current safety issues in CMR. NMR Biomed 2000; 13(3):109–115.

20

CMR: The Future

Gerald M. Pohost

Department of Medicine, Division of Cardiovascular Medicine,
Keck School of Medicine, University of Southern California,
Los Angeles, California, U.S.A.

Krishna S. Nayak

Departments of Electrical Engineering and Medicine, Division of Cardiovascular
Medicine, Viterbi School of Engineering, Keck School of Medicine, University of
Southern California, Los Angeles, California, U.S.A.

While this book provides a practical approach to the applications of CMR, the present and concluding chapter contains a concise description of the editors' view of the future of CMR. We believe that CMR is actually early in its evolution, and that there are several impending developments that will lead to the evolution of CMR becoming the noninvasive diagnostic modality of choice for cardiovascular imaging and potentially for the guidance of cardiovascular interventions. Major advances in hardware, software, and contrast agents, will lead to several new and improved applications. Indeed, CMR will become the "one-stop shop" for diagnostic imaging.

Already, many CMR centers have adopted new higher field magnets (Food and Drug Administration (FDA)-approved 3 T magnets) that have the potential to provide superior quality images and depict spectra from nuclei such as ^{31}P and ^{13}C. The future is even more dramatic when one considers the potential applications of new contrast agents, molecular imaging, and nanotechnology.

HARDWARE

One of the most important hardware changes over the past decade has been the evolution of the gradient subsystem, which has allowed rapid CMR imaging using pulse sequences such as fast gradient-echo imaging, and most recently, the use of steady–state free precession (SSFP) imaging. While SSFP is a pulse sequence that was developed decades ago and was responsible for a high resolution and remarkable tomographic image of a lemon on the cover of *Nature* in 1976 (1), it has now become among the most important pulse sequences used for CMR imaging. The early version of SSFP required a "steady-state" and accordingly was highly degraded by motion and resonant frequency variations. In those days some predicted that cardiac imaging would not be possible due to the requirement of the "steady-state". However, virtually anything seems to be possible with this amazing technology. Virtually every component of a CMR system can be improved and development of new software expands the flexibility virtually infinitely. Thus, the development of hardware and software leading to short repetition times has allowed high-resolution CMR with SSFP.

Advanced magnet technology has allowed the development of higher field whole-body systems and magnets with remarkably short bore lengths making the technology more patient-friendly by reducing the possibility of claustrophobia. Since the FDA's approval of whole-body 3T clinical magnets in 2001, 3 T magnets have become increasingly adopted for CMR (2,3). The higher field strength allows increased signal-to-noise ratio (SNR), which provides higher spatial resolution and greater speed of acquisition. The increased field strength is particularly important for improvement in myocardial perfusion imaging, coronary artery imaging (currently limited at 1.5 T by inadequate spatial resolution), and spectroscopy (currently limited at 1.5 T by inadequate SNR). Compared to 1.5 T, 3 T has already demonstrated improvement in myocardial perfusion imaging (using the first-pass of paramagnetic contrast agent) and myocardial scar (using delayed-enhancement).

The length of the magnet bore used for whole-body magnetic resonance imaging (MRI) has traditionally been as long as 2.0 m (2.3 m including the outside covers). Magnet bore lengths have become as short as 1.53 m for both 1.5 and 3 T (or 1.67 m including the outside covers). In this shorter system design, the body gradient coil is also shorter leading to more of a funnel-shaped bore and an even more patient-friendly system. This more "open" design further reduces the incidence of claustrophobia, and provides greater ability to interact with the patient. Also, it might be possible for patients to undergo leg exercise while positioned within the magnet bore.

There is also a clear trend in the direction of parallel imaging using receiver coil-arrays. Current systems are equipped with eight to 16 receiver channels, which are essential for "parallel imaging" with an increase in acquisition speed from three to eight times (for example, with a commercial eight-channel cardiac coil-array, one can typically increase imaging speed threefold in short-axis views with no loss of image quality). We expect further increases in the number of coil elements and receiver channels to further improve image quality and speed. At some point, there will be diminishing returns (i.e., when coil noise exceeds body noise), but at least 32 channels have been demonstrated to further improve CMR speed and quality (4).

A problematic consideration, especially at higher field strengths, is tissue heating related to the necessary increase in radiofrequency (RF) levels. The reduction of tissue heating (SAR) is being explored by the use of parallel excitation with arrays of transmit coils (5). This approach should allow greater flexibility in the use of RF in CMR pulse sequences. The use of CMR was contraindicated in patients with pacemakers and implanted cardiac devices (ICDs). Recent work and changes in pacemaker design have demonstrated that it is possible to use CMR as a diagnostic tool in patients with such implanted devices (6).

SOFTWARE AND PULSE SEQUENCES

The two most important developments in software and pulse sequence design have been parallel and, as described above, SSFP imaging. Parallel imaging provides a robust method for accelerating image acquisition, which has been successfully adopted by CMR instrument vendors, replacing methods based on echo–planar and spiral imaging approaches. The key feature is that parallel imaging accelerates the use of 2DFT acquisitions, which are the sequences that are the most robust to artifacts. SSFP imaging provides the highest signal-to-noise efficiency of any pulse sequence, and optimal relaxivity-related contrast (T2/T1) that is useful in cardiovascular imaging. Accordingly, SSFP provides excellent contrast between blood and myocardium, and between blood and vessel wall. SSFP-based techniques can be combined with other techniques to suppress fat, create oxygen level dependent and encode flow (among other functions). In our opinion, SSFP and parallel imaging will ultimately allow coronary artery imaging with resolution as good as that of multislice CT without the need for radiopaque, potentially nephrotoxic, contrast agents, and without ionizing radiation.

Real-time imaging using the above techniques is important for rapid localization and for the performance of studies in patients with irregular cardiac rhythms and less capable of holding their breath for the ~20 seconds required (roughly 20% of cardiac patients we see in practice). The incorporation of interactive scanning reduces examination times, which is important for stress and vasodilator studies. We believe that the future of CMR will involve real-time image reconstruction (generating image sequences analogous to X-ray fluoroscopy and 2D and 3D echocardiography allowing real-time visualization of cardiac motion), and real-time operator control of the scan plane and various sequence parameters with intuitive input devices. In this way the system of the future will be able to access the full power of MRI with optimal image contrast, with high spatial resolution and with high acquisition speeds.

The great power of CMR is its ability to perform many types of imaging in one examination. Today, cardiac morphology, function, and delayed enhancement are frequently performed in a single study. With improvements in perfusion and coronary artery imaging, these will also become part of the comprehensive CMR cardiac examination. In our opinion, with the development of appropriate software infrastructure, the performance of the comprehensive CMR examination will be routinely feasible in less than one hour.

APPROACHES TO ENHANCE CONTRAST

Conventional Contrast Agents

Better paramagnetic-based contrast agents and ultimately the use of nanotechnology will lead to improvement in image contrast and to targeted detection of specific pathologies. For example, Mn^{2+}, could provide improved contrast for perfusion imaging as compared with gadolinium-based agents. To deal with the toxicity of ionic manganese, the future portends the use of nanotechnology to encase the manganese that would allow the nontoxic use of the strong paramagnetic properties of $MnCl_2$. It would also allow the use of higher doses of gadolinium. In addition, the use of nanotechnology would allow the administration of lanthanides such as dysprosium (Dy^{2+}) that induce chemical shift. When dysprosium remains within the interstitial space, the extracellular sodium ($^{23}Na^+$) peak would be shifted differentiating between inter- and intracellular molecules. What this means is that imaging of sodium-23 would provide a clinical approach for testing the integrity of the myocardial cell membrane (7).

Finally, paramagnetic contrast agents have been developed that remain largely within the blood pool. Such agents have been touted as allowing better imaging of the coronary arteries and other vascular systems. Again, nanotechnology should provide a means for improving the imaging of the lumen of the coronary arterial and other vascular beds.

Molecular Imaging and Nanotechnology

Molecular imaging allows targeting of specific disease states (8). In order to allow paramagnetic agents to enter the cell, they must have molecular specificity and they must be small enough to move through the cell and nuclear membranes. Nanotechnology uses extremely small nanoparticles that can enter the myocardial or endothelial cell. A resultant and revolutionary new class of contrast agents based on nanotechnology could, for the first time, allow MRI of individual cells and subcellular organelles. As described, new contrast agents could be created by encasing gadolinium or manganese inside fullerenes. Fullerenes are single molecules of carbon atoms arranged in spherical or tube-shaped structures. By enclosing the gadolinium/manganese inside the carbon molecules, the toxicity of the paramagnetic metals can be eliminated and increasing its effectiveness as a contrast agent. It is even possible to create a "buckyball" that encases a single atom of gadolinium or manganese. More recently, a method for encasing as many as 100 atoms of the metal inside a short length of carbon nanotube has been developed. The resulting "gadonanotubes" are 100 times more effective than traditional metallochelates as contrast agents for optimal clinical use.

Hyperpolarized ^{13}C

Naturally abundant carbon is largely comprised of ^{12}C, which is not useful for magnetic resonance observations (imaging and spectroscopy). Approximately 1.1% of naturally abundant carbon is ^{13}C, which exhibits clinically relevant magnetic resonance properties. Carbon-13 has been used in many basic studies, since carbon is part of the molecular structure of all biologically relevant materials. However, ^{13}C can now be used as a highly sensitive MRI tracer. To make ^{13}C highly sensitive, requires the use of hyperpolarization. Hyperpolarization must be performed external to the body, and improves the level of ^{13}C polarization from roughly 0.0003% to 20–50%, which represents an increase in signal-to-noise by four to five orders of magnitude (9). The loss of polarization, and thus signal, occurs rapidly, at the rate of the T1 of ^{13}C (roughly 40–50 seconds), however, the extremely high starting signal level, and opportunity to image with practically zero background signal, leads to a host of improved imaging possibilities. Clinically important CMR applications that benefit from the use of hyperpolarized ^{13}C, include vessel lumen and wall imaging, and perfusion imaging (10).

APPLICATIONS

High-Speed Imaging of Morphology, Ventricular Function, Perfusion, Viability and Metabolism

It is already possible to image cardiac morphology, ventricular function, and viability within about 30 minutes. With higher field magnets, one should be able to add diagnostic perfusion imaging within that 30-minute time frame. Diagnostic assessment of myocardial ^{31}P metabolism could be added within another 30 minutes.

Advanced Perfusion Imaging

Clinical CMR perfusion imaging is presently comparable to radionuclide perfusion imaging. Looking forward we can anticipate CMR perfusion imaging to have higher spatial resolution, and greater volume coverage, which will help with the evaluation of smaller territories of perfusion defect. This includes the detection of subendocardial ischemia, and ischemia related to microvascular disease. In addition, quantitative approaches are presently being developed and implemented. Quantitation will provide more reproducible results; thus the application of CMR perfusion imaging in evaluating the results of therapeutic approaches to myocardial ischemia will be more reliable among multiple centers (11).

Coronary Angiography

Catheter-based coronary angiography has been performed since its inception in the 1970s. More recently, CMR and X-ray CT-based "noninvasive" approaches have provided a fair means of detecting CAD using imaging of the arterial lumen particularly of congenital anomalies and occlusive disease of coronary arterial bypass grafts. Even more recently, high-speed multislice X-ray CT (MSCT), has allowed high-resolution 3D imaging of the coronary arteries, albeit with relatively high doses of radiopaque contrast agent and X rays. It is anticipated that imaging of the coronary arteries comparable to that of MSCT will be possible with expected improvements in CMR during the next few years. The present trend for improved MR coronary angiography involves the use of 3D acquisitions in combination with fat-suppressed SSFP imaging at 3 T, and using large receiver coil-arrays and parallel imaging (4,12).

Characterization of Vessel Wall and Plaque

With more in vivo studies of the vasculature in patients with coronary artery and other vascular disease, our understanding of the mechanism of arterial occlusion (leading to MI and stroke) has improved. Using CMR approaches it is possible to evaluate the composition of atherosclerotic plaques, which is different in "vulnerable" and stable plaques (13). Knowledge of plaque vulnerability can provide a means of assessing risk for MI or thrombotic stroke. Such plaque characterization will improve with the application of higher field CMR. Thus, CMR studies in the future will provide improvement in risk stratification and in the effects of various treatment strategies. While much of the work characterizing arterial plaque has been performed in the aorta and carotids, several new methods have been developed for plaque characterization in the smaller and more mobile coronary arteries (14).

Microvascular Disease or Dysfunction

Patients (especially women) with chest pain or other syndromes suggestive of heart disease have no significant coronary artery disease using traditional coronary angiographic approaches that depict only the arterial lumen (15).

Nevertheless, the symptoms in such patients can become very concerning for both patient and physician. Myocardial perfusion imaging, especially at higher fields, can demonstrate the appearance of global multifocal or subendocardial defects with the administration of adenosine or the performance of cold-pressor testing compared with imaging in the basal state. Furthermore, similar patients have shown a decrease in phosphocreatine (PCr)/ATP ratios with handgrip stress (16). These CMR findings suggest microvascular disease or dysfunction. The diagnosis of disease at the microvascular level can explain bothersome symptoms related to myocardial ischemia in patients whose diagnosis was uncertain for years. While it may be comforting to know the explanation for symptoms, the treatment for the symptoms of microvascular disease remains uncertain.

Spectroscopic Imaging

Commercially available 3 T and even more recently developed 7 T magnets will enable improvement in spectroscopic methods, because of increased signal-to-noise and improved separation of spectral peaks (17). For example, ^{31}P spectroscopy studies of myocardium had substantial noise at 1.5 T, which did not allow easy visualization of intracellular inorganic phosphate. At 3 T, inorganic phosphate can be seen, even in the absence of ischemia. On a conventional spectrum, the resonance position of inorganic phosphate shifts to the right when the intracellular milieu becomes more acidic and to the left when the intracellular milieu becomes more alkaline. Accordingly, the resonance position of the inorganic phosphate peak can be used to determine the intracellular pH, providing an additional approach to evaluating the relative concentrations of PCr and ATP for studying the pH changes induced by myocardial ischemia (and thus the severity of ischemia).

Interventional Guidance

Cardiovascular interventions including those for electrophysiology, regenerative medicine, and revascularization are typically guided by X-ray fluoroscopy. Substantial progress is being made merging prior MR data with X-ray guidance of such procedures.

In addition, the development of MR-compatible interventional devices and real-time imaging is allowing entire procedures to be performed solely under MR guidance (18). Recent technical innovations include automatic coil selection based on catheter position, automatic tracking of catheters, and forward-looking coils to guide the crossing of total vascular occlusions.

SUMMARY

The future of CMR includes major hardware advances (e.g., short high-field magnets and RF coil-arrays), major software advances (e.g., different types of contrast combined with SSFP and parallel imaging, and integrated cardiac examinations performed in less than one hour), and novel contrast-enhancing agents (e.g., hyperpolarized ^{13}C and nanotechnology-based approaches). Clinical applications to look forward to, will include high-resolution and quantitative imaging (perfusion, coronary lumen, and wall), methods to target disease (molecular), spectroscopic imaging of metabolism, and real-time monitoring of cardiovascular interventions.

The present chapter describes several aspects of what we envision as the future of clinical CMR. There are undoubtedly techniques not described here, and some not yet thought of, which will have profound impact on clinical CMR. The future of CMR is bright.

REFERENCES

1. Hinshaw WS. Image formation by nuclear magnetic resonance: the sensitive-point method. J Appl Phys 1976; 47:3709–3721.
2. Forder JR, Nayak KS, Pohost GM. Cardiac imaging at 3T: new pulse sequences and strategies for cardiac imaging must be developed. Diagnost Imaging 2002; 24(13):65–73.
3. Forder JR, Pohost GM. Cardiovascular nuclear magnetic resonance: basic and clinical applications. J Clin Invest 2003; 111:1630–1639.
4. Hardy CJ, Cline HE, Giaquinto RO, Niedorf T, Grant AK, Sodickson DK. 32-element receiver-coil array for cardiac imaging. Magn Reson Med 2006; 55(5):1142–1149.
5. Katscher U, Bornert P. Parallel RF transmission in MRI. NMR Biomed 2006; 19(3):393–400.
6. Martin ET, Coman JA, Shellock FG, Pulling CC, Fair R, Jenkins K. Magnetic resonance imaging and cardiac pacemaker safety at 1.5 Tesla. J Am Coll Cardiol 2004; 43(7):1315–1324.
7. Miller SK, Elgavish GA. Shift-reagent aided ^{23}Na NMR spectroscopy in cellular, tissue, and whole-organ systems (special issue: in vivo spectroscopy, ed. by Berliner LJ and Reuben J). Biol Magn Reson 1992; 11:159–240.
8. Caruthers SD, Winter PM, Wickline SA, Lanza GM. Targeted magnetic resonance imaging contrast agents. Methods Mol Med 2006; 124:387–400.
9. Golman K, Axelsson O, Johannesson H, Mansson S, Olofsson C, Petersson JS. Parahydrogen-induced polarization in imaging: subsecond ^{13}C angiography. Magn Reson Med 2001; 46:1–5.
10. Olsson LE, Chai CM, Axelsson O, Karlsson M, Golman K, Petersson JS. MR coronary angiography in pigs with intraarterial injections of a hyperpolarized ^{13}C substance. Magn Reson Med 2006; 55(4):731–737.
11. Jerosch-Herold M, Seethamraju RT, Swingen CM, Wilke NM, Stillman AE. Analysis of myocardial perfusion MRI. J Magn Reson Imaging 2004; 19(6):758–770.
12. Nehrke K, Bornert P, Mazurkewitz P, Winkelmann R, Grasslin I. Free-breathing whole-heart coronary MR angiography on a clinical scanner in four minutes. J Magn Reson Imaging 2006; 23(5):752–756.

13. Yuan C, Kerwin WS. MRI of atherosclerosis. J Magn Reson Imaging 2004; 19(6):710–719.
14. Fayad ZA, Fuster V, Fallon JT, et al. Noninvasive in-vivo human coronary artery lumen and wall imaging using black-blood magnetic resonance imaging. Circulation 2000; 102(5):506–510.
15. Special issue: challenging existing paradigm in ischemic heart disease: the NHLBI-sponsored Women's Ischemia Syndrome Evaluation (WISE). J Amer Coll Cardiol 2006; 47(3 suppl 1):S1–S72.
16. Buchthal SD, den Hollander JA, Merz CN, et al. Abnormal myocardial phosphorus-31 nuclear magnetic resonance spectroscopy in women with chest pain but normal coronary angiograms. N Engl J Med 2000; 342(12):829–835.
17. Schaefer S. Cardiovascular Magnetic Resonance Spectroscopy. Springer, 1992.
18. Lederman RJ. Cardiovascular interventional magnetic resonance imaging. Circulation 2005; 112(19):3009–3017.

Abbreviations

2D	two-dimensional
3D	three-dimensional
3T	3 Tesla
AC	air-conditioning
ACLS	advanced cardiac life support
AHA	American Heart Association
Ao	aorta
ARVC	arrhythmogenic right ventricular cardiomyopathy
ARVD	arrhythmogenic right ventricular dysplasia
ASD	atrial septal defect
ASE	American Society of Echocardiography
ATP	adenosine triphosphate
AV	atrioventricular
B_0	polarizing magnetic field (usually 1.5 or 3 T)
B_1	radiofrequency magnetic field
Balanced FFE	balanced gradient fast field echo (see bSSFP)
BB	black blood
BB-FSE	black blood-fast spin echo
BH	breath-hold
BRISK	block regional interpolation scheme for k-space
bSSFP	balanced steady-state free precession (also known as true-FISP, balanced FFE, and FIESTA)
CABG	coronary artery bypass graft
CAD	coronary artery disease
CE	contrast enhanced
CE-MRA	contrast enhanced magnetic resonance angiography
CI	confidence intervals
CM	cardiomyopathy

(*Continued*)

CMR	cardiovascular magnetic resonance
CMRI	cardiovascular magnetic resonance imaging
CMRS	cardiovascular magnetic resonance spectroscopy
CNR	contrast-to-noise ratio
CT	computed tomography
DRESS	depth-resolved surface-coil spectroscopy
DTPA	diethylene-triaminepentaacetic acid
ECG	electrocardiogram
EDD	endothelium dependent dilation
EDV	end-diastolic volume
EF	ejection fraction
EKG	electrocardiogram
EPI	echo-planar imaging
ESV	end-systolic volume
FB	free-breathing
FDA	Food and Drug Administration
FIESTA	fast imaging employing steady-state acquisition (see bSSFP)
FLASH	fast low-angle shot
FMD	fibromuscular dysplasia
FMRI	functional magnetic resonance imaging
FOV	field of view
FS	fat saturation/saturated
FSE	fast spin-echo
Gd	gadolinium
Gd-DTPA	gadolinium-diethylene-triaminepentaacetic acid
GRAPPA	generalized autocalibrating partially parallel acquisitions (parallel imaging)
GRE	gradient-recalled echo
G_x, G_y, G_z	linear magnetic field gradients
HASTE	half-Fourier single-shot
HCM	hypertrophic cardiomyopathy
ICD	implantable cardiac device
IMH	intramural hematoma
IR	inversion recovery
IRAD	International Registry of Acute Aortic Dissection
ISIS	image-selected in vivo spectroscopy
IVC	inferior vena cava
IVS	interventricular septum
IVUS	intravascular ultrasound
LA	left atrium
LAD	left anterior descending coronary artery
LAO	left anterior oblique
LBBB	left bundle branch block
LCx	left circumflex coronary artery
LM	left main coronary artery

(*Continued*)

LV	left ventricle
LVH	left ventricular hypertrophy
LVOT	left ventricular outflow tract
MDE	myocardial delayed enhancement
MFR	myocardial flow reserve
MHD	magneto-hydro-dynamic
MI	myocardial infarction
MIP	maximum-intensity projection
Mo	equilibrium magnetization
MPR	multiplanar reformat
MR	mitral regurgitation
MRA	magnetic resonance angiography
MRCA	magnetic resonance coronary angiography
MRI	magnetic resonance imaging
MRSI	magnetic resonance spectroscopic imaging
MS	mitral stenosis
MSCT	multislice computed tomography
MTC	magnetization transfer contrast
NIH	National Institutes of Health
NMR	nuclear magnetic resonance
NSTEMI	non-ST-segment elevation myocardial infarction
NYHA	New York Heart Association
OM	obtuse marginal coronary arteries
PAU	penetrating aortic ulcer
PC	phase contrast
PCA	phase contrast angiography
PCr	phosphocreatine
PD	proton density
PET	positron emission tomography
PFO	patent foramen ovale
PG	plethysmograph
PISA	proximal isovelocity surface area
PRESS	point-resolved spectroscopy
PVM	phase velocity mapping
RA	right atrium
RAS	renal artery stenosis
RCA	right coronary artery
RF	radio-frequency
ROC	receiver-operating characteristic
ROI	region of interest
R-R	interval between R-waves in the electrocardiogram (i.e., duration of one heartbeat)
RV	right ventricle
RVOT	right ventricular outflow tract
SE	spin echo

(*Continued*)

SENSE	sensitivity encoding (parallel imaging)
SMASH	simultaneous acquisition of spatial harmonics (parallel imaging)
SNR	signal-to-noise ratio
SPECT	single-photon emission computed tomography
SR	saturation recovery
SSFP	steady-state free precession
STEAM	stimulated-echo acquisition mode
SV	stroke volume
T_1	longitudinal relaxation time (also known as spin–lattice relaxation time)
T_2	transverse relaxation time (also known as spin–spin relaxation time)
T_2^*	transverse relaxation time including the effects of intravoxel dephasing
TE	echo time
TEE	transesophageal echocardiography
TI	inversion time
TOF	time of flight
TR	repetition time
TRICKS	time-resolved imaging with contrast kinetics
True-FISP	true fast imaging with steady precession (see bSSFP)
UNFOLD	unaliasing by Fourier-encoding the overlaps using the temporal dimension
VEC	velocity-encoded cine
VENC	velocity encoding/encoded
VOI	volume of interest
VPS	views per segment
VR	volume rendering/rendered
VSD	ventricular septal defect
WHO	World Health Organization
WISE	women's ischemia syndrome evaluation

Index